A TREATISE

ON

HOMŒOPATHIC

PRACTICE OF MEDICINE:

COMPRISED IN

A REPERTORY FOR PRESCRIBING,

Adapted to Domestic or Professional use.

Third Edition, Improved and Enlarged.

BY

HUNTING SHERRILL, M. D.

MEMBER OF THE HAHNEMANN ACADEMY OF MEDICINE;
THE HOMŒOPATHIC SOCIETY OF THE STATE OF NEW YORK; AND
THE AMERICAN INSTITUTE OF HOMŒOPATHY:

Author of a Treatise on Epidemics; and an Essay on the Cholera of 1832.

NEW YORK:
WILLIAM RADDE, PUBLISHER,
322 BROADWAY.

1854.

JOHN POLHEMUS, Printer,
66 Courtlandt Street, New York.

PRELIMINARY REMARKS.

In this, now the third edition of the Repertory for prescribing, great pains have been taken during twelve years' study and investigation of the subject, to make it as complete as possible.

From all the various authors on Homœopathy we have been able to consult and examine, we have collected facts, and selected medicines according to their virtues; and we rejoice to give credit to such works, from which selections have been made, and which have been of use to aid our own observation and experience.

In this manner, we trust this Repertory will be perfected to such a degree, that for arrangement and convenience, and domestic use, and ready reference, it has not been exceeded by any other work of the kind.

We purpose to show that generally a number of medicines are set down for each disease, or for the various grades and features of it. It is however to be understood, that these medicines are not all equally useful in the case, but some are more so in one feature or stage of the case, and others in another.

The peculiar stage or character of the disease for which a medicine would be most useful, or homœopathic to the present symptoms of the case, may be discovered by persons having some expeperience in the art, and by following the directions here given at the place where the disease is named. In doubtful cases, close observation must be the best teacher. Much also may be learned by examining the Repertory and studying the pathogenitic effects of the drugs mentioned in some work on pure materia medica.

It is also very important (particularly in chronic and complex cases) to obtain an accurate history of the case, to ascertain what previous ailments the patient has had, and what medicines have been used in the treatment.

It happens often that the patient's illness is owing to some previous disease which has not been well cured, or to the injurious and poisonous effects of a drug he may have taken.

This work being intended merely as a Repertory, for a ready reference to aid in prescribing, the description and the pathology of diseases are omitted; also, we have not thought it advisable to examine into remote or proximate causes, which are generally very hypothetical, and often unsatisfactory.

In the Homœopathic mode of treatment, the symptoms presented by morbid action are the principal guide for prescribing—more so than a pathological knowledge, which may be very uncertain; it is therefore presumed that the prescriber will know the general name of the affection, or can comprehend the symptoms set down in the work, and the remedy indicated, and connected with them.

ARRANGEMENT OF THE REPERTORY.

Divisions or parts of the body are selected, and placed in an alphabetical order as heads of affections or symptoms peculiar to them, though some diseases which do not properly come under one of these heads, are set in their alphabetical place.

GENERAL DIVISIONS.

Abdomen, followed by diseases of this part of the body.
Abscess.
Ague.
Angina, the various species.
Apoplexy.
Appetite and Taste.
Apthea—Thrush.

Back, and various affections of this part.
Bladder, and diseases of the Urinary organs.
Brain.
Bones.

Cancer.
Chest, and diseases of the Respiratory organs.
Cholera.
Colic.
Cold.
Constipation.
Consumption.
Coughs, various species.

Diarrhœa.
Dropsy.
Drunkenness.
Dysentery.
Dyspepsia.

Ears, and diseases of these organs.
Emotions, the great variety.
Erysipelas.
Eruptions.
Eyes, and their diseases.
Extremities, general diseases of.

Face.
Fever, varieties and species.

Genitals, and diseases of them.
Gonorrhæa.

Hæmorrhage.

Hæmorrhoids.
Head, and affections of it.
Heart, " "
Hernia.
Herpes.
Hoarseness.

Injuries mechanical.
Inflammation of various parts.

Jaws and Gums.

Liver, and its diseases.

Mania.
Measles.
Melancholia.
Mind and Memory.
Mouth.

Nausea and Vomiting.
Neuralgia.
Nose, and disease of it.

Pain.
Palsey.

Rheumatism.

Scalp, diseases of it.
Scrofula.

Skin, affections of.
Sleep.
Small Pox.
Spasms, various kinds.
Stomach, and diseases of it.
Syphilis.

Teeth.
Throat.
Tumors.

Ulcers.

Vertigo.

Wounds.
Worms.
Women—diseases peculiar to them.
——— Pregnancy.
——— Accouchment, & diseases succeeding.

Infants, diseases of.

Poisons, and remedies for them.

MODE OF SELECTING THE MEDICINE.

The plan we have pursued throughout this work, will be very convenient to determine and fix on a medicine most proper to use. If a patient complains of fever, headache, pain in the stomach, nausea, &c. by turning to Fever in the Repertory, you will find that Bell. is a prominent remedy for fever. Then look at Headache, and Bell. will be seen to be a leading remedy for headache; turn to Stomach and Nausea, and Bell. is there named for those affections. Thus it will appear, that Bell. is the leading remedy for four of the prominent symptoms of the case; consequently, Bell. will be a proper remedy to be used. Acon. Ipec. or Nux V. would also be appropriate, and do very well, and in some cases better.

Again, suppose a patient has acute inflammation, fever, sore throat, pain in the chest, and cough, by examining the Repertory it will be seen, that for fever of an inflammatory type, the prominent remedy is Aconite—turn to Angina (sore throat,) and there you have Acon.; for pain of the chest or acute inflammation of the lungs, Acon. will be found to be a prominent remedy;

for cough, with its concomitant symptoms, Acon. is a prominent medicine. Thus, the remedy which covers the greatest number of symptoms, is Acon. and will be the best to use. Other medicines would not be amiss, such as Anti. Bell. Bryo. Ipe. &c.

A prominent combination of symptoms affecting females, for which we are often consulted, are headache, disordered stomach, costiveness, bearing down pains of the womb, irritation and distensions of the uterus; difficulty in urinating, piles and hæmorrhoidal tumours, and bleeding from the hæmorrhoidal vessels.

By examining the Repertory, it will be perceived, that for headache, Nux V. is a remedy; for disorder of the stomach, Nux V. is also a proper remedy; for costiveness, you will find Nux V. an indicated medicine—for the affections of the womb mentioned, Nux V. is a valuable medicine, and for the Piles and the other Hæmorrhoidal affections, Nux V. holds a prominent rank. Therefore in a case comprising all or a portion of those symptoms, Nux V. will be a useful and leading remedy, but not to the exclusion of other articles, such as Bell. Bryo. Puls. Rus. T. Sepi. Stramo. &c.

This plan being pursued in other cases will lead to a tolerably correct course of prescribing a proper remedy.

In administering medicine on this plan it is

proper to give but a very minute dose of those specific remedies at a time, so as to produce only a gentle aggravation at first, or a quieting equilibrium in the system, or an antidotal operation to vitiating or psoric or poisonous material lurking in the body, rather than a harsh, irregular commotion or counteracting operation.

Therefore, a minute dose which produces no injurious operations nor poisonous effects and that does no injury, if it does not cure, is found to be best, and all that is necessary to produce the desired effect, and bring about a cure of the disease.

In a few cases only, Bloodletting is mentioned in this Repertory. The Homœopathic practitioners commonly dispense with the use of it. They generally hold that disease may be cured as well and as safely without its use; and experience has also shown that by the use of Homœopathic medicine it is seldom necessary to resort to it. Some, however, are of opinion that the use of it may be sometimes compatible with Homœopathic medicine with great advantage—and no doubt cases do occur in which bleeding may be used with great benefit.

A congress of Homœopathic physicians from all parts of Europe was held in Paris, in 1852, when a committee was appointed to examine into the subject, and report upon the use of Bloodletting in connection with Homœopathic treatment.

In the *Homœopathic Examiner*, for August, 1846, new series, vol. i. p. 4, Dr. Gray states:

"Among the means which we must, as I think, use empirically, I will cite, in addition to those introduced into Jahr's new Manual, the *polypodium filix mas* and the cowhage (against intestinal worms,) the Mesmeric passes (Chyropathy), and the external and internal application of heat and moisture (Hydropathy.)

"To this list, which I consider indispensible to a successful practice of medicine at the present day, I will add BLOODLETTING, an agent which I have not ceased to apply during the eighteen years of my acquaintance with Homœopathy, albeit much less frequently than I did as an Allopathist.

"At first, by advice of my learned and lamented predecessor Dr. Gram, it was continued upon purely empirical grounds, but now, and for many years past, I apply it upon the Homœopathic basis, having acquired, partly by experiments on myself, and partly by reading Allopathic authorities to that end, a tolerable pathogenesis of it, which it is my purpose to elaborate for the Examiner."

"With this frank advertisement of views, which I should like to see adopted and acted upon throughout the ranks of our school, because I entertain them with perfect sincerity, I tender my editorial services to the readers of the journal, with a pledge to them to follow where Truth leads, even if to-morrow it should make me retrace every position I now maintain."

"JOHN F. GRAY."

In a work written by Hull or Laurie on Homœopathic practice, Bloodletting in connection with Homœopathic treatment is recommended in some cases.

In Dr. Peter's work on Headaches, we find this remark: "It is well known that the excessive loss of blood frequently produces violent congestion to the head." Agreeably to the Homœopathic law of cure, if the loss of blood produces congestion, it would be proper and necessary to resort to that remedy to cure such condition of the system, when it exists as the effects of disease.

We are of opinion that any plan or system of treating diseases which totally excludes Bleeding is very injudicious, and must necessarily, in many instances, subject the case to a fatal termination, when by a judicious use of this remedy it might have been cured. We are well informed of and have witnessed many, very many, such cases.

This remedy is more particularly recommended in this Repertory in cases of compound inflammation, or congestion, in which it has proved eminently successful—(see Appendix A.)—more advantageously so under Allopathic treatment, but it is not devoid of its benefits connected with Homœopathic practice. When there takes place in the early stage of the case, as it does in Epidemic diseases, an overloaded fullness of some of the vital organs and internal blood-vessels, and a congestive accumulation of fluids in those parts, the circulation is slow, the pulse small and flaccid, the countenance dingy and lurid, the respiration labored and slow. There is a dull, aching, painful sensation in the body and limbs. In such conditions, by lessening the quantity of fluids in the vessels, the heart is relieved of a part of its load, by which it is enabled to act more freely, and to propel the blood through the lungs with greater facility, which will be the means of removing congestion, and an increased quantity of vital air is added to the blood in the lungs—which in such conditions is the best excitant that can be used. In cases of congestive depression, this course aids very much to bring about reaction.

An objection has been made to taking blood from the body as a remedy for disease, for the reason that it is the support and life of the system. So is the life of the body or flesh owing to the oxygen introduced into the body through the lungs, and life is more immediately dependant upon it than upon the blood. It has often been urged that the loss of blood produces a state of debility and lasting weakness. It is replied to this, that the blood is not the life of the body, but one of the agents by which life is supported and kept up, and that the effects of a moderate loss of blood are sometimes the very reverse of causing weakness or lasting debility.

In some states and conditions of disease, the blood which in ordinary cases is the agent to preserve life, sometimes is the agent to destroy it, and that very soon unless means are used to prevent that result by lessening the quantity in the system. We have not been able to discover that the drawing of blood when indicated, does or can interfere with the operation of Homœopathic medicine which may be adapted to the case, as there is not a counteracting or neutralising agent to the medicine introduced into the system. In several cases of severe inflammation of important parts and in congestive conditions of the body, we have observed that the proper Homœopathic medicines which were applied to the condition of the disease have not afforded sufficient relief; when recourse was had to a judicious abstraction of blood and the Homœopathic remedies were continued, a decided favorable change soon took place, the disease yielded, and the patients readily recovered.

It was by the application of this pathological and physiological law, which led to a successful mode of treating the Epidemic of 1812, and which has proved very successful in treating the compound inflammatory or congestive states of Epidemic Cholera.

For authorities on this subject, we may refer to

Leo Wolf, of Russia; Brussias, of France; Clot Bey, of Egypt; the British Medical Board at Bombay; Dr. Corbyn, British Military Surgeon in Bengal; Sir J. Baker, British Consul General to Egypt; Professor Chapman, and Drs. Bell and Conde, of Philadelphia; and Dr. Ferris, of New York.

In such congestive, depressed states of the system, by the abstraction of blood sometimes in small quantities, and that repeated, the pulse uniformly rises, becomes more full and firm, the blood changes its color from a dark, carbonated hue, to a florid, healthy color, which we have witnessed in numerous instances. Facts corroborating this statement are set forth in the writings of Rush, Donaldson, Armstrong, Mann, Gallup, Jno. Bell's Anatomy, Bell, Conde, &c. &c.

The small, flaccid pulse, the sunken, prostrated weakness, the difficulty of breathing, the dingy, leaden color of the face—the symptoms of Asphyxia, &c. which sometimes take place on the first attack of the disease, and particularly in Epidemic diseases, are not the effect of direct debility or exhaustion, but those symptoms are generally the effect of depression, compound inflammation, or congestion. This condition is very different from direct or real debility, exhaustion, and weakness, which takes place in advanced states of disease. The general remedies which would be proper for one of those conditions would be very improper and injurious in the other: and where one set of remedies would be proper and useful in the same condition of disease the other would be fatal.

The custom of giving freely of opiates and vegetable irritants and alcoholic libations in the early stage of the cases, when bleeding judiciously used with other remedies corresponding with it would have been more adviseable, no doubt has been the cause of the great fatality attending Epidemics as, well as Epidemic Cholera in particular. [See Appendix A.]

MODE OF ADMINISTERING THE MEDICINE.

The rule for giving the medicine as directed by Hahnemann is as follows: In acute or severe cases, to give the stronger preparations or those of the low dilutions or triturations, and to repeat the dose often—more so than in milder or more protracted cases. In very severe cases, such as Croup, Spasms, Convulsions, Colic, and in acute inflammations, the medicines ought to be given at first every fifty, forty, thirty, twenty, or ten minutes. After a few doses being given in this way, the periods should be lengthened, or, if there is decided mitigation of the symptoms, it should be entirely suspended for a time, until its effects are observed; for sometimes a few doses in this manner will entirely check or cure the case. Or, it may be proper to give a different medicine; and in this stage the dose ought not to be repeated more than once in two or three hours.

In less acute cases, the dose should be given once in two, three, or four hour; or administered at longer intervals; in lingering cases, it is best to extend the time to two or three times in twenty-four hours. In chronic diseases, and those of long standing, it is considered best to give the doses at much longer periods, such as once in a day, or once in two, three, or four days, or even at longer intervals. These are essentially Hahnemann's directions.

In chronic diseases and those of long standing, it is considered best to use the high triturations or dilutions; and in the acute diseases, the stronger or lower preparations.

Medical Potences.—"The majority of the Homœopathists may be said to have decided hitherto in favor of the lower potences, such as 3d, 6th, 8th, in acute cases—and higher, such as the 18, 24 to 30, in chronic diseases. The main point to be attended to, is the correct selection of the remedy. In Fevers, the directions are, to give half a drop of the medicine chosen every two or three hours." Hull's Laurie.

The quantity of the dose is very much governed by the fancy and opinion of the prescriber, and this is not of so much importance, as it is to select and use the article the most Homœopathic to, or corresponding with the case. If dilutions are used, one to three drops are about a dose. If triurations are selected, about gr. 1 will be a proper dose, or two or three grains may be dissolved in a wineglassful of water, and a teaspoonful of it given at a time.

When the globules are chosen, they may be put on the tongue and dissolved in the mouth or swallowed, or there may be six or eight of them dissolved in a wine glass of water, and a teaspoonful of it given as often as may be desirable.

The readers attention is particularly called to these specific directions about using and giving doses, as the whole of the directions throughout the Repertory for giving the medicine are based on these directions.

Rules for Diet, while taking the Medicine recommended in this work.

Articles which ought *not* to be used are Coffee, Green Tea, Cocoa, Chocolate, Pepper, Mustard, Catsup, Malt Liquors, Wine, Spirits, Lemonade, or other acids, Alkalies, Mineral Waters, Spices of all kinds, Cabbage Sour Krout.

In animal food, avoid Pork and meat generally, or take of it moderately. It is best boiled or stewed. Smoked or salt meat is objectionable; also old cheese. Avoid spicy vegetable articles, confectionery, and whatever contains medical matter. Let the diet be plain and simple; use black tea or water, or milk and water, as a drink.

Aliments allowed.—Those are Soup and Broth, made plain, without seasoning with pepper or spices, to which plain vegetable, mucilagenous, or farinaceous articles may be added.

Meats, plainly cooked, stewed or boiled are preferable, and may be taken in moderate quantities.

Fish, plain, common fish may be used; they had better be boiled.

Vegetables, plain, common vegetables—well prepared, avoiding those of a spicy nature, are always useful as a diet.

Eggs, lightly prepared, and bread, are uniformly useful and admissible articles of food.

Puddings, from all the farinaceous articles, made plain, and used with plain, simple dressing, are useful and proper.

Fruit, of good quality, used in moderation, is always admissible and useful.

Drinks, should be water, milk, black tea, toast water, mucilage and water, rice water, or any similar mild article.

Some writers are much more lengthy on the subject of rules for diet; but those I have mentioned contain all that are particularly necessary.

When there is a severe attack of Fever, nature fixes the best rule. She entirely impairs the appetite, particularly in children, except a longing for cold water, which is the best drink to be taken along with the medicine, and the use of it should be indulged in.

A REPERTORY FOR HOMŒOPATHIC PRESCRIBING.

ABDOMEN.

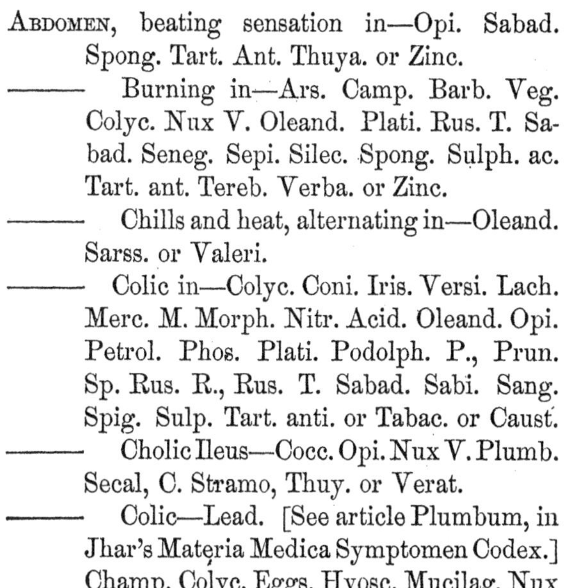

ABDOMEN, beating sensation in—Opi. Sabad. Spong. Tart. Ant. Thuya. or Zinc.

—— Burning in—Ars. Camp. Barb. Veg. Colyc. Nux V. Oleand. Plati. Rus. T. Sabad. Seneg. Sepi. Silec. Spong. Sulph. ac. Tart. ant. Tereb. Verba. or Zinc.

—— Chills and heat, alternating in—Oleand. Sarss. or Valeri.

—— Colic in—Colyc. Coni. Iris. Versi. Lach. Merc. M. Morph. Nitr. Acid. Oleand. Opi. Petrol. Phos. Plati. Podolph. P., Prun. Sp. Rus. R., Rus. T. Sabad. Sabi. Sang. Spig. Sulp. Tart. anti. or Tabac. or Caust.

—— Cholic Ileus—Cocc. Opi. Nux V. Plumb. Secal, C. Stramo, Thuy. or Verat.

—— Colic—Lead. [See article Plumbum, in Jhar's Materia Medica Symptomen Codex.] Champ. Colyc. Eggs. Hyosc. Mucilag. Nux

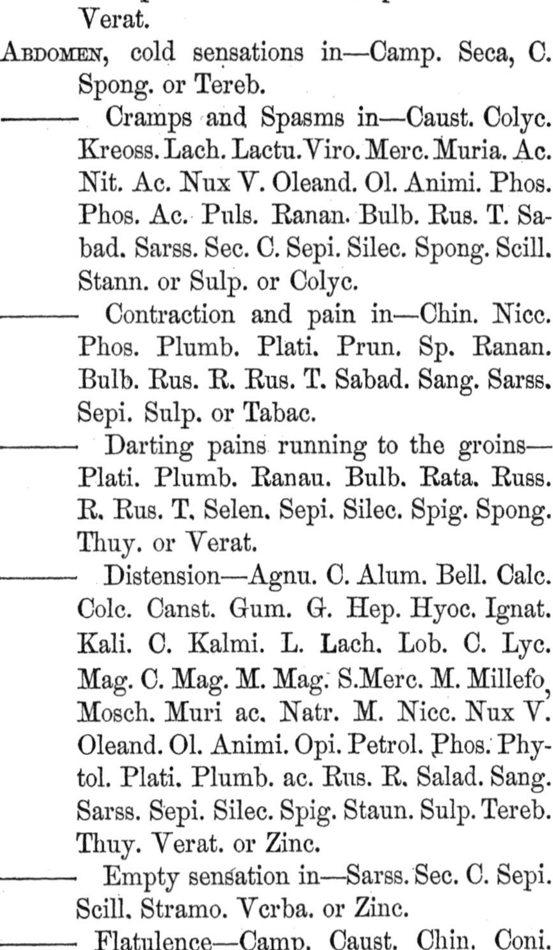

V. Opi. Phos Plumb. Sapo. Stramo. or Verat.

ABDOMEN, cold sensations in—Camp. Seca, C. Spong. or Tereb.

——— Cramps and Spasms in—Caust. Colyc. Kreoss. Lach. Lactu. Viro. Merc. Muria. Ac. Nit. Ac. Nux V. Oleand. Ol. Animi. Phos. Phos. Ac. Puls. Ranan. Bulb. Rus. T. Sabad. Sarss. Sec. C. Sepi. Silec. Spong. Scill. Stann. or Sulp. or Colyc.

——— Contraction and pain in—Chin. Nicc. Phos. Plumb. Plati. Prun. Sp. Ranan. Bulb. Rus. R. Rus. T. Sabad. Sang. Sarss. Sepi. Sulp. or Tabac.

——— Darting pains running to the groins—Plati. Plumb. Ranau. Bulb. Rata. Russ. R. Rus. T. Selen. Sepi. Silec. Spig. Spong. Thuy. or Verat.

——— Distension—Agnu. C. Alum. Bell. Calc. Colc. Canst. Gum. G. Hep. Hyoc. Ignat. Kali. C. Kalmi. L. Lach. Lob. C. Lyc. Mag. C. Mag. M. Mag. S. Merc. M. Millefo, Mosch. Muri ac. Natr. M. Nicc. Nux V. Oleand. Ol. Animi. Opi. Petrol. Phos. Phytol. Plati. Plumb. ac. Rus. R. Salad. Sang. Sarss. Sepi. Silec. Spig. Staun. Sulp. Tereb. Thuy. Verat. or Zinc.

——— Empty sensation in—Sarss. Sec. C. Sepi. Scill. Stramo. Verba. or Zinc.

——— Flatulence—Camp. Caust. Chin. Coni.

Morph. Natr. M. Nitr. ac. Nux Mosch, Nux V. Ol. Anini. Opi. Petrol. Phos. Plati. Plumb. Acet. Rus. R. Rus. T. Tart. Ant. Thuy. Verb. or Zinc.

ABDOMEN, Flatus fœtid—Carb. V. Staph. Verat. or Zinc.

——— Gangrene in—Ars. Caps. Carb. V. Kreoso. Lyc. Merc. Phos. Sulp. ac. or Verat.

——— Griping in—Colyc. Merc. M. Nat. M. Nicc. Nitr. ac. Nux V. Oleand. Ol. Animi. Petrol. Rus. R. Sabi. Sepi. or Stron.

——— Groin and Inguinal Rings, pressure on—Natr. M. Nux V. Petrol. Phos. Plati. Plumb. Prun. Sp. Rus. R. Rus. T. Sepi. Spig. Spong. Stramo. Tereb or Zinc.

——— Groins, Glands in Swelled or Ulcerated Merc. Nitr. Ac. Petrol. Silec. Stron. Thuy. or Zinc.

——— Hernia, sensations of pressing out—Arum. Nux V.—Spig. Spong. Stramo. Sulph. ac—Sulph. Tart. ant—Thuy. Verba. Verat or Zinc.

——— Hernia, beating in—Nux V. or Sulph. ac.

——— Induration in groin—Coni. Sang. Sep. or Silec. (See Glands, Induration of.)

——— Intestines, pain in great—Cham. Merc. Spig. Stann. Verat. or Verba.

——— Inflammation in Secondary — Hyosc. Merc., Merc. Iod.—Nux V.—Ol. Animi.—Sec. C. Scill. Stann. Stramo. or Sulp.

ABDOMEN, itching sensation in—Ol. Animi. Sabad. Sabi. Spig or Stramo.

——— Live animals in, sensation of—Sabad. Stramo. Sepi. Sulp. or Thuy.

——— Liver, pain and darting in—Sabad. Sang. Spong. Tereb or Verat. (See Liver.)

——— Pains, periodical in—Coni. Ox. ac.—Phos. Rhodod. Sang. or Sepi.

——— Paralytic pushing sensation.—Nux V.—Rus. T.—Sabi. Sabid. Sang or Stramo.

——— Pressure and pain in—Ammo. Caust. Anacord. Anisi. Baryt. Bell. Calc. Camp. Cann. S.—Coni. Hep. Ignat. Iodi. Kali. C. Kalmi. Lat.—Kreoso. Lach. Lauroc. Merc. Nicc. Opi. Oleand. Ox. ac.—Phos. Rus. T.—Sobad. Silec. Spig. Scill. Sulp ac., or Tart. Anti.

——— pressing outward.—Sulp. Tabac. or Tereb.

——— pressing as though filled with stones.—Sabad. or Tart. ant.

——— Puffed—Opi. Petrol. Rus. T.—Sepi. Scill. Stramo. Sulp. Tereb. or Zinc.

——— Quivering sensation. — Lach. Lauroc. Lyc. Nux V.—Plati. Rhodod. Sabad. Sepi. or Staph.

——— Rash over.—Selen. or Sulp.

——— Rumbling in.—Bismuth. Borax. Bromi. Camp. Canth. Coni. Colyc. Gum. G. Ignat. Iodi.—Kali. C. Kali. Jod. Kalmi.

Lat.—Lact. Viro. — Lauroc. Lyc. Mosch. Mur. ac. — Nit. Ac. — Nux V. — Olead. Phos. Plati. Plumb..—Podoph. P.—Puls. Ranan. Bull.—Rus. T.—Sabad. Sabi. Sarss. Sepi. Spig. Staph. Stramo. Sulph. Tart. Ant. or Tabac.

ABDOMEN, Sensitiveness—Iodi. Lyc. Merc. Petrol. Phytoll. or Stramo.

——— Spleen, enlarged and painful—Ars. Hep. Iodi. Rhodod. Sabad. or Sepi.

——— Stitches in.—Camp. Sarss. Sepi. Spong. Stann. Stron. Sulp. Tart. Anti. or Zinc.

——— Trembling sensation. Staphys. or Verat.

——— Tympanites. Colyc. Rus. T. Tereb. or Tart. Ant.

ABSCESS.

ABSCESS, or inflammatory swelling inclining to form an abscess or suppuration—to discuss it, the best remedies are, Acon. Bell. Bryo. Ipe. Silec. or Sulph. Externally, apply cold water, in which a little tincture of Arnica is mixed, or use a cold solution of Acetate of lead, or the latter may be used in the form of cold poultice.

——— To promote suppuration — give Ars. Baryt. Cham. Hep. Lach. Merc. or Opi. Externally, use warm emmollient poultices or fomentations.

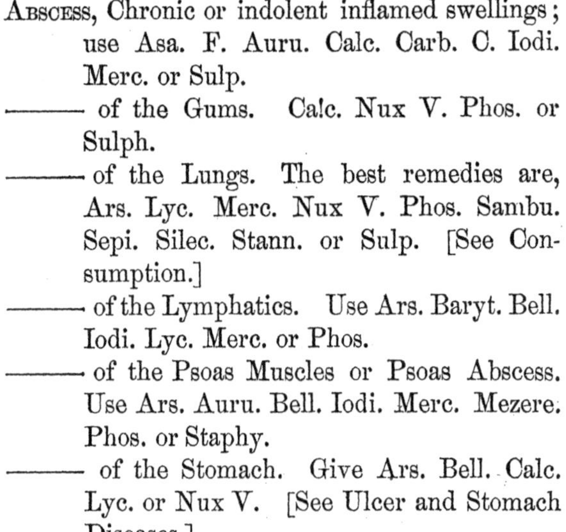

ABSCESS, Chronic or indolent inflamed swellings; use Asa. F. Auru. Calc. Carb. C. Iodi. Merc. or Sulp.

——— of the Gums. Calc. Nux V. Phos. or Sulph.

——— of the Lungs. The best remedies are, Ars. Lyc. Merc. Nux V. Phos. Sambu. Sepi. Silec. Stann. or Sulp. [See Consumption.]

——— of the Lymphatics. Use Ars. Baryt. Bell. Iodi. Lyc. Merc. or Phos.

——— of the Psoas Muscles or Psoas Abscess. Use Ars. Auru. Bell. Iodi. Merc. Mezere. Phos. or Staphy.

——— of the Stomach. Give Ars. Bell. Calc. Lyc. or Nux V. [See Ulcer and Stomach Diseases.]

AGUE, &c.

AGUE CHILLS AND SHUDDERING—They generally occur at the commencement of febrile diseases, and they take place in a variety of ways, and under various conditions. They are sometimes of very short duration, at others, they continue a long period before reaction takes place, and the subsequent fever is established. A very long continued chill generally is succeeded by a severe fever, or state of disease somewhat in proportion to the severity of the ague. The most useful and appropriate remedies for Ague and Chills, are Acon. Agar. Ammo. C. Angust. Ars. Caust. Camph. Dulcam. Hell. Ignat. Ipe. Lauroc. Merc. Mosch. Nux V. Puls. Rus. R. Rus. T. Sabad. or Verat.

AMAGDALITIS.

Amagdalitis. Tonsils inflamed and enlarged. Use Baryt. Bell. Calc. Caps. Canth. Cham. Hep. Iodi. Ignat. Lyc. Nux V. Puls. Sep. or Sulph. [See Angina Tonsilitis.]

ANEURISM.

Aneurism, a diseased enlargement of an artery. The remedies most useful to relieve or cure this affection, are Arnic. Caust. Carb. V. Calca. Hep. Ignat. Lyc. Nux V. Silec. or Thuy.

In the North American Homœopathic Journal, No. 9, p. 68, some cases are related as having been cured by Lycopodium.

ANGINA.

Under this name, a variety of diseases of the throat and tonsils are arranged and treated of as follows:

ANGINA, Quinsy or Sore Throat. The proper remedies are Acon. Bell. Bryo. Dulcam. Ignat. Ipe. Nux V. Puls. Samb. Sang. Sepi. Sulp. or Tart. Antimo.

—— Catarrhal (common cold.) Acon. Bell. Cham. Dulcam. Hyosc. Ipe. Merc. Viv. Nux V. Natr. M. Puls. Rus. R. Rus. T. Samb. Sulp. or Verat.

The medicine should be used in the following order. In the first stage, when there is obstruction in the head and nose, or snuffling, use Dulcam. Hyosc. or Puls. When there is fever and soreness of the throat or upper part of the chest, and dry cough, give Acon. Bryo. Ipec. or Tart. A. If the throat is sore and red or swelled, and there is cough, use Bell. Lyc. Merc. or Samb. If there is dry cough, inclining to spasmodic efforts, give Droser. Hyosc. Nux V. or Verat. In the various stages of the case, the other medicine named will often be useful.

ANGINA, Gangrena. If this state should appear to be approaching, the best remedies are Ars. Caps. Carb. V. Kreoso. Lyc. Merc. Sol. Nig. Phos. Sulph. ac. or Verat.

——— Laryngitis. This is an inflammation of the membrane lining the throat and larynx. It resembles croup considerably in many cases—it is also connected with a common cold or catarrhal sore throat. The remedies for it in the first stage arc Bell. or Acon.; in the more advanced state, or when there is hoarseness, use Anti. Seneg. or Dolecho. The treatment proper is about the same as for Angina Catarrhalis. (See also Hoarseness.)

——— MEMBRANA (Croup.) This is a very serious disease, affecting infants and young children: if it is not soon arrested, it may prove fatal.

CROUP—It is an inflammatory affection of the glottis and upper part of the wind pipe; sometimes it attacks very suddenly. It produces a short difficult breathing, a shrill, whistling, squaling cough—a ringing sound, sometimes resembling the barking of a dog; the child throws back the head, to endeavour to breathe more easy—in some cases, a spasmodic action takes place in the part—from a secretion of mucus in the inflamed part a tough membrane forms, which closes up the passage, and causes a fatal termination, if the disease is not early checked. Frequently a croupy cough takes place, which need not be very serious—this may be cured by a few doses of Acon. Bell. or Ipe. In Croup, more or less fever sets in. A prompt use of remedies is required to check and cure it. The first medicine to use is Aconite. A suitable and proper mode of giving it, is to mix about 5 to 10 drops of the third or sixth dilution in a half gill of water; or use 8 or 10 pellets of the same attenuation, in that quantity of water; some use much higher attenuations, and they say with success; this mixture ought to be given often; the dose should be repeated according to the severity of the case, say a teaspoonful every 30, 20, 10, to 5 minutes. By using it in this way, a few hours, the force of the disease will be generally checked, the fever and cough moderated. Then give the medicine at longer periods, or stop using it. It may then be best to omit the Aconite, and give Hep. or Spong. alternately about every hour or half hour, or give one of these in alternation with Acon. In the more advanced stage, if the symptoms are severe with rattling, give Phos. Anti. Kali. Bicc. or Iodi. Samb. or Seneg. From the beginning, let the patient often sip cold water, and apply a cloth wetted in cold water to the neck and chest. By this course, the case will generally be checked or cured. We have had no failure under it, when fully and properly followed.

In the North American Journal of Homœopathy, No. 2, page 252, it is stated, that Acon. and Bryona, given alternately, is a sure mode of treatment for Croup.

It was stated in the Hahnemann Academy of Medicine, by Dr. Gray, that to dissolve one grain of Tart. Anti. in four ounces of water, and give a teaspoonful every 20 or 30 minutes, had generally cured under this prescription.

ANGINA, Membrana, or Rattling or Spasmodic stage, give Bromi. Kali. Bic. Kali. Iod. or Phos.

—— Palati. Bell. Phos. Samb. Ammo. C. Baryt. M. Merc. Phos. Puls. Rus. R. or Rus. T.

—— Pectoris. Acon. Ars. Arg. N. Petrol. Samb. Stramo. Verat. Let oxygen be inhaled, or use electricity passed through the chest.

—— Pharyngea. Acon. Bell. Merc. Puls. Sulp. Tart. Ant. or Verat.

——— Syphilitica. Kali. Iod. Merc. Mezere. or Nitr. ac.

——— Tonsilitis. Use Acon. Bell. Baryt. Canth. Hep. Ignat. Merc. Nux V. Petrol. Samb. Staphy. Sulp. or Thuy. [See Amagdylitis.]

——— ——— A chronic enlargement. Give Bell. Baryt. C. Iodi. Ignat. Merc.

APHONIA.

APHONIA, or loss of the Voice, or Hoarseness (which see.) The remedies for this affection are Acon. Arnic. Ars. Bell. Carb. V. Tart. Anti. or Nux V. Oleand. Plati. Phos. or Thuy.

——— Of Infants. Use Chin. Opi. Tart. Anti. or some of the preceding remedies.

APOPLEXY.

APOPLEXY. This is a disease which attacks the brain, and generally produces a sudden falling down and a state of insensibility—it is commonly produced by an unnatural or increased determination of blood or fluids to the brain.

There are a variety of diseased states of the brain which results in this disease. We avail ourselves of the use of Dr. Peters' work on Homœopathic Treatment of Apoplexy for some explanations on this subject; the variety of ways in which the affection appears are enumerated as follows:

(1.) Apoplexy from excess of blood in the whole system. (Plethoric state.)

(2.) ——— from retention or rush of blood to the head. (Congestive.)

(3.) ——— from rupture of some blood vessel in or about the brain. (Hæmorrhagic.)

(4.) ——— from debility or other nervous disorder of the brain or nervous system. (Nervous.)

(5.) ——— from an increased quantity of watery or other fluids on the brain. (Serous.)

(6.) ——— from primary disease or enlargement of the heart. (Cardiac.)

(7.) ——— from diseased or disordered liver. (Hepatic.)

(8.) ——— from Bright's disease of the kidneys. (Nephritic.)

(9.) ——— from febrilé or inflammatory state.

(10.) ——— from debility or loss of blood. (Asthenic.)

(11.) ——— from indigestion, repletion or other disorder of the Stomach. (Gastric.)

(12.) ——— from convulsions in general or epilepsy. (Convulsive or spasmodic.)

(13.) ——— from the effects of pregnancy. (Puerperal.)

(14.) ——— from injuries and blows on the head. (TRAUMATIC.)

It is said "sufficient has been done (here) to give a fair view of the many different causes which are capable of producing Apoplexy, as to justify a protest against a routine of treatment of Apoplectic conditions.

It must be confessed that it will be very difficult in many cases to determine accurately which kind of the disease exists, and some of them cannot be known until it is ascertained by post mortem examination. Enough, however, may be discovered by a judicious mind to learn that among the varieties there is such a difference as to require a remedy to be adapted Homœopathically to the symptoms.

For the first, second and third variety, the first remedy should be Acon. If there is a full flushed face give Bell., or use Bell after the Acon., or after the first stage is passed give Cocc. or Hyosc. To these varieties of the disease we infer the following judicious remarks in Dr. Peter's book will apply:

"Even if it be admitted that allopathic physicians bleed too much in Apoplectic attacks, it is generally supposed that Homœopathic physicians bleed too little—if the strength and vascular condition of the patient permit of it, or seem to require it, it seems very certain that bleeding will not interfere with the action of Homœopathic remedies—and it is even supposed that in some apoplectic and congestive affections of the brain, the pressure upon it and the nervous system may be so great, that they are as it were benumbed, and unable to respond to the action of any remedy until the pressure be relieved by blood-letting—hence I will endeavor to state as fairly as possible the advantages and disadvantages of blood-letting in Apoplexy."

Wood says: "If the strength of the pulse admit, blood should be drawn from the arm; but bleeding is not to be indiscriminately resorted to, or pushed to an unlimited extent."

Solly says: "Blood-letting is the most dangerous remedial agent in some cases of Apoplexy; —many a valuable life has been saved by the prompt and free use of the lancet; but more have been hastened into eternity by its indiscriminate employment."

As near as the remedies can be arranged in a concise way for a Repertory, they should be used as follows:

If the stupor continues, give Opi. or Rus. T.

If convulsive motions take place, Ignat. or Nux V

If the disease is growing out of debility or nervous weakness, give Cupr. Fer. or Nux V. or China.

If it seems to have been brought on from an increased quantity of serous fluids on the brain, we refer to the article Dropsy of the Brain for the remedies.

If from disease of the liver, the remedies pointed out under Liver will be indicated.

If from febrile inflammatory affection, please to examine Inflammation of the Brain for the treatment.

For the other varieties, reference is made to the heads of the affection named, for the remedies.

It may be difficult to point out the condition in cases of Apoplexy, where bleeding would be proper and when not. In the work just referred to, it is in a measure confined to those of full plethoric habit, with full tense pulse: and not in congestive cases, for these Opium in small or full doses is proposed.

In several instances in this work, we have pointed out the benefits of bleeding, in Congestion of the head and chest, when Apoplexy did not exist, and when the pulse is small and flaccid. It seems reasonable, that when congestion of the brain takes place so as to produce Apoplexy, that blood-letting might be useful; and if opium is given in large doses, it will be safer to precede it by the abstraction of blood: after which, opium in many cases acts more effectually.

In the somewhat advanced stage, if the stupor or impaired state of the mind continues, give Cocc. Hyosc. or Opi. or Rus. R. or Sec. C.

When Apoplexy is produced by mechanical injury, give Arnic. succeeded by Bell. Bathe the injured part with a lotion of Arnica; in an advanced state, if the symptoms continue, give Iodi. or Hell. In severe cases, blood-letting is recommended by Laurie and Hull.

"I am fully convinced that blood-letting is safe and useful in some cases."—(*Peters.*)

Copeman, an opponent to bleeding, says, "The only cases in which bleeding is proper, are those in plethoric habits." And Copeland admits the benefit of blood-letting, where there is slowness and fullness of the pulse. Rau says bleeding may be necessary in cases of true plethora.

It is stated on good authority, that Apoplexy may be brought on by a softening of the brain.—The remedies recommended for this variety, are Nux V. or Strychine.

APPETITE AND TASTE.

Appetite and Taste.—Aversion to bread or wine or coffee—give Rus. T. Sabad., Sep. or Sulp. ac.

——— Aversion to salt—Selen. Verb.

——— Bitter and insipid taste.—Give Caust. Colyc. Lach. Mag. C. Mag. M. Merc. Nicc. Nitr. ac. Phos. ac. Phytoll. Plati. Puls. Ranan. Bulb. Rus. R. Sec. C. or Stann.

——— Bloody taste.—Tarax.

——— Coppery taste.—Ranan. Bulb. or Russ. T.

——— Flat taste.—Sec. C. Seneg. Sulp. Thuy. or Valeri.

——— Greasy taste.—Sabad. Sang. or Sulp.

—— Horrid unpleasant—Lach. Lauroc. Lact. Viro. Mag. C. Mag. M. Merc. Nitr. ac. Phos. ac. Plumb. ac. Podopyl. Rus. T. Scill. Sep. Stramo. Sulp. or Sulp. ac.

—— Metalic—Merc. Rus. T. Sarss. Seneg.

—— Pappy—Sulp. or Sulp. ac.

—— Pepperminty sensation—Verat.

—— Putrid—Camp. Rhodod. Sep. Silec. Sulp. Sulp. ac. Thuy. or Verat.

—— Saltish or sweet—Rhodod. Sulph. Tart. Ant. or Valer.

—— Sour—Caust. Chin. Merc. Muri. ac. Nuc. Phos. Plati. Rus. T. Sarss. Scill. Silec. Sulp. Sep. Spig. Stron. or Staphy.

—— Thirst, very great—Acon. Camp. Sec. C. Silec. Stramo. Sulp. Verat. or Zinc.

—— Wanted or loss of—Chin. Sec. C. Silec. Spig. Stramo. Sulp. Verat. Zinc. or Ferr. or Caust.

—— Taste deficient—Arnic. Baryt. Bryo. Chin. Caps. Ferr. Hep. Ignat. Iodi. Kali. Bic. Lact. Vero. Lauroc. Lobel. Mag. M. Mosch. Morph., Nux V. Puls. Sep. Sang. Tereb. or Verat.

—— Hunger, excessive,—Caust. Chin. Lach. Mag. C. Natr. M. Opi. Oleand. Phos. Plati. Rus. T. Seneg. Spig. or Silec.

—— Voracious—Cam. Iodi. Lobel. Lach. Merc. Nitr. ac. Phytoll. Puls. Sabad. Sep. Spong. Sulp. or Verat.

—— Loathing of food—Chin. Mag C. Merc. M. Mosch. Muri. ac. Natr. M. Nux V. Prun. Sp. Puls. Sol. Nig. Stramo. Sepi. Silec. Sulp. ac. Tart. A. or Thuy.

APTHEA.

APTHEA.—Thrush, or Sprue.—The proper remedies are Bell. Borax, Camp. Hell. Iodi. Kali. Bic. Merc. Nux V. Petrol. Sepi. or Sulp., the best are Borax and Merc.

ASPHYXIA.

ASPHYXIA.—A state of the body during life in which the pulsation of the heart cannot be perceived, and the breathing is interrupted or irregular. There are several varieties of it, produced from different causes. Some of the principal ones are noticed here: Swooning, or common fainting.—The remedies for it are Acon. Ambr. Canst. Camph. Lauroc. Ammo. Aqua. or Ammo. Spts. Place the patient in a horizontal posture, and dash a little cold water in the face, apply the fumes of hot vinegar to the nose, or Camp. or Aqua. Ammo.

—— Apparent death from hunger—give the patient food in extremely small quantities, such as milk by the drop, beef tea and milk; or milk and water by injection in small quantities. When there is some improvement, the quantity of nourishment may be increased so as gradually to aid the reacting powers of life; and as there is a further improvement, the food may be increased.

——— Apparent death from a fall or mechanical injury—Keep the patient quiet; let the head be a little raised; place a very small dose of Arnica in the mouth. Repeat it in a short time; as soon as reaction begins, take BLOOD from the arm, but do it cautiously.—*Hull's Laurie.* Give injections of Arnica. *Note.* We have often witnessed the good effects of bleeding, as here directed.

——— Apparent death from hanging or suffocation—Place the patient in a straight position, the shoulders and head raised; rub the skin gently; give an injection of two or three drops of laudanum in a little warm water; apply warm cloths to the skin; inflate the lungs; furnish the fumes from hot vinegar to the nose for breathing. Give a little more Arnica or Camphor. When a person recovers to this state, he should be laid in a quiet position, and such remedies used as may best promote respiration, and reaction of the circulation of the blood, by the use of pure air or a gentle application of diffusible stimulants to the face—warmth to the skin, a little mild nourishment, &c.

——— Apparent death from lightning.—Place the subject in a current of cool air—dash cold water on it—after this, if the body gets cold, apply warm cloths or other hot applications to the surface, with friction. Put a little Nux V. on the tongue. This should be repeated in 15 or 20 minutes. Also give Nux V. by injection. After they revive, treat them similar to the preceding direction.

——— Apparent death from drowning.—1st. avoid rough usage. 2d. don't hold the body up by the feet. 3d. don't roll it over a cask. 4th. don't rub it with salt or spirits. 5th. don't inject smoke or tobacco; though warm water and spirits or salt and water may be used by injection. Rub the skin moderately with warm flannel—cover the body warm in bed, clear out the mouth and nose, give a little Lachesis, Solanum Nigrum or Solanum Mimosa—distend the chest by artificial means, as breathing—inflate the lungs—apply oxygenous air, if possible to the nose, to be breathed in.

——— Apparent death from freezing—Place

the body in a cold place, away from a fire —cover the frozen part with snow or ice, or apply cold water to it. When the parts get softened, they should be gently rubbed steadily till the skin is red; if they don't revive by this time, a small injection of about ten drops of spirits of camphor should be given. After this, give coffee and milk by injection: and a little coffee and milk may be given by the mouth.—*Hull's Laurie.*

ASTHMA.

ASTHMA.—By medical authors this disease is described as an affection of the lungs, producing difficulty of breathing, coming on at intervals, attended with a suffocative sensation, wheezing, a short contracted cough, languor, headache, flatulence, and a great oppression at the chest. The patient is unable to be in a recumbent position, or laying down; he has to sit up or be raised up in bed. He is anxious to obtain a full admission of air to supply a more increased quantity of vital air into the lungs. If the paroxysm is severe, the face becomes lucid, the hands and feet cold, the surface covered with a cold sweat, the pulse small and irregular.

Some persons are subject to almost continued symptoms of this disease, and liable to have it increased into a severe paroxysm from exposure or irregularity. This condition, sometimes is connected with a peripneumonic affection, which makes aggravated cases.

——— The remedies generally most useful for this distressing affection are Acon. Ambr. Ammo. C. Ars. Arg. N. Bell. Cann. I. Caust. Coni. Colch. Cupr. Digital. Ipe. Iodi. Kreoso. Lauroc. Lyc. Mosch. Muri. ac. or Nitr. acid. The last is said to have superior efficacy in relieving this disease. Or Nux V. Prus. acid, Phos. Puls. Sabi. Sang. Stann. Stramo. Sulp. Tart. A. Thuy. or Verat.

——— The dry or nervous form—The remedies are Acon. Bell. Bryo. Cupr. Ipe. Nux V. Opi. or Sulp. or Mosch. or Hyosc. Lyc. Samb. Silec. or Tart. Anti.

——— If a severe stricture or cramps take place, give Ambr. Nux V. Ipe. or Mosch.; after using these, if the cramps continue protracted, it will be better to give Hyosc. or Cupr. Samb. or Ars. Caust. or Stann.

——— Should the attack appear to arise from vapours, or some matter that has irritated the lungs, give Ipe. Hep. Merc. or Camp. Cupr. or Ars.

—— If it is brought on by convulsions or eruptions, or erysipelas receding, use Ars. Bryo. Carb. V. Phos. or Puls.

—— If the attack proceed from suppression of perspiration, or cold, or catarrh, give Ipe. Nux V. or Ars. or Puls.

—— When a congestion of blood in the chest seems to have brought it on, give Acon. Nux V. or Bell. Coni. or Auru. Folio. Puls. or Sulp. or Ipe.

When some of the above remedies have been used without affording relief, and the stricture continues severe with dyspnœa, or connected with pneumoniac affection, the advisable and best course to pursue is to mix about grs. 20 of Ipecac in a half-pint of warm water, and give a table spoonful every fifteen minutes, or at longer periods, till nausea and gentle vomiting is produced. By this course, the stricture is at once relieved and the breathing is more free; a perspiration comes out on the skin which affords great relief. When the late Dr. David Hosack resided at his country residence near Poughkeepsie, his wife had a severe attack of asthmatic pneumonia. I attended her as associate counsel. A variety of remedies were used, which afforded some relief, but did not effect a cure. On the progress she was seized with stricture at the chest and dyspnœa. Dr. Hosack declared the case was about hopeless, and that she would die. At

7 P. M. I proposed the use of Ipecac. as above detailed, like to what I had used in a number of similar cases with success. The Dr. objected to the proposal; but after a short reflection, he directed me to prepare the medicine and give it, and stay and watch its operation. I did so; the anticipated effect was produced. The breathing was relieved; a sweating came on by 12 o'clock; the next morning Dr. H. pronounced the patient safe. She recovered.

In severe cases of congestion of the lungs with Dyspnœa and labored breathing, we have frequently used this remedy in such a way, with great and decided benefit.

Asthma Humida.—The most useful remedies for this form of the disease, are Bryo. Bell. Coni. Coff. Colchi. Dulcam. Lobeli. or Ferr. Hep. Merc. Puls. Sepi. Samb. Sulp. or *Nitric acid.*

In a paper inserted in the North American Journal of Homœopathy on Nitric acid in Asthma, it is said to possess superior virtues to cure this disease.

——— If there is fever and pain in the chest, give Acon. Bryo. Ipe. or Tart. Ant.

——— If the attack comes on suddenly with stricture and a suffocating sensation, use Ipe. or Amb.

——— When the case does not yield to the remedies used, and the respiration continues laborious, with extreme anguish and deathly appearance or cold skin, Ars. Prussic acid or Veratrum are the proper remedies.

Should the case prove stubborn and some other remedy besides those named be necessary, a very good one may be found among those mentioned in general at the head of this article.

——— Hystericum—Agar. Ambr. Asa. F. Bell. Caust. Coni. Puls. Samb. or Stann.

——— Infantum—Acon. Asa. F. Bell. Cham. Camp. Cupr. Lobeli. Merc. Nux V. or Samb. (See Infants.)

——— Millar. (See Infants.)

BACK.

Back, bruised sensation in it. Natr. M. Nux V. Sabi. Sabad. Seneg. Silec. Sulp. ac. Tabac. or Tart. A.

——— Burning and Itching on it, Sabad. Scill. Senega. Spig. Stann. Sulp. ac. Tabac. or Tart. Antimo.

——— Coccygis, pain in it, Thuy. or Verat.

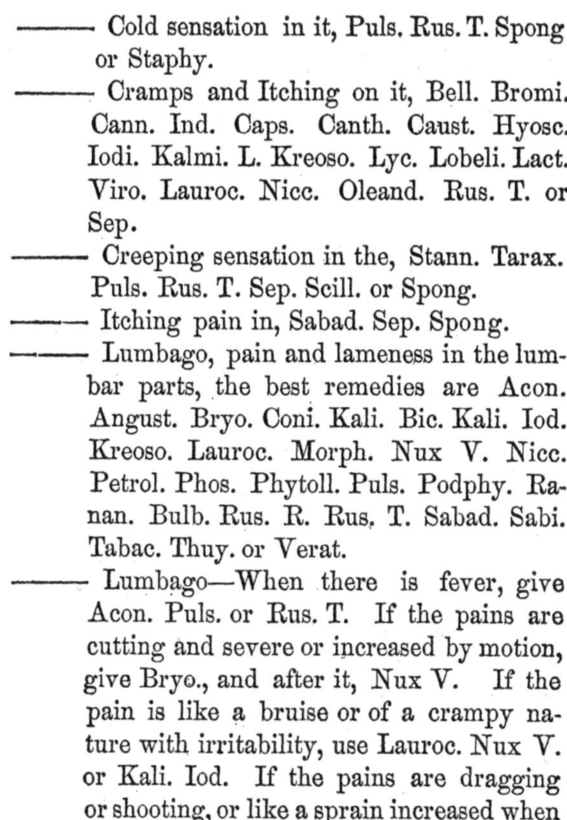

——— Cold sensation in it, Puls. Rus. T. Spong or Staphy.

——— Cramps and Itching on it, Bell. Bromi. Cann. Ind. Caps. Canth. Caust. Hyosc. Iodi. Kalmi. L. Kreoso. Lyc. Lobeli. Lact. Viro. Lauroc. Nicc. Oleand. Rus. T. or Sep.

——— Creeping sensation in the, Stann. Tarax. Puls. Rus. T. Sep. Scill. or Spong.

——— Itching pain in, Sabad. Sep. Spong.

——— Lumbago, pain and lameness in the lumbar parts, the best remedies are Acon. Angust. Bryo. Coni. Kali. Bic. Kali. Iod. Kreoso. Lauroc. Morph. Nux V. Nicc. Petrol. Phos. Phytoll. Puls. Podphy. Ranan. Bulb. Rus. R. Rus. T. Sabad. Sabi. Tabac. Thuy. or Verat.

——— Lumbago—When there is fever, give Acon. Puls. or Rus. T. If the pains are cutting and severe or increased by motion, give Bryo., and after it, Nux V. If the pain is like a bruise or of a crampy nature with irritability, use Lauroc. Nux V. or Kali. Iod. If the pains are dragging or shooting, or like a sprain increased when at rest, use Arnic. or Rus. T. If the pains are deep seated with a dullness, give Acon. or Bell. After the pain is relieved and stiffness remains, use Phytoll. or Angust or Coni., or Rus. T.

If the pain proceeds from a sprain of the back or a wrench forming that disease termed crick or strain of the back, use Arnic. Bryo. Nux V. or Rus. T. Avoid hot and irritating applications to the part; apply cloths wet in cold water or ice to the small of the back.

——— Lancing, pain in it, use Bryo. Lyc. or Rus. T. or Caust.

——— Sprained dragging sensation, increased when still, give Scill. Rus. R. or Rus. T.

——— Stiff, deep, grinding pains, use Bell. Puls. Rus. T.

——— Tired, bruised feeling, give Arnic. Merc. Nux V.

——— Psoas Muscles inflamed, give Acon. Bell. Canth. Colyc. Uva. Urs. or Tereb.

——— Psoas region to prevent suppuration there, give Acon. Hep. Scill. Silex. or Sulph.

——— Pus discharged from the Psoas part, use Auru. Asa. F. Arg. N. Plumb. Sulp.

——— Nates, (Buttocks,) Cramps in them.—Bryo. Scill. Spong. Staphy or Thuy.

——— Neck cramps in the nape, Iodi. Lyc. or Zinc.

——— Sprained and stiff.—Arnic. Lyc. Sep. Silec. Staphy.

——— Stiff and painful, give Caps. Coni. Hyosc. Iodi. Lach. Lauroc. Lyc. Mosch. Nux V.

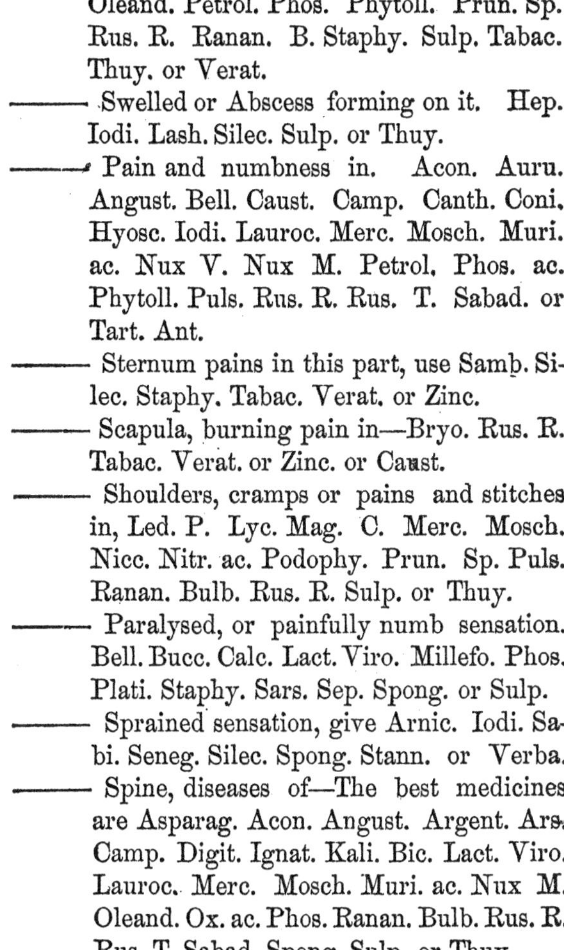

Oleand. Petrol. Phos. Phytoll. Prun. Sp. Rus. R. Ranan. B. Staphy. Sulp. Tabac. Thuy. or Verat.

——— Swelled or Abscess forming on it. Hep. Iodi. Lash. Silec. Sulp. or Thuy.

——— Pain and numbness in. Acon. Auru. Angust. Bell. Caust. Camp. Canth. Coni. Hyosc. Iodi. Lauroc. Merc. Mosch. Muri. ac. Nux V. Nux M. Petrol. Phos. ac. Phytoll. Puls. Rus. R. Rus. T. Sabad. or Tart. Ant.

——— Sternum pains in this part, use Samb. Silec. Staphy. Tabac. Verat. or Zinc.

——— Scapula, burning pain in—Bryo. Rus. R. Tabac. Verat. or Zinc. or Caust.

——— Shoulders, cramps or pains and stitches in, Led. P. Lyc. Mag. C. Merc. Mosch. Nicc. Nitr. ac. Podophy. Prun. Sp. Puls. Ranan. Bulb. Rus. R. Sulp. or Thuy.

——— Paralysed, or painfully numb sensation. Bell. Bucc. Calc. Lact. Viro. Millefo. Phos. Plati. Staphy. Sars. Sep. Spong. or Sulp.

——— Sprained sensation, give Arnic. Iodi. Sabi. Seneg. Silec. Spong. Stann. or Verba.

——— Spine, diseases of—The best medicines are Asparag. Acon. Angust. Argent. Ars. Camp. Digit. Ignat. Kali. Bic. Lact. Viro. Lauroc. Merc. Mosch. Muri. ac. Nux M. Oleand. Ox. ac. Phos. Ranan. Bulb. Rus. R. Rus. T. Sabad. Spong. Sulp. or Thuy.

——— Spine. The diseases of it may be acute or chronic inflammation, which may terminate in softening of the parts, or in induration of the spinal column, or in suppuration, or in gangrene, or in effusion of blood or watery fluid.

——— Disease of the spine—In the stage of acute inflammation, Acon. should be used with great perseverance; the person should be kept still in bed. This should be followed by Bell. Dulcam. Digital. or Ars. Puls. or Nux V. Rus. T. or Verat.

——— Spine in chronic inflammation—For the protracted type, give Asparag. Arg. Ars. Hyosc. Ignat. Merc. Nux V. Phos. Ranan. Bulb. Rus. R. Rus. T. Staphy. Sulp. or Thuy.

——— Spine, cracking sensation in.—Give Sulp. Tabac. or Verat.

——— Spine, curvature of.—Calc. Kali. Iod. Rus. T. Staphy. Silec. or Thuy. A mechanical apparatus may be necessary to support the parts.

——— Stiff, enlarged glands or tumors on.—Use Hep. Iodi. Nicc. Nux V. Phos. Prun. Sp. Rus. R. Rus. T. Sang. Spong. Sulp. ac. or Tereb.

——— Trembling sensation in—Rata. Rhodod. Sabad. or Tarax.

——— Weakness in—Angust. Sep. Scill. Sulp. ac. (See Rheumatism.)

BLADDER.

Bladder, the diseases of it and the urinary organs. —Calculus (gravel.)—The remedies are Ammo. M. Asparag. Calc. Canth. Cann. S. Lyc. Natr. C. Nux V. Petrol. Phos. Silec. or Uva. Urs.

——— Catarrh of the, or simple gleet—Borax. Caps. Colyc. Kali. C. Kreoso. Phos. or Nux V. Puls. Petrol. Sulp. Tart. A. or Tereb.

——— Diabetes Millitus—The remedies found most useful for this difficult disease are Carb. V. Led. P. Merc. Natr. M. Phos. ac. or Benzo. acid. Other remedies are also indicated, and have been used with more or less success. They are Ammo. C. Ammo. Caust. Arg. Nit. Baryt. C. Coni. Colyc. Iodi. Nux Jug. Rus. R. or Muri. ac. or Asclepias Vincet. Ars. or Alum. Tereb. Verat. When there is great desire to urinate, drawing up of the testicles, pain in the kidneys, dryness of mouth, &c. use Merc. Solub.

If the countenance is pale, of a deathly appearance, swelled gums, dry mouth or throat, excessive discharge of urine, give Verat.

When there is an absence of thirst, the urine milky, Muriatic ac. The diet should be nutritious. The other remedies are to be used in the various features of the disease, according to the symptoms presented and effects produced. (Examine the Materia Medica.)

—— Dysuria and Stranguary—Give Acon. if there is fever, use Arnic. Ars. Bell. Cann. I. Canth. Hep. Iodi. Kali. C. Lyc. Natr. C. Nux V. Phos. Prun. Sp. Puls. Rus. T. Sec. C. Silec. Sulp. Tereb. or Uva. Urs.

—— Inflammation of—The remedies are Acon. Bell. Camp. Canth. Cann. S. Digital. Nux V. Phos. Puls. Rus. R. Sep. Sulp. or Tereb.

—— Ischuria, (suppression of urine,) Apis. Mell. Canth. Cann. S. Cann. Ind. Coni. Hyosc. Nux V. Puls. Plumb. ac. Rus. T. Staphy. Stramo. Tart. A. or Tereb.

—— Itching and pain in neck of.—Stann. Tarax or Canth. Petrol.

—— Purulent discharge from the—Acon. Ars. Bell. Canth. Hyosc. Lyc. Lauroc. Muri. ac. Nux V. Opi. Petrol. Phos. or Tereb.

—— Spasms in the—Cann. S. Colyc. Prun. Sp. Puls. Sep. or Tereb.

—— Stone in the—Cann. S. Cann. I. Caust.

Kali. C. Lauroc. Nux V. Petrol. Phos. Sec. C. Tart. A. Uva. Urs. or Calc. aqua.

——— SYMPHISIS pain under—Tereb.

——— TENESMUS of—Sarss. Scill. or Tereb.

——— URETHRA burning, itching and pain in—Give Arg. N. Auru. Baryt. M. Cann. S. Camp. Caust. Colyc. Ignat. Kali. Bic. Lach. Petrol. Prun. Sp. Puls. Rus. R. Rus. T. Sabad. Staphy. Sulp. Tabac. Tart. A. Tereb. or Thuy.

——— URETHRA, bleeding from, Arnic. Auru. Bell. Coni. Iodi. Mann. Millifo. or Nux V.

——— BURNING pain in, Ammo. Caust. Camp. Canth. Hep. Kali. Bic. Kali. C. Kreoso. Lach. Lyc. Phos. Ac. Rus. T. Sabad. Sep. Stramo. or Tereb.

——— ITCHING in or pressing on, Ammo. C. Ammo. M. Ars. Arg. N. Arnic. Auru. Cann. I. Cann. S. Lyc. Petrol. Phos. Sulp. Ac. Tart. A. or Zinc.

——— URINE BLOODY, Arnic. Canth. Caps. Calc. Caust. Coni. Hep. Lobel. Mann. Merc. Millefo. Nux V. Opi. Prun. S. Phos. Sabad. Scill. Sep. Tereb. Thuy. Uva. Urs. or Sec. C.

——— BURNING pain in passing the urine—Cann. S. Petrol. Rus. R. Uva. Urs. or Verat.

——— Urine too copious. Caust. Kali. Iod. Kalmi. L. Kreoso. Lact. Viro. Mag. C. Mosch. Nicc. Nitr. ac. Ox. ac. Petrol. Rus. R. Rus. T. Sabi. Spong. Staphy. Sulp. ac. or Tarax.

——— DIFFICULT passing it. (See Dysuria.)

——— ENURESIS and wetting the bed, Acon. Bell. Baryt. C. Benzoic. acid. This is of superior efficacy; or Canth. Camp. Caust. Hyosc. Lobel. Muri. ac. Nitr. ac. Rus. T. Sep. Silec. Staphy. or Sulp. or Caust.

——— MICTURATION or dribbling, Canth. Caust. Lach. Lauroc. Millefo. Morph. Nitr. ac. Oleand. Petrol. Phos. Sabad. Scill. Stramo. Sulp. Thuy. or Verat.

——— MUCUS in, or milky appearance, Lach. Natr. C. Natr. M. Nux V. Nitr. ac. Petrol. or Seneg.

——— SEDIMENT in brown, dark or redish, Petrol. Puls. Sec. C. Selen. Sulp. Sulp. ac. Tart. Ant. Tereb. Thuy. or Zinc. or Caust.

——— SMELL of Ammonia or Iodine, Stron.

——— SMELL sour or fœtid, Natr. C. Natr. M. Puls. Rhodod. Rus. R. Sabad. Selen. Silec. or Thuy.

——— Yellow, redish and various colours, Bromi. Cann. S. Kali. Bic. Phos. Plate. Selen. Spong. Tereb. Verat.

BOILS.

BOILS.—To disperse them, use Acon. Bell. Rus. T. or Silec. To promote a suppuration, give Ars. Baryt. Hep. Merc. Opi. Externally use warm emmolient applications. (See Abscess.)

BONES.

Bones.—Caries, or curvature, or Nodes, &c. The remedies most useful in these affections are Arnic. Asa. F. Angust. Calc. Kali. Iod. Lach. Merc. Sol. Nig. Phos. ac. Sabad. Staphy. Sulp. Sulp. ac. or Phosphate of Iron;—in caries, we have observed great benefit from this article.

BRAIN.

Brain.—This organ is subject to various diseases, and those are often of a serious nature. They are mostly treated of under headache in this work.

Inflammation of the brain is noted under that article. A consideration of this will be found in its alphabetical place. A determination of blood to the head sometimes takes place, termed a rush of blood to the head, producing congestion, or an increased fulness of the vessels; sometimes this amounts to apoplexy. In persons who are predisposed to this affection, they should avoid the use of full, hearty, stimulating food, and all kinds of spirituous drinks; avoid extremes of exposure or excitement. It will be beneficial for them to take once a day or so, *a small dose* of Bell. Cocc. or Hyosc.

If there is an attack of Congestion somewhat severe, give Acon. or Bell.; after using one of these medicines, and the disease continues, give Arnic. Camp. Cann. I. Colyc. Digital. Hell. Hyosc. or Lauroc. Merc. or Nitr. acid.

If there continues stupor or indifference of the mind, use Coni. Hyosc. Nux V. Phos. or Stramo.

——— Concussion of—This morbid state of the brain is frequently produced by mechanical injuries. In the first place, the proper remedy is Arnic. Cold water should be applied to the head. If the affection is severe, and relief is not early obtained, the subsequent remedies should be Camp. Iodi., or if fever comes on, Acon.

For other affections of this organ, reference is made to them in their proper place.

BREATH FŒTID.

Breath Fœtid, and offensive, the medicines are Argent. Ars. Arnic. Bell. Carb. V. Cham. Hyosc. Iodi. Kali. C. Merc. Nux V. Puls. Petrol. Silec. Spig. or Sulp.

BRONCHITIS.

BRONCHITIS, Inflammation and raw soreness of the throat, Fauces and upper part of the chest or Bronchial Tubes. It may be an acute or a chronic disease. In the first or early stage, when there is some fever and soreness and pain of the throat, with dry cough, use Acon. Bell. or Ipe. If the fever is lessened, but soreness and cough continues, give Bryo. Digital. Ipe. or Tart. A. If there is cough and rattling, use Hep. Ipe. Spong. or Merc. If the throat is sore with head-ache or irritating cough, use Bell. Hyosc. or Sulp. If the cough is worse at night, give Hyosc. or Nux V. If there is tightness of the chest with dry cough, hoarseness &c., Nux V. Spong. Tart. A. Phos. or Iodi. The other remedies mentioned, will be useful in many conditions of the case, according to symptoms presented.

—— Chronic or advanced stage, give Ammo. C. Ammo. M. Caust. Hep. Iodi. Puls. Phos. Spong. or Sulp.

General remedies are Acon. Ars. Ammo. L. Ammo. M. Iodi. or Hep. Merc. Spong. or Sang. Seneg, Canth. Carb. V. Digital. Hep. Hyosc. Iodi. Lact. Viro. Nux V.

Petrol. Puls. Rus. R. Sep. Scill. Spong. Stophy. Sulp. or Tart. A. (See Chest, Angina, Cough, and Consumption.

BRONCHOCELE.

Bronchocele.—This is a morbid enlargement of the fore part of the neck, commonly called Goitre; the thyroid gland is generally the seat of the disease. In many cases, these tumours become very large and inconvenient; we have seen them as large as the head. In Cooper's Surgery, they are described "an indolent enlargement of the thyroid gland, with a swelling of the upper part of the neck." The remedies for this affection are very similar to those for Scrofula, such as Iodine, Spongia or Phosphate of Iron.

BURNS.

Burns.—At first, give Acon. or Arnic. afterward use Caust. or Sulp. For external use, put 10 drops of Tinct. of Arnic. to a half-pint of water, apply it, bathing with it cold; or add a teaspoonful of Alcohol to a gill of water, and use it in the same way; or wet a cloth with it, and lay it on the burned or scalded part; or use Spts. of Turpentine diluted in the same manner, so as to cause but little pain. It is recommended to apply moderately dry heat for a length of time, by holding the part near the fire, or holding a hot iron near it. An excellent remedy is soap, so much diluted as to cause very little pain; or at first to cover the part with dry flour dusted on; this quiets the pain directly. It is best to keep the part cool,—let it be exposed to the air as much as possible.

After the first stage is over, and the inflammation and pain have abated, the sore should be treated as an ordinary sore or ulceration, according to circumstances.

Internally, give Caust. Rus. R. Rus. T. or Sulp.

CACHEXIA, OR DYSCRASIA.

CACHEXIA, or DYSCRASIA.—This is a depraved, bad habit of body. An impaired state of the solids and fluids. This condition is generally connected with some general diseased action, producing emaciation, feebleness, and a want of action, such as scrofula, dropsy, marasmus, or chronic affection of some organ; of course, the remedies should be used in accordance with the immediate exciting cause. The general useful remedies are: Arnic. Ars. Calca. Carb. V. Coni. Ferr. Merc. Muria. acid. Sulp. or Iodi.

CARBUNCLE.

Carbuncle.—An inflammatory tumour, of the nature of a boil or abscess, inclining to run into a state of gangrene or mortification. In the first stage, it should be treated the same as an inflammatory swelling, by giving Acon. Bryo. Ipe. or Anti. and using means to disperse it. If the disease progresses and increases, use warm emollient remedies to procure suppuration. When symptoms of gangrene appear, give Ars. Carb. V. Chin. Kreoso. Rus. R. or Sec. C. Externally, apply yeast or charcoal poultices. When these ulcerate and break, several openings form of a honeycomb appearance. Then a free opening should be made in them.

CANCER.

CANCER.—This disease is defined by writers, "an ulcer proceeding from a previous scirrhous indurated tumour." Those tumours may form and remain a long time, even many years, without becoming very large or painful. At length, darting or twinging pains run through them. They grow and become more painful, and if means are not used to arrest their progress, they ulcerate, and form an open CANCER. They are seated in the glandular structure of the body. When ulceration takes place, it forms a painful sore, very difficult to cure. Various parts of the body are subject to them, but they are generally located on the nose, lips, cheeks, neck, stomach, and breast and womb of females; and the testicles of males. The treatment of this disease should be early directed to the occult or indurated state. The remedies most useful at this period, are Ars. Aster. Rub. Caland. Cicuta. Coni. Lauroc. By an early and steady use of some one of these medicines, the disease may often be arrested in its progress, and cured. When it has advanced so as to become an open ulcer, the above remedies are still recommended under various conditions of the ulcer. In addition to these, others are proper, such as Carb. Veg. Carbo. Ani. Kreoso. or Arnic. Clemat. Argent. Lyc. Petrol. Phos. or Phosphate of Iron. We have seen very happy results from this last medicine; by its use, the pain is lessened, and the ulcer placed in a more favourable way of healing.

CANCER of the breast of females. The appropriate remedies are Ars. Coni. Calend. and others of the above named medicines.

——— chimney sweep's Cancer. The proper remedies are Ars. Calend. Rus. T. or Thuy. or Kreoso.

——— of the lips. Ars. Arnic. Argent. Kreoso. or some of the preceding medicines.

——— of the stomach. This affection is attended with great difficulty and danger. The remedies recommended for it, are Ars. Baryt. C. Coni. Lyc. Nux V. Petrol. or Phos. High attenuations of medicine are adviseable. (See Diseases of the Stomach.)

——— of the uterus. This affection is veiled in a great deal of obscurity. The proper remedies for it, are Ars. Coni. Calend. Cicuta. Kreoso. and others of the preceding.

——— When it is attended with burning pain, give Ars. Bell. or Phos. Ferr. When the ulcer has a tingling, throbbing sensation, use Clematis. Lauroc. or Phos. If the ulceration is deeply seated, or there are sinouses running to the bone, use Auru. or Phos. Ferr. If they become fistulous, use Lyc. Baryt. or Argent. If the discharge become fœtid or offensive, use Carbo. V. internally and Carbon externally. A great number of remedies have been proposed and introduced as external applications for the cure of Cancers, but they have almost uniformly consisted of some corroding or caustic material, intended to destroy the texture of the part, and as it is termed, "eat them out." This is a painful process, and a very uncertain mode of curing. By their use, the adjoining substance becomes inflamed, the disease is apt to spread and affect the surrounding parts; if a portion of the indurated body is removed, some of the disease, or roots, as it is termed, may remain—which are almost sure to spring up and grow again. When caustics are used to an open cancerous ulcer, it is rendered irritable and painful, fungus excrescences spring up, and they may grow as fast as the caustic corrodes them down. Sometimes the patient is desirous of having the tumefied mass removed by a surgical operation; when it is situated in a favorable part, so that there is no material danger from wounding surrounding parts, it may be done with safety—in fact this is the shortest and best course. When they are removed they had better be done early, before the adjacent parts are seriously affected. Surgical writers agree that the operation for the removal of Scirrhous, Cancerous Tumours often fails from its being done after the disease has far advanced—when, if it was performed early it would have succeeded. This has been the result of our observation.

When a Scirrhous Gland is situated in a part where there is no danger of injuring surrounding organs, if it is removed early by an operation, we have observed, the patient has not been troubled with it afterwards.

CARDIALGIA.

Cardialgia, (Heartburn.)—A disordered state of the stomach producing a burning, uneasy sensation, attended with unpleasant exhalations, such as flatulence, oily or acid eructations, &c. The remedies for it are Ambr. Bell. Chin. Coff. Carb. V. Nitr. ac. Natr. C. Nux V. Plati. Puls. Petrol. Sang. Stann. Sulp. Sulp. ac. Tart. A. or Verat.

or Ferr. If there is acidity, this is one of the best remedies. Small doses of simple iron filings is a preferable form to give it.

CARIES AND NECROSIS.

CARIES AND NECROSIS. — From various causes the bones become diseased with this affection, forming what in common language is termed a *fever sore*. This condition of disease has generally, by Allopathic practitioners been left to nature—except the use of local remedies, and there has been plenty of these conjured up. They cannot produce much good, further than to keep the part comfortable, and the removal of detached pieces of bone. It must be by the internal use of remedies that a cure can be expected, and by this course important benefits are produced. By such remedies, we have witnessed very favorable results. For this disease, use Asa. F. Angust. Auru. Calca. Iodi. Merc. Nitr. acid, Phos. or Sulp. or Phosphate of iron. We have succeeded in curing Caries by the long continued use of this last medicine. Also nitric acid may produce excellent effects in this disease.

CHAPS OR CRACKS.

Chaps or Cracks on the hands.—With some, this is a very troublesome affection. The remedies for it are Arnic. Calca. Hep. Lach. Petrol. Avoid using soap in cold weather for washing. Indian meal or bran is more preferable for keeping them soft. (See Rhagades.)

——— Of the Nipples.—Use Arnic. Borax, Hép. Sulp. (See Woman, article Nipple.)

CHEST AND RESPIRATORY ORGANS.

Chest and Respiratory Organs.—This portion of the body is one of the most important departments in regard to the operations of the vital functions, and the diseases to which they are subject. They have furnished a theme for numerous discussions and examinations, to endeavor to arrive at a knowledge of their nature, and the means by which they may be relieved or cured. The symptoms produced by many of those morbid affections as are presented to view, will here be enumerated, and the Homœopathic remedies which are indicated and found most useful for them detailed.

——— Anguish sensation in it.—Give Acon. Bryo. Ipe. or Verat

——— Anxiety in.—Sulp. or Thuy.

——— Back and Shoulders, pain in.—Bryo. Baryt. Iodi. Lach. Lact. Viro. Lauroc. Lyc. Phos. or Rus. R.

——— Bloody expectoration from.—Give Bell. Millefo. Sabad. Scill. or Ipe.

——— Breathing irregular.—Use Tabac. or Verat.

——— Bruised sensation.—Arnic. Bryo. or Iodi.

——— Burning pain or stitches in.—Ammo. C. Anacard. Arg. Baryta. M. Borax. Caust. Ipe. Ignat. Kalmi. L. Lach. Nitr. ac. Phos. Puls. Rus. R. Rus. T. Sang. Stann. Sulp. Tart. A. or Verat.

——— Congestion of the Lungs.—Give Acon. Hyosc. Lact. Viro. Millefo. Nitr. ac Nux V. Phos. Puls. Sabad. Seneg. Spong. or Zinc. and perhaps Vena Section will be adviseable.

——— Hepatized Lungs, or Tubercles in them. —Give Kali. Iod. Iod. Merc. Muria. ac. Phos. or Sulp. See (Consumption.)

——— Hollow sensation in it.—Seneg. Stron. or Sulp.

——— Inflammation of the Lungs—Acon. Bell. Bryo. Ipe. Tart. Anti. See inflammation of the Lungs.

——— Inflammation, chronic—The suitable remedies are Bryo. Iodi. Nux V. Phos. Sang. Spong. or Sulp.

——— Itching sensation in—Nicc. Phos. Plumb. ac. Rus. T. Staphy. or Zinc.

——— Itching and Herpes over the chest—give Lach. Sepi. Tabac. or Sulp.

——— Itching and stitches increased on motion —Lach. Seneg. Sep. or Sulp.

——— Lungs gangrened or inclined to it—use Ars. Carb. V. Sec. C. or Silec.

——— Oppression of the lungs—give Ambr. Bell. Caust. Coni. Lyc. Petrol. Phos. ac. Puls. Rus. T. Staphy. or Verat.

——— Pain in it, intermittent—Arnic. Ars. Oleaned. Ranan. Bulb. Tart. Ant. or Verat.

———Parylitic or typhoid state—Nicc. Nux V. Phos. Seneg. or Ars. Carb. V. or Chin.

——— Pleurodynia—Ammo. C. Arg. N. Bryo. Camp. Caust. Coni. Iod. Kali. Bic. Kali. Iod. Lach. Lauroc. Lyc. Petrol. Puls. Rus. R. Rus. T. Sang. Silec. Sulp. ac. Tart. A. Verat. or Zinc.

——— Pressing outward sensation--Camp. Spig. Thuy.

——— Pulse and beat of heart irregular—Lach. Opi. Phos. or Seneg.

——— Rattling sensation—Natr. M. Natr. C. Nux V. Petrol. Phos. Sabad. Scill. or Stann. or Caust.

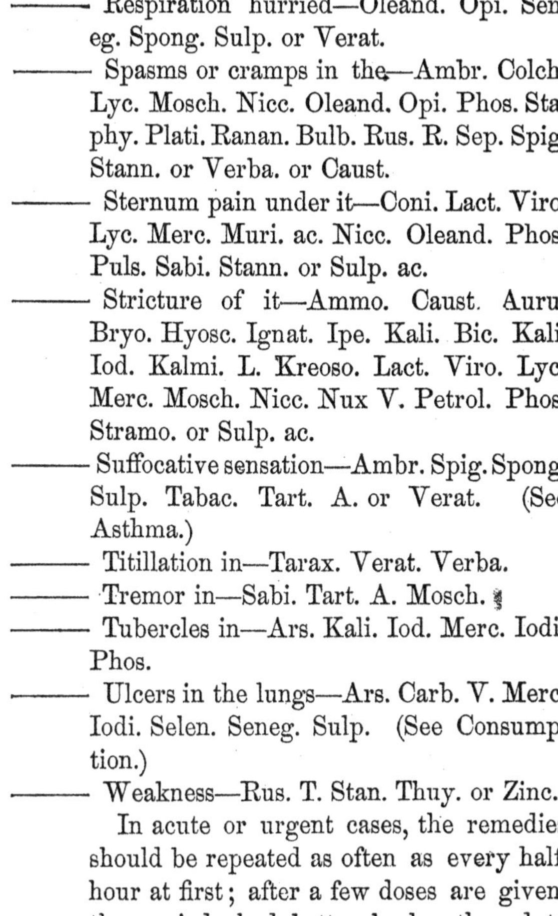

——— Respiration hurried—Oleand. Opi. Seneg. Spong. Sulp. or Verat.

——— Spasms or cramps in the—Ambr. Colch. Lyc. Mosch. Nicc. Oleand. Opi. Phos. Staphy. Plati. Ranan. Bulb. Rus. R. Sep. Spig. Stann. or Verba. or Caust.

——— Sternum pain under it—Coni. Lact. Viro. Lyc. Merc. Muri. ac. Nicc. Oleand. Phos. Puls. Sabi. Stann. or Sulp. ac.

——— Stricture of it—Ammo. Caust. Auru. Bryo. Hyosc. Ignat. Ipe. Kali. Bic. Kali. Iod. Kalmi. L. Kreoso. Lact. Viro. Lyc. Merc. Mosch. Nicc. Nux V. Petrol. Phos. Stramo. or Sulp. ac.

——— Suffocative sensation—Ambr. Spig. Spong. Sulp. Tabac. Tart. A. or Verat. (See Asthma.)

——— Titillation in—Tarax. Verat. Verba.

——— Tremor in—Sabi. Tart. A. Mosch.

——— Tubercles in—Ars. Kali. Iod. Merc. Iodi. Phos.

——— Ulcers in the lungs—Ars. Carb. V. Merc. Iodi. Selen. Seneg. Sulp. (See Consumption.)

——— Weakness—Rus. T. Stan. Thuy. or Zinc.

In acute or urgent cases, the remedies should be repeated as often as every half hour at first; after a few doses are given, the periods had better be lengthened to one or two hours, or at longer periods; in moderate or lingering cases, at still longer times.

CHILBLAINS.

Chilblains or Frost-Bite—Give internally, Agar. Ars. Carb. V. Lach. Nitr. ac. Nux V. Petrol. Phos. Rus. T. Sulp. Thuy. Zinc. Externally, bathe the feet with lotions of Arnic. Iod. or Rus. S.

CHOLERA.

Cholera Simplex or Simple Cholera Morbus.—The most adviseable and useful remedies for it, are Acon. Ars. Camp. Ipe. Merc. Nux V. Tart. Anti. or Colyc. Cupr. Plumb. or Opi. or Puls.

Should the disease have been brought on by cold or exposure, give Cham. Ipe. Ars. Puls. or Verat.

Where there is vomiting or diarrhœa, give Ipe. Anti. or Camph.; if there is fever, use Acon. in alternation with one or the other of these medicines.

If there is griping or cramps. give Nux V. or Ignat.

If colicy pains come on, use Colyc. Cham. Merc. Nux V. Puls. or Cuprum. or Opi.

If vomiting is a prominent symptom, give Camp. Ipe. or Anti. Should the disease continue after these remedies have been used, and there is griping pains, give Cupr. Colyc. or Verat. or Merc. Sol.

If there is a good deal of Tenesmus, give Lobel. or Nux V.

If in the progress of the case, there should be prostration, great thirst, or heat of the stomach, or a clammy state of the skin, give Ars. Cupr. or Verat. After the painful symptoms are over, if the diarrhœa continues, Cupr. Plumb. or Zinc. will be useful.

CHOLERA (EPIDEMIC.)

Cholera (Epidemic.)—In order to furnish some authority for the mode of treatment here recommended, it is proper to state that from the history of the Cholera, in all parts of the world, it appears that from dissections made, it has been discovered, that "the cells and cavities of the brain were filled and stuffed with dark blood, the lungs were injected and filled with dark or black blood." "The vessels of the stomach were injected with blood, showing traces of inflammation and congestion." Dr.

Cruvellier, of France, who had charge of an hospital, made extensive post mortem examinations; and discovered evidences "of inflammation of the stomach and intestines, and the brain was injected with blood."

In the description of simple inflammation of the villous coat of the stomach and intestines, without regard to cholera, Dr. Donaldson and Dr. Abercrombie say "it is attended with vomiting and diarrhœa of a watery nature, the skin is cold, the eyes are sunken in, the fingers are withered, the pulse is small and flaccid." Well does this description of inflammation of the internal surface of the alimentary canal show symptoms similar to those presented in Epidemic Cholera. With diffidence, we here lay down a plan of treatment of this fearful disease, which appears to be well adapted to the nature of the affection, and one which has proved more successful than any we have known. The remedies most useful are, Acont. Ars. Bell. Camphor. or Canth. Cuprum.—and Guaco. has lately been introduced as a remedy in Central America where it grows. It is stated to have superior efficacy to cure this disease. Other remedies are, Ipe. Phos. or Veratum.

The adviseable mode of using the remedies, is this. After the attack, first give Acon., about 3 or 4 drops of the 3d to 6th dilution, alternately with Camphor, or about one tenth of a drop of Camphor, may be used instead of the first dilution, every 5, 10, 20, to 30 minutes, or at longer intervals according to the violence of the case. When there is severe vomiting, Spirits of Camphor given in drop doses as recommended by some, is evidently too much, in severe cases, where the stomach is very irritable. These remedies should be used in the manner above stated. Even if there is a cold skin, or cramps have set in, let the patient often take small drinks of cold water, or small pieces of ice may be taken and held in the mouth, or swallowed.

There is in many cases a great demand for these cold articles to allay the burning and excessive heat and thirst which takes place; the water will be frequently vomited; but this is not an objection to it, for this removes the acrid irritating matter from the stomach, if such should happen to be there. It restrains and quiets the inflammation and burning of the internal surface of the stomach, and tends to stop the vomiting; cases are recorded which have been cured by cold water only. This course of treatment pursued early after the attack, will in a great number, or a majority of cases, check, control, or cure the case. This has been the result of our observations.

If it continues and spasms come on, or having set in, they continue with a cold skin, give Veratrum. If this does not check the symptoms, and afford relief after giving a few doses, and waiting a reasonable time, give Cuprum. either alone, or in alternation with Verat.; these remedies in this condition of the case, exert a very favorable influence over the disease. If there continues or takes place, a burning at the stomach, or a retching, give a high attenuation of Ars., a few doses alone, or alternately with Cupr. or Verat. (See the remarks on the specific properties of copper, in this disease, at the end of this article.)

When there are symptoms of congestion of the brain or lungs, attenned with a dingy leaden hue of the face, dull headache, sunken eyes, a tight short breathing, and small flaccid compressible pulse, spasms and a cold skin, in some cases these are among the first symptoms that occur.

In this condition, draw about four ounces of blood from the arm, or any part where it can be obtained. Blood may generally be obtained by placing the arm or feet in very warm water, and there rub them a while; a large vessel should be used for this, so as to immerse the hand and arm in the water—a large milk pan is a good article for the purpose.

When a vein should be opened, the blood at first will run very slow, perhaps only drop. By rubbing the arm in the warm water, it will moderately flow. In such cases, the blood is very dark and carbonated; it becomes more florid directly after a portion of it is abstracted, and there is a more free introduction of vital air admitted into the blood in the lungs.

If the symptoms are not considerably relieved in four or five hours, the operation of bleeding should again be performed; and this may be done to great advantage three or four times, in this small Homœopathic way. We have drawn blood more than this number of times, in this manner, and when blood could be obtained, by its aid with other remedies, we have almost invariably succeeded in curing the case.

In some cases, Ipe. in high attenuations will answer the purpose to allay the nausea or vomiting. If the stools are black or have a gangrenous fætor, Carb. V. will be a very suitable remedy.

If the attack is severe, and the pulse continues distinct and pretty firm, a full ordinary quantity of blood had better be taken at once, which generally directly tends to cure the case. In 1832 we had, and witnessed several cases which were checked and cured by the abstraction of blood, in which little or no medicine was given. It is stated that under the direction of Sir John Baker, British Consul General to Egypt in 1832, the feet and legs of those attacked with Cholera were put into a hot foot bath, and a vein was opened on either of those parts, the blood slowly run into the water so that the quantity lost, could not be determined, when the desired effect was produced.— The feet were wiped and rubbed dry. The next day or two, they (the patients) returned to their post in the army, or to their labor, none died!— *New York Morning Star*, *Dec.* 12*th*, 1848.

In such a congestive condition of the system taking place in the early stage of disease, on the abstraction of blood, the pulse rises, becomes more full and firm, the patient has an increased energy, and reaction is very much aided by it. We might quote authorities and cases in favor of this maxim, for they are abundant.

We have almost uniformly observed in this depressed state of cholera, that by this course, the vomiting and spasms have soon ceased, and the diarrhœa is checked, or very much lessened.

This result we have witnessed dozens of times. We have pursued this course, somewhat modified during three seasons, while the Epidemic cholera was raging, with very favorable results.

In 1849 in this city, under the course of treatment detailed here, the fatal cases did not exceed two per cent. A Register containing the result of the cases, was included in an Essay we published on that Epidemic in 1849. This Register contains the name of each patient, the residence, manner of attack, remedies used, with the termination. It corroborates the statistical result above named.

A similar register is contained in our treatise on the Epidemic cholera of 1832. This shows that the fatal cases in that Epidemic, were only five per cent.

During the sinking collapse stage, if the course above detailed does not relieve it, give Cupr. Guaco. or Veratrum, according to the judgment and opinions of the prescriber, or Arsenic—or Prus. acid according to the peculiarity of the symptoms; or if there are symptoms of asphyxia, or deep sinking takes place, Phos. will be a very proper remedy.

A very important agent which ought not to be omitted in low congestive, or collapse state of cholera, is Oxygen Gas or vital air, furnished for the patient to breathe. This may be supplied in a measure on an emergency, by the fumes of hot vinegar being brought near the nose so as they may be inhaled; experience and chemical knowledge may furnish better oxygenous articles.

It will be very important in the collapse state to keep away from the patient, mustard, liniments, chloride of lime, and all articles which by their volatile nauseous fumes will vitiate the air, and render it unfit for breathing. By inhaling such fumes, the blood in the lungs will be deprived of pure vital air, which is very much needed, and is one of the most efficient agents to bring about reaction.

In this is shown an important Physiological reason for blood-letting in the congestive state of this disease. It enables the dark black deoxydated blood to pass through the lungs with more facility; there to receive a supply of oxygen from the atmosphere, by a more free respiration, and this is the best stimulant to restore vitality that can be introduced into the system.

When the skin is cold the best external applications, according to our experience are hot water, or hot bricks placed about the patient, or fomentations of hot alkaline solutions and friction with hot dry flannel.

Note.—We have with pain seen patients struggle, and gasp for breath or vital air, from being enveloped in those fumes and nauseons exhalations alluded to, which filled the lungs, and deprived the blood of the ordinary oxygen, blended in the atmosphere. In such cases the patient requires all the natural oxygen of the atmosphere, and as much more as can well be supplied.

Medical readers may recollect the noted story related by SYDENHAM, that in 1660, among other calamities, an Epidemic plague raged in England, where many died suddenly.

A surgeon who had travelled much in foreign parts, was in the service and applied to the Governor, for leave to assist his fellow soldiers who were afflicted, which being granted, he took away so large a quantity of blood at the beginning of the disease, that they were ready to faint and drop down; for he bled them all standing and in the open air, and had no vessel to measure the blood, which falling on the ground, the quantity each person lost could not be known.

He gave no remedy except water after the bleeding; yet of the numbers treated in this way, not one died!!

DIRECTIONS

to prevent an attack of Cholera when it is prevailing in a place. It is best not materially to change the diet, or mode of living; but diminish the quantity of food usually taken. A moderate and steady use of good vegetables and fruit is adviseable, and will contribute very much to ward off an attack. There is a very great error in prohibiting these articles of diet.—On the contrary, avoid the use of stimulating peppery and spicy articles; also avoid spirits and all Alcoholic material—wash often and keep clean; avoid excessive bodily and mental exercise. It is best not to take Cathartic medicines.

As a general medicine or preventive Cuprum or Veratrum, is found to be the best. They are the great antidotes for cholera. The following is the proper method of using them; take the third, or higher attenuation, dilution, or trituration of Cupr. and Verat., one dose of each a day, or take a dose of one on one day, and the other the next, and so continue on.

It is stated on good authority, that in 1832, 150,000 persons in Vienna and 80,000 in Poland took these medicines in this way, that few of them took the disease, and that none of them died.

In the tenth No. of the North American Journal of Homœopathy, page 241, there is a paper, noticing a discovery made by Dr. Buro, of the Prophylactic powers of Copper, in preventing cholera, also indicating it as a remedy in the cure. In favor of this remedy, the following important facts are stated.

In 1832, in a copper foundary in Paris, out of 1300 workmen only 8 died, and one of those was a drunkard.

In 1849, out of 1300 workmen in a copper foundary in Paris, there were only 8 deaths; the most of these were drunkards. In a bronze manufactory where a large quantity of copper was used, in Paris,, there were employed 7000 workmen, out of them there were not over 10 deaths.

In Naine, in 1832, 500 men were engaged in copper works, there was only one death; the cholera prevailed severely in the vicinity.

In Russia, in a district containing 46,000 inhabitants in which were numerous copper mines, "the cholera did not penetrate the mines, though it was very prevalent in the neighborhood."

"In the use of copper," says Hahnemann, "it is the most certain and efficacious preventive of cholera." Dr. Buro, who made some discoveries and improvements on this subject, proposes using a chain of 20, 30, or 40 little plates of copper to go round the body to be fastened together by steel rivets and iron, during the prevalence of cholera.

A COMMITTEE of the New York Homœopathic Physician Society, in 1849, recommended the following regimen and medicine; and as far as is known, those who observed the directions, escaped the cholera.

"If there is an uneasiness of the stomach, or laxity of the bowels, take a drop of Spts. of Camphor 2, 3, or 4 times a day," this is Hahnemann's direction. The doses of Camphor ought to be very small.

Should there be a retching or nausea, which the Camphor does not check, give the 3d or 6th dilution or trituration of Ipe.

If there is heat or burning of the stomach, give Acon. or let it be given in alternation with Camphor; this course carefully pursued during the premonitory stage is tolerably sure to cure, or at least check the disease.

Avoid using stimulating and exciting remedies and nostrums, to prevent or cure the cholera; generally they are injurious, and large doses of

Opiates and Stimulants are very likely to produce the disease or increase it, and produce congestion of the brain and lungs, in consequence of which *the case may become fatal.*

Drugs of this description being injudiciously used to prevent and cure Epidemic Cholera, have, no doubt, been the means of rendering hundreds of cases fatal!!

From a large number of cases recorded in our treatise on the Epidemic Cholera of 1832, we select an abstract from three cases, which will show the influence of moderate and repeated bleeding, to remove congestive depression, and its aid in raising the pulse, and of bringing about reaction of the artereal and vital functions.

At this time we were not informed on the Homœopathic mode of cure, the way of treatment then pursued was moderate and repeated vomiting, and means of bringing about sweating, a free use of cold water as a drink in the first stage, and in the congestive prostrated cases, blood-letting; the detail of the remedies is omitted here.

The cholera was prevailing with great violence at Poughkeepsie, and many deaths had occurred.

Case first.—1832, July 26th, G. P. aged 14, was severely attacked; he had vomitings and diarrhœa of rice water consistence, sinking prostration, pulse nearly imperceptible; extremities cold, skin purple, eyes sunken in, tongue cold, burning heat at the stomach, urine suppressed, with spasms severe.—The arm was put in a pan of very warm water, a vein was opened, four ounces of blood taken; this was very thick and black; the patient was faintish, but soon roused up, the pulse was more full and free; liquids were rejected and ice was given, which was retained a while; in three hours, he was bled again, to four ounces; blood still dark, the pulse rose to more firmness, and the warmth of the skin increased.

July 27th—In five hours the spasms and vomiting abated, tongue still cold, the pulse had risen and increased to 100 in a minute: Vena. Section again to eight ounces. The pulse now rose, and became firm and full.

July 28th—The pain and spasms are gone, sweats freely, and passed urine for the first time since the attack.

July 29th—Inclined to sleep and stupor, is faintish, countenance dull and blueish, pulse obstructed, took six ounces of blood; after this bleeding, the faintishness and blueness entirely left him; the breathing was free and easy, pulse firm and regular.

July 31—Dismissed—cured.

This is the first cure of cholera we ever saw.

Case second, July 29th, 1832.—S. M. T. aged 14. Was attacked with vomitings and diarrhœa of a rice watery consistence and spasms; 9 A. M. suddenly prostrated, and nearly motionless, except the spasms; pulse imperceptible, burning heat at the stomach, respiration laborious, skin and tongue cold; leaden color of the face, eyes sunken, voice sepulchral, and urine suppressed

Aether was given a dose or two, the arm was placed in very warm water, and rubbed, as soon as possible a vein was opened, the blood came only by drops,—by perseverance, three ounces were obtained which was thick and black; it remained unchanged in the bowl, and had so far lost its vitality, as not to attract oxygen from the air, as blood generally does, to give it a more florid color on standing.

12, M.—She is becoming a little warm, pulse still nearly imperceptible, three ounces of blood more taken.—3 o'clock, P. M.; she had got into a warm sweat, pulse more full, but depressed, took four ounces of blood.

July 30th—6 o'clock, A. M.; pulse gaining in fullness and firmness, but oppressed, and difficulty of breathing—took four ouuces more of blood. 11, P. M.; sweats freely, breathing improved; tongue a lively red, (a mark of an inflammatory state of disease,) pulse still depressed; skin inclining to coldness, and is dull and purple—bleeding four ounces.

The blood now ran freely, and was of a florid lively color.

July 31st—Has improved considerably, still has symptoms of depressions, and suppressed inflammatory condition—took four ounces more of blood.

Aug. 1st—The disease is entirely broken up—cured.

Case third, July 27th, 1832.—C. M. aged 15. Was attacked with severe rice watery evacuations. In two hours, he became extremely cold and purple, and was insensible; violent spasms took place, so that it took several persons to hold him, he was speechless; his eyes were sunken in, his fingers withered.

The arm was immediately immersed in almost boiling water, ten ounces of blood were taken; it was very thick and black, some relief followed, and in three hours he was bled again; the blood ran more freely and was more florid; now the vomiting, spasms, and diarrhœa ceased; in six hours, a genial warmth was perceptible over the skin, the pulse raised tolerably fair, and the bleedings, in a small way, were several times repeated; so that in all, in forty-eight hours, he lost forty-four ounces of blood, at the end of which time, his senses returned, then, by a moderate use of sudorifics, nourishment, &c. he recovered.

These persons all have enjoyed good health and are now living—1853.

Those inclined to examine the authorities for this mode of treating this peculiar character of disease, are referred to Sydenham's Works, the elegant History of the Epidemic of 1793, by Dr. Rush, the essay on the epidemic of 1812, by Dr. Mann, do. by Professor Gallup, Donald's History of Epidemics, and to our humble History of the Epidemic of 1812, as it prevailed in Dutchess County, New York.

"Riverius describes an epidemic which prevailed in 1623, which carried off one half of all those who were attacked; finally, he prescribed the loss of three ounces of blood; the pulse rose, with this small evacuation; three hours afterwards, he drew six ounces more with the same good effect; and this course, he says, rescued the patients from the grave."

CONGESTION.

Congestion—This state of the body frequently takes place when it is affected with disease. It often presents an obscure set of symptoms, and a condition which may lead to errors in the mode of treatment.

By writers congestion is defined "a collection of blood or fluids in vessels or parts more than is natural when they are over distended, and the motion through the part is slow;" there seems to be an interruption of the regular balance of the circulation, and there is a determination of fluids to a part. This condition takes place at the attack of violent diseases, such as epidemics; an appearance of weakness and sinking frequently occurs, which in reality may be prostration, from excess of morbid excitement, and produces an overpowering of the corporeal and vital functions, instead of direct debility. It has obtained various names by different writers. Sydenham termed it oppression or depression; Dr. Brown called it indirect debility; Dr. Rush termed it debility from action or over action; Dr. Donaldson gives it the name of compound inflammation, or inflammation combined with congestion. Armstrong adopted the term CONGESTION, by which it appears now to be understood; when there is a severe attack of disease, and when this state takes place, there is frequently an acheing tired sensation, a dull heavy headache, a nausea and vomiting, or diarrhœa, and a dingy lurid countenance; the eyes are dull, or loose their natural brilliancy, there is a torpid doughy feel of the skin, it is sometimes very cold; there is often a small and flaccid, or what is termed by writers, a compressible pulse, the breathing is short and labored, particularly so when the congestion is located on the lungs. In the first stage, the tongue is covered with a light whitish fur, soon after the attack, the edges of the tongue show a lively redness; Dr. Rush says this appearance of the tongue is a sure indication of an inflammatory condition of disease; this appearance of the tongue, when the depression was removed and reaction permitted to come out, was exhibited in the epidemic of 1812, 1832, 1834 and 1849. The symptoms are frequently more severe and violent than here detailed; this set of symptoms with others are described as having ushered in a great portion of the cases of the violent and malignant epidemics of our country.

An error of treatment of this state of disease seems to have been, in the early use of cordial, stimulating articles, exciting sudorifics, or opiates and mercurials, from an opinion that those symptoms indicated a state of direct debility, or an approximation to a typhoid and gangrenous condition of the system; opinions of this kind led to the use of those remedies in the Allopathic practice, intending to support the action, and, as we have heard it expressed, *to keep the system from running down.* Experience shows that such a plan of treatment has not been the most successful, —and generally has been very fatal.

It appears that, from the facts disclosed in the histories of those diseases, and from the effects of remedies used, those symptoms of congestion do not indicate a state of direct debility or exhaustion, but on the contrary, they attend a condition of compound inflammation or depression; that at the attack of those violent diseases the morbid condition is one of phlegmasial action; congestion is more likely to take place in full plethoric habits, and on the sudden attack of disease, though it may be connected with a state of weakness. The foregoing remarks allude mostly to opinions and practice of the Allopathic school.

When this condition of disease is to be treated by Homœopathic means, the remedies should be selected and used according to the symptoms presented; generally, the first remedy is Acon. or Bell.; after these, if there is stupor, or pressure on the head, use Cocc. or Opi. or Hyosc.; when there is a great depression and apparent obstruction to the circulation, it will be adviseable to take a small quantity of blood, if the pulse rises and becomes more firm, as it generally does, and the symptoms are not relieved, the operation may be repeated to advantage. In such cases the blood is dark or black, and deoxydated; in some severe cases of depression and languid circulation, the blood is so dark and deprived of vitality, that it has lost the property of absorbing oxygen from the air, to give it a more florid color while standing in the vessel, which it generally does; yet, by pursuing the course here indicated, the circulation has improved, reaction taken place, and the patients have recovered from such a condition as above described.

On the abstraction of blood early in a small Homœopathic way, (and this is a Homœopathic remedy for such a state of disease,) the pulse uniformly rises, becomes more full and firm, the blood changes its dark, carbonated appearance to that of a more florid color, and exhibits more evidence of vitality: when the depression is removed in this way, reaction sometimes comes out with a full bounding pulse.

In illustration of this subject, an extract is introduced from our History of the Epidemic Cholera of 1832: "bleeding ought to be confined to the first twenty-four or forty-eight hours. There is an important rule respecting bloodletting which is of the utmost importance, where there is great depression—the pulse is small, obscure, or imperceptible; the quantity of blood drawn at a time should be small, and the operation often repeated, until a more full and firm pulse comes out." In such cases taking large quantities of blood would be injurious; this was an important point in practice in the Epidemic of 1793, noticed by Dr. Rush; also in that of 1812, noticed by Drs. Mann and Gallup.

To show the reactive powers of the system, in closing this article, we introduce a case taken from our history of 1832, just referred to. Mrs. B—had a violent attack of cholera, attended with spasms, depressd state, cold blue skin, almost pulseless; rice watery evacuations,—by three small bleedings and other means, reaction came out; when it was so active and violent, that it required three more bleedings to subdue the inflammatory action; in all, she lost about seventy-five ounces of blood, when she soon recovered, and enjoyed good health afterwards.

In the advanced stage, if the symptoms are somewhat moderate, it will be adviseable to use Millefo. Merc. Nux V. Nitr. ac. Rus. T. or Colyc. Tart. A. or Sulp.

CONGESTON of the brain—Give Acon. Bell. Cocc. or Hell. and some of those remedies above mentioned. At first, apply cold water or ice to the head; when the first or urgent stage has somewhat passed, warm water and spirits should be applied to the head, as directed by Hahnemann and Teste.

COLIC.

COLIC.—The remedies most useful for this class of diseases are the following; they are arranged so as to be used according to the various symptoms. Acon. Bromi. Camph. Caps. Cham. Colyc. Ipe. Lobel. Merc. M. Nicc. Nux V. Opi. Phos. Rus. R. Stophy. (See this article under Abdomen.)

——— Flatulent—give Anis. Ars. Caps. Carb. V. Cham. Muri. ac. Nux V. or Phos.

——— Hæmorrhoidal, or griping at the anus.—Use Acon. Aloe. Lobel. Nux V. Puls. or Sulp.

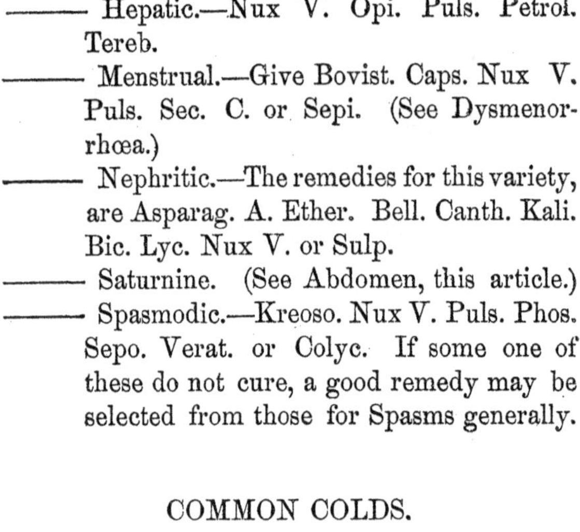

——— Hepatic.—Nux V. Opi. Puls. Petrol. Tereb.

——— Menstrual.—Give Bovist. Caps. Nux V. Puls. Sec. C. or Sepi. (See Dysmenorrhœa.)

——— Nephritic.—The remedies for this variety, are Asparag. A. Ether. Bell. Canth. Kali. Bic. Lyc. Nux V. or Sulp.

——— Saturnine. (See Abdomen, this article.)

——— Spasmodic.—Kreoso. Nux V. Puls. Phos. Sepo. Verat. or Colyc. If some one of these do not cure, a good remedy may be selected from those for Spasms generally.

COMMON COLDS.

Common Colds.—The treatment for those affections, is detailed under Angina Catarrhalis, which see.

——— To prevent taking them, by those very subject to it, every day or two, or at longer periods, take a dose of 4 or 5 globules, of the 1st or a low attenuation, or a powder of a low trituration, of Calca. C. Ferri. Ignat. Nux V. or Sepi. By following this course, persons may guard the body against the frequent taking cold, or of being affected with quinsy.

COMA.

Coma.—The remedies proper for this affection, are Ars. Bell. Bromi. Cocc. Coff. Hyosc. Ignat. Lach. Mosch. Opi. Sabad. Sola. Nig. Tart. Anti. or Verat. (See Stupor.)

CONSCIOUSNESS.

Consciousness, loss of.—The suitable remedies for this condition of disease are Camph. Bell. Phos. Stramo. (See Asphyxia.)

CONSTIPATION.

Constipation, or Costiveness and Stool.—This is a very common and troublesome state of disease. It often requires a good deal of care and perseverance to afford relief in those cases, or to cure the inactive torpid state of the bowels. The common practice of the Old School practitioners is to give purgatives in such cases, and to direct their constant repetition. This course only affords a temporary relief, and rather increases the difficulty. A constant use of drastic purgatives frequently brings on Hæmorrhoids and other diseases in and about the rectum. The object of the

Homœopathic practitioner ought to be to afford present relief, also to use remedies to enable the bowels to respond to the calls of nature, by their inherent peristaltic action, so as to procure regular natural evacuations. There are a great number of medicines which are useful for this purpose. They should be used according to the symptoms and condition of the case. Those most useful are Alum, Ammo. C. Asteria. Rubens. Bryo. Carb. V. Colyc. Gum. Gtt. Hyosc. Iodi. Ipe. Kali. Bicc. Kreoso. Lach. Lyc. Ignat. Narcissus. Nux V. Nitr. ac. Opi. Petrol. Phos. Podophylline. —this is very efficacious,—Puls. Ranan. Bulb. Rus. R. Rus. T. Sabad. Sepi. Sulp. Tart. Anti. Tereb. Thuy. or Verat.

The remedies should be used in this manner: In recent cases, Opi. Nux V. Sulp.

——— In old people.—Use Bryo. Lach. Tart. A. Phos.

——— In torpid conditions of the bowels.—Use Alum. Opi. Plumb. Podophilin.

——— Rheumatic cases.—Use Bryo. Puls. Rus. T. Lyc. Podophylin. or Rus. T.

——— Dyspeptic subjects alternating with Diarrhœa.—Use Ignat. Nux V. Puls. Rus. R. Stramo. or Sulp.

——— When Hæmorrhoids are attending.—Use Sulp. Ignat. Nux V. Petrol. or Sabad.

——— If attended with dry skin or determination of fluid to the head.—Use Tart. A. Ipe. Bryo. Puls. or Verat.

——— In females, who have irregular Catamenia.—Use Nux V. Sepi. Puls. Sulp. or Tereb.

——— When there is in the anus burning and pain and irritation.—Use Colocy. Kali. C. Mag. M. Natr. Muria. Nicc. Nux V. Oleand. Phos. ac. Plumb. ac. Puls. Rus. T. Sabad. Staphy. Stron. Tereb. or Thuy. (See Hæmorrhoids.)

——— If the patient has ascarides discharged.—Aloe. Chin. Mag. C. Sepi. Spong. Scill. or Sabad.

——— If it is in consequence of over quantities of food.—Nux V.

——— If it is the effect of fat greasy food—give Puls.

——— If the expulsion requires great straining–use Opi. or Platina.

——— If the case is obstinate, with contraction of the anus—use Plumbum. Met.

——— When there seems to be a loss of action of the rectum, with dry skin and cold feet—give Verat.

——— If it becomes habitual—use Sulp.

——— If it is accompanied with Colic—give Silecia.

——— If there is flatulence, and a pressure of blood to the head—give Lyc.

——— Bloody stools.—Give Caust. Kali. Bic. Lyc. Millefo. Merc. Natr. C. Nux V. Oleand. Puls. Rus. R. Sabi. Sarss. Scill. Stramo. Tart. Ant. or Thuy.

——— Bloody and pus passing.—Give Lach. Lobel. Natr. C. Nitr. ac. Sabad. Sulp. ac. Thuy. or Verat.

——— Anus contracted.—Give Lach. Lauroc. Mag. C. Nux V. Nicc. Plumb. Acet. Rus. R. Rus. T. Sulp. (See Hæmorrhoids.)

——— Fissure of anus.—(See Hæmorrhoids.)

——— Anus, pressing on.—Give Sabad. Sulp. ac. Tabac. Valeri.

——— Anus prolapsus.—Give Aloe. Merc. Nux V. Opi. (See Hæmorrhoids, this article.)

——— Anus, spasms in.—Lach. Nux V. Phos. Rus. R. Spig. Sec. C. Seneg. Sulp. Thuy. Verat.

——— Anus, sensation of crawling in.—Give Aloe. Spig. Thuy or Zinc.

——— Expulsion power, loss of.—Give Aloe. Nux V. Silec.

——— Flatus, excessive and fœtid.—Carb. V. Seneg. Sec. C. Sepi. Spig. Scill. Stann. Sulp. or Zinc.

——— Rectum and anus burning or paralyzed

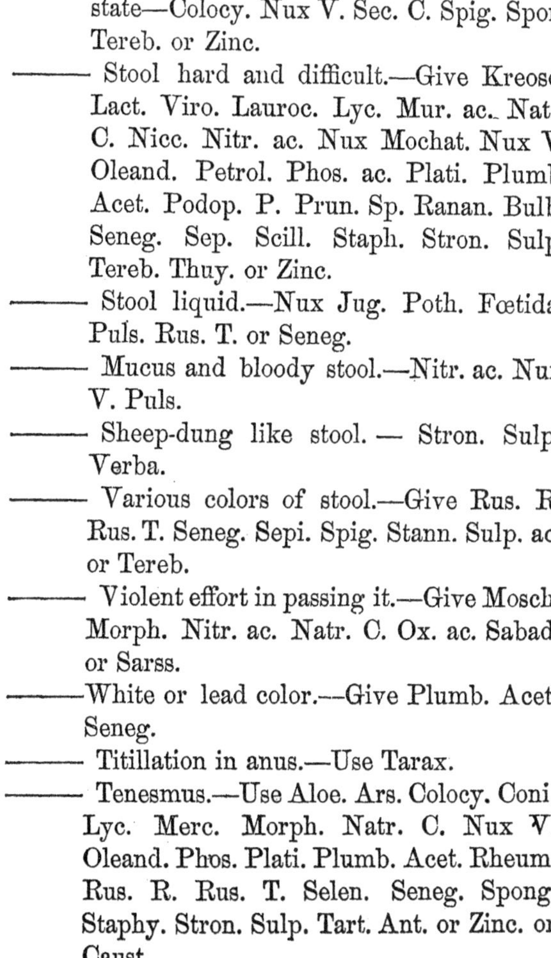

state—Colocy. Nux V. Sec. C. Spig. Spon. Tereb. or Zinc.

——— Stool hard and difficult.—Give Kreoso. Lact. Viro. Lauroc. Lyc. Mur. ac. Natr. C. Nicc. Nitr. ac. Nux Mochat. Nux V. Oleand. Petrol. Phos. ac. Plati. Plumb. Acet. Podop. P. Prun. Sp. Ranan. Bulb. Seneg. Sep. Scill. Staph. Stron. Sulp. Tereb. Thuy. or Zinc.

——— Stool liquid.—Nux Jug. Poth. Fœtida. Puls. Rus. T. or Seneg.

——— Mucus and bloody stool.—Nitr. ac. Nux V. Puls.

——— Sheep-dung like stool. — Stron. Sulp. Verba.

——— Various colors of stool.—Give Rus. R. Rus. T. Seneg. Sepi. Spig. Stann. Sulp. ac. or Tereb.

——— Violent effort in passing it.—Give Mosch. Morph. Nitr. ac. Natr. C. Ox. ac. Sabad. or Sarss.

———White or lead color.—Give Plumb. Acet. Seneg.

——— Titillation in anus.—Use Tarax.

——— Tenesmus.—Use Aloe. Ars. Colocy. Coni. Lyc. Merc. Morph. Natr. C. Nux V. Oleand. Phos. Plati. Plumb. Acet. Rheum. Rus. R. Rus. T. Selen. Seneg. Spong. Staphy. Stron. Sulp. Tart. Ant. or Zinc. or Caust.

CONSUMPTION.

CONSUMPTION.—The important nature of this disease, and its frequency in affecting individuals, and in hastening the termination of life, renders it worthy of consideration, to give it careful attention, but as it is not the object here, to dwell upon descriptions, or detail symptoms of diseases, the reader who has a disease of the lungs, is advised to apply to a Homœopathic physician. For if those cases are carefully and judiciously treated in the early stage, they may generally be relieved, or cured, or the disease very much arrested in its progress. There is no disease affecting the human system for which there are so many nostrums, specifics, and certain cures offered, as for that of the delicate, intricate, and important organ, the lungs; and for which no one general medicine can effect a cure, and a combination of many medicines in a mass or syrup, and nostrums, are still more uncertain, absurd, and dangerous. Numerous, very numerous cases of diseases of the lungs are rendered fatal, and the patient hastened out of time, by the use of those advertised, ignorantly and criminally recommended medicines.

By medical writers, this disease is divided into three stages; in reference to this division, the medicine will be given herein. The remedies which are generally recommended and used to the best advantage, are the following. But these are useful or not, according to the stage of the disease, or situation and peculiarity of the individual or patient: Acon. Ambr. Ars. Bell. Calc. Dulcam. Ferr. Ferr. Iod. Guaco. Iodine. Kali. Iodi. Kreosot. Lach. Lact. Viro. Lyc. Merc. Merc. Iod. Naptha. or Jucor or cod liver oil. This last remedy has lately become a hobby in Allopathic practice; if a patient has a disease of the lungs, *cod liver oil* seems to be a standard remedy, and patients are induced to swallow this *nauseous, disgusting drug*, by the bottle frequently, to their very great injury,—often hastening death.

There are, however, some peculiar conditions of diseased lungs for which this remedy would be useful; and this may be ascertained by examining the pathogenesis of the drug, in a work on pure Materia Medica. The other suitable medicines are, Bryo. Ipec. Hep. Puls. Nux V. or Hyosc. or Nitr. acid. In the second stage, when there is less fever and inflammatory symptoms, but harassing cough, moderate expectoration, slight pains in the chest, night sweats, loss of appetite, and diminution of strength, the proper remedies are, Nitr. acid, Spong. or Kali. Iod. Merc. or Lach. Lyc. Phos. or Calc. Coni. Iodi. Samb. or Ammo. M. or Zinc. In the third stage, or when purulent expectoration takes place, night sweat, emaciation, or debility, &c. some of the aforementioned medicines will be proper: or use Guaco. Sepi. Staphy. Iodi. of mercury, phospate of iron. This last medicine frequently produces very happy results.

The symptoms of this disease runs into each other so, that it is impossible to point out a very definite line between the stages. (Please to examine Chest diseases, Cough, Hectic, &c.)

CORDE.

Corde.—See Genitals, Penis, and Priapnism.

CORNS.

Corns—The remedies most useful to effect a cure of this troublesome complaint are, Arnic. Ammo. C. Calc. and Iodi. This last may be given and used with great benefit externally, or give Lach. Petroleum. Silec.

Sulp. or Thuya. By the continued use of some of these remedies, those annoying excresences may generally be cured.

COUGH.

Cough—This affection is a very common general disease, produced by a variety of causes, and connected with many states of morbid action; therefore, it will be apparent that there are a great number of remedies which may be used to advantage for it, under different conditions; always endeavoring to select the one most Homœopathic to the case.

Those generally most useful and proper are, Acon. Ammo. C. Ambr. Arnic. Ars. Bell. Bryo. Baryt. Bromi. Calc. Cham. Carb. V. Dolich. Droser. Dulcam. Hep. Hyosc. Ignat. Kali. Iod. Lach. Lyc. Mag. M. Merc. Nitr. ac. Nux V. Oleand. Opi. Petrol. Phos. Phytol. Prun. Sp. Puls. Prus. ac. Rus. R. Sang. Sabad. Sambu. Seneg. Sepi. Stann. Scill. Sulp. or Verat.

——— With fever and pain—Acon. Bell. Ipe.

——— Dry sore throat, or barking cough—Bell.

——— Nervous irritable state, hoarseness—Ignat. Hyosc. Nux V. Opi.

——— Increased in cold air—Ars. Lach. Phos.

——— Increased with twitching in the throat—

Cham. Arnic. Bryo. Lyc. Phos. Drose. Puls. Merc. or Sulp.

——— Raw feeling in the throat—Nux V. Puls.

——— Dryness in the throat—Puls. Lach. Carb. A. or Petrol.

——— If there is burning in the chest—Ammo. C. Ephorb. Natr. C. or Phos.

——— Mucus accumulating in the throat and chest—Ars. Anti. Caust. Kreoso. Stann.

——— If worse when lying down—Ars. Lach. Hyosc. Puls. Merc. Nux V. or Sulp.

——— Cough catarrhal—Bell. Bryo. Hep. Spong. Spig. Scill. Sulp. or Verat.

——— Chronic—Ammo. C. Ars. Lach. Stann. Stron. Sulp. or Sulp. ac.

——— Expectoration bloody—Led. P. Lyc. Merc. Millefo. Muri. ac. Natr. C. Nux M. Puls. Prus. ac. Phos. Rus. T. Sabad. Sabi. Scill. Spong. Staphy. Sulp. or Zinc.

——— Expectoration green—Lach. Stann.

——— Of mucus—Ammo. C. Ammo. M. Ars. Lach. Ipe. Scill. Sulp. Stann. Staph. Stron. or Tart. Anti.

——— Of pus—Calc. Sabi. Stann. Prus. ac. Sulp.

——— Hollow—Spig. Spong. Staphy. Stron. Sulp. or Tart. Anti.

——— Night—When it is worse in the night than in the day time, give Caust. Coni. Hyosc. Nux V. Phos. Puls. Rus. T. Scill.

Sabad. Seng. Sep. Silec. Spong. Sulp. Verat.

——— Spasmodic—Coni. Lact. Viro. Lauroc. Merc. Opi. Phos. Rus. T. Sabad. Sepi. Scill. Stramo.

——— Suffocating—Coni. Dolich. Ipe. Lauroc. Lach. Lact. Viro. Lobel. Lyc. Puls. Rus. T. Samb. Sepi. Silec. Spig. Spong. Stramo. Tabac.

——— Throat ulcerated—Lach. Lyc. Natr. C. Nitr. ac. Seneg. Silec. Spong. Stann. Sulp. or Zinc.

——— Tingling and dry sensation of the throat —Kreoso. Lact. Viro. Lyc. Lauroc. Muria. ac. Nicc. Nux M. Rhodod. Rus. T. Sabi. Scill. Seneg. Silec. Spong. or Sulp.

COUGH (HOOPING.)

Cough, Hooping. — This is considered to be a contageous disease; it generally attacks children, though there are cases reported where adults have had it. It prevails in some districts almost every year, and still more frequently in cities. It spreads more in the cold season than in the warm. Sometimes the cases are very numerous and violent, being like an epidemic, at others they are scattering and not very violent. It has hitherto been a severe, baffling disease, and often has proved fatal either from the severity of the attacks, or more commonly from the violent remedies used in the treatment; "now, however, we have it in our power to give remedies specific to the affection," (Hull.) In this way, the symptoms are quietly subdued, and the patient generally passes safely through the disease.

The general remedies are, Acon. Ambr. Ammo. M. Ars. Bell. Bryo. Cham. Caps. Drose. Dulcam. Hep. Ipe. Iodi. Merc. Nux V. Opi. Prus. ac. Phos. Puls. Sambu. Sang. Sepi. Sulp. Tart. Anti. or Verat. They should be used as follows. If it proceeds from wet or exposure, attended with Snuffling, use Dulcam. or Puls.

——— If there is lacrymation, rheumy eyes, Sneezing, or hoarseness, give Droser. Dulcam, or Puls.

——— If the patient is hoarse, and has a sore mouth or nostrils—Merc.

——— When there is a dry barking cough, or hooping, give Bell. or Hep. or alternate these with Rus. T. or Seneg.

——— Should there be severe cough with hooping, use Nux V. or Phos.

——— If there is much fever, give Acon. Anti. or Ipe.

——— In the second or convulsive stage, use Drose. Verat. Cupr. Arnic. or Coni.

——— If the child is reduced, having cold, or has involuntary emissions from the bowels, Ars. Cupr. or Verat. are proper.

——— If there is a hollow sensation, use Nux V. Phos. Puls. Sambu. or Verat.

——— If the case is attended with convulsions, give Carb. V. Cupr. Coni. Drose. Hyosc. Mosch. or Nux V.

——— If spasms more severe come on, give Ambr. Bell. Hep. Lach. Nux V. Phos. Prus. ac. or Verat.

——— When vomiting is troublesome, use Carbo. V. Camph. Ipe. Nux V. Opi. Petrol. or Sulp.

CROUP.—See Angina Membrana.

COXALGIA.

Coxalgia—The general remedies for this disease are, Bell. Bryo. Calca. Rus. Tox. Sulp.; though others may be required, as various symptoms present themselves. See Hip-joint disease, under head Extremities; also Rheumatism, Scrofula, &c.

DEBILITY.

Debility.—This proceeds from a variety of causes; the remedies generally useful for it, are Ars. Argent. Calca. Carb. V. China. Ferr. Iodi. Nux V. Phos. Puls. Ranan. Bulb. Rus. R. Sang. Stann. Stramo. Sulp. ac. Thuy. or Verat.

DELIRIUM.

Delirium.—An impaired and deranged state of the mind takes place from various causes, and is connected with a variety of diseases. It sometimes appears when there is a plethoric or inflammatory state of the system; at others when there is a state of exhaustion, weakness, and typhoid debility. For the first state, the appropriate remedies are those calculated to reduce arterial action, subdue the attending fever, and remove the morbid excitement from the brain, such as Acon. Bell. Bryo. Cocc. Ipe. Tart. Anti. or Nux V. When the first or active state is moderated, or in a measure removed, the proper remedies then are Hell. Hyosc. Opi. Phos. Puls. Staphys. Stramo. or Verat. When it takes place under a condition of debility or exhaustion, the last named remedies would be proper, and, in some instances, cordial stimulant remedies, to give tone and reaction to the system, would be adviseable.

Delirium Tremens.—This form of delirium is confined to drunkards and opium eaters. It is attended with great derangement of the stomach and the brain; a state of agitation of body and mind takes place, with a trembling, quivering of the limbs, hence the name Trembling Delirium. The mind gets impaired, cramps and spasms often set in. As the case proceeds, the most strange and harassing ideas affect the mind, and frightful horrifying spirits are presented before the imagination. The patient is generally affected with distress or burning pain of the stomach, a dull headache, or a darting pain in the head; the eyes are glairy and wild, sometimes bloodshot; the face is a dull yellow or of a dingy hue.

The remedies most useful for attacks of this disease are Acon. Camp. Bell. Ipe. Hyosc. Opi. or Nux V. This last is one of the most useful when there are spasms and tremors. Those named are principally the useful medicines.

When there is fever heat and burning at the stomach, give Acon. either alone or in alternation, with Camph. The doses should at first be repeated every half hour, then at longer periods, according to the severity of the symptoms. There is generally a great thirst and a desire for cold water, as a drink, which should be indulged. We have known patients drink six or eight quarts of water in about twelve hours, and with benefit. Part of it may be vomited, but that need not prevent its use. Cloths, wet in cold water, should be applied to the head, or bags of ice used instead thereof.

After the fever and heat of the stomach has in a measure subsided, give Hyosc. Nux V. Opi. Stramo. or Verat.

If the case continues protracted, as it often does with wakefulness and raving, it becomes very necessary to procure sleep. We have witnessed cases where a continued wakefulness and raving lasted six or seven days. If by the use of the above named remedies, sleep is not produced, recourse should be had to opiates, in free doses, until this effect is brought about. In some cases, morphine in solution has been given, 15 drops every hour, until 150 drops were used before it had the effect, when the patient fell asleep and slept soundly eight hours, then woke up calm, rational, and cured!

Note.—Generally in this state of disease, in plethoric habits, before giving large quantities of opiates, blood-letting should be used to avoid producing congestion of the brain. Opiates after the free use of this remedy frequently operates very favorably in quieting irritation and subduing disease.

DIABETES. See Bladder.

DIARRHŒA.

Diarrhœa, or Diseased Looseness of the Bowels.—The suitable remedies are Acon. Arg. N. Ars. Bell. Bryo. Calc. Cupr. Camp. Cham. Cann. S. Cinnamo. Coff. Dulc. Ferr. Guaco. Gum. Gtt. Hyosc. Ignat. Iris. Versic. Ipe. Kali. C. Lauroc. Merc. Sol. Nux V. Opi. Phos. Puls. Rus. R. Rus. T. Sang. Stramo. Sulp. Tart. A. or Verat.

——— Chronic.—Diarrhœa sometimes takes on chronic forms, and proves very troublesome and difficult of cure. In such cases the following are the most useful remedies: Ars. Canth. Camp. Chin. Colocy. Nux M. Nitric. ac. Phos. Phosphate of Iron, Samb. Sulp. Sulp. ac. Tabac. or Sulphate of Iron excicated.

——— with burning tenesmus.—Lauroc. Natr. M. Nux V. Phos. Rus. T. Rhodod. Sabi. or Sulp.

——— Itching at the Anus.—Aloe. Sulp. ac. or Sulp.

——— Lientery.—Use Ars. Canth. Chin. Coni. Ferr. Hyosc. Ignat. Nux V. Oleand. Phos. Sang. Sulp. or Verat.

——— Putrid discharges.—Ars. Carb. V. Chin. Coni. Kreoso. or Sepi.

——— Rectum contracted.—Caust. Phos. Sep. or Sulp.

——— Evacuations black.—Kreoso. Carb. V. Sulp. Verat.

——— Mucus and Sour.—Chin. Coni. Plumb. Phos. Sec. C. Silec. Sulp. ac. Verat. or Merc. or Colyc.

——— Watery.—Camp. Rus. R. Sec. C. Verat.

——— White.—Camp. Spong. Verat.

——— If the discharges are bilious, use Puls. or Bryo. Nux V. or Cham. Merc. Ipe. or Ars. Chin. Digital. Ignat. or Phos. ac.

——— In obstinate cases the more proper remedies are Nux V. Ammo. M. Seneg. Rheum. or Cham. or Sulp. ac. or Sulp. or Ferr. Exicat.

——— If the discharges are like common excrements, use Ipe. Puls. Nux V. or Bryo. Cham. Tart. A. or Ars. or Sulp.

——— When the discharges are serous, use Ars. Cham. Chin. Puls. or Lach. Rus. T. Ferr. or Hyosc.

——— When it affects a person of intemperate habits, give Carb. V. Nux V. or Bell. Coni. or Ars.

——— If attended with colic pains or tenesmus, give Ars. Cham. Colocy. Puls. Rus. T. Sulp. ac. or Hep.

DISEASES OF A CHRONIC KIND.

Conium and Silecia are generally useful for them.

DREAMS AND WAKEFULNESS.

See SLEEP, and these affections there.

DROPSY.

Dropsy.—This disease consists in a preternatural collection or deposition of water or serous fluids, in the cellular tissue or some cavity of the body. It receives different names from the nature of the collection of the material, or the part affected. In this manner, when the cellular membranes seated under the skin generally are the seat of the disease, it is termed Anasarca or Œdema.

If the cavity of the *Chest* is the part affected it is named *Hydrothorax*. If the Abdomen is affected and filled or partially so with water, it is *Acites*. Should the disease be seated on the brain filling the cavities or cells with serous or watery fluid, it is termed *Hydrocephalous*.

When the collection of water is in the Scrotum, it is *Hydrocele*. If the Womb is the seat of a dropsical disease, it is *Hydrometra*.

The general remedies for this disease are Ammo. C. Apis. Mell. Apocynum. Ars. Arni. Camp. Cann. S. Clemat. Coni. Colich. Colocy. Digit. Dulcam. Ferr. Hell. Kreoso. Kali. Iod. Lach. Lact. Viro. Lyc. Merc. Prun. Sp. Podophy. Puls. Scill. Sola. Nig. Tart. Anti. or Zinc.

——— of the brain, *Hydrocephalous*.—In the first stage if there is fever, pain or pressure on the brain, give Acon. at first, and this may be followed by Digital. Ipe. Bell. or Tart. Anti.—in the somewhat advanced stage, if the disease has moderated and there are symptoms of dullness or torpor, give Hell. Lach. Merc. or Ars. or Nux V.

If there is stupor or slight delirium—Stramo. Sulp. or Verat.

——— of the brain. In some cases the acute condition is moderated, but the disease is not fully removed, or the case forms a slow insiduous type, and the disease assumes a protracted chronic form. In such cases the remedies are Camph. Ars. Colocy. Merc. Iodi. Stramo. or Sulp. or Hell., and it would be well to examine the record of some of the other remedies for dropsy in a pure Materia Medica for a remedy.

——— of the Chest, *Hydrothorax.* The deposition of the fluid may take place in one side of the Thorax, or in both—or it may be deposited in the cellular substance of the Lungs, or in the cavity of the Chest exterior to the Lungs. The disease is commonly a long time in forming, it is often the effect of previous inflammation of those parts—or the result of general disease. The leading symptoms in the early stage are shortness of breathing, increased by exercise, cough, pressure on the chest, slight expectoration of mucus, the feet swell, as the disease advances, it is difficult to lay in a recumbent posture, the skin is pale, there is thirst and some other general symptoms of dropsy.

The remedies found most useful are Acon. Ars. Carb. V. Hell. Ipe. Lyc. Colch. Digitalis. Spig. or Dulcam. or Sulp.

In the early stage when there is fever, Acon. or Digital. or Ipe.

If there is difficult respiration, pain in breathing, palpitation of the heart, coldness of the extremities, Ars. or Colch.

If the liver is diseased, use Merc. Iodi. Spig. or if there is considerable weakness or œdema, Ferr. or Chin.

If the sufferings are increased in foggy weather, with symptoms of common cold, Dulcam. Puls. or Nux V.

If it is subsequent to inflammation, give Ars. Carb .V. Lyc. Kali. C.—to palliate the disease some of the other remedies named will be useful and may aid in the cure.

——— of the Abdomen, *Ascites.* This disease comes on insidiously, and there is an obscurity about it. The fluid may be confined to a particular part or encysted—at others the fluid may be diffused in the cavity. The abdomen becomes prominent and distended, the patient is feverish, the digestion is impaired, there is a scanty high-colored urine, the feet and legs swell, and general debility ensues.

——— The remedies for this form of the disease are Acon. Ipe. Apocynum. Merc. or Bryo. Led. P. Kali. C. Lyc. Sulph. or Scill.

In the early stage, if there is fever, thirst and pains in the abdomen—give Acon. Bryo. Camph. or Apocyn.

If any particular organ is the seat of the disease or been the cause of it, the remedy should be given which has a specific action on the part. If the disease seems to have been caused by repressed eruptions—give Digital. Rus. T. or Sulp.

If it is preceded by intermittent fever—Chin. Ferr. Merc. Sola. Nig. or Sulp. are proper remedies.

If it occurs in drunkards, give Ars. Hell. or Nux V.

Should it be the result of a large use of mercury, give Chin. Ferr. Nitr. ac. or Sulp.

If there are shooting pains, suppressed urine—Hell. If there is anasarca and great weakness—Ars.

In chronic cases connected with a disease of a viscus, such as the liver, use Merc. or Lach. Sulp.

——— of the Scrotum, *Hydrocele.* There are two varieties of this disease; in one the water is deposited in the cellular tissue of the bag, it is of the nature of anasarca and connected with it, and may be cured by similar general remedies that are useful for anasarca. In the other variety, the watery fluid is collected in the tunia vaginalis, the membrane immediately enclosing the testicle. In this case, the fluid is in immediate contact with the testicle—the remedies for this form of the disease, are Graph. Nux V. Puls. Rhodod. or Sulp.

Sometimes the disease is not cured by the remedies used, the collection of water becomes large, attended with pain; and in such cases it may be necessary to have recourse to an operation to remove the fluid, called puncturing the sac for hydrocele; during this affection, the part should be suspended by a bandage.

——— of the Womb. It is a matter of doubt whether a dropsy of the womb takes place as a primary disease, this seems to be an opinion of some authors, for many of them do not even notice it. If it does take place, it is generally a symptomatic affection. Encysted dropsy of this organ is noticed—also hydatids are described as forming in the organ. The remedies for those affections, would be some of those for dropsy, mentioned above.

DRUNKENNESS.

Drunkenness.—If there is stupor and fever so as to prove to be dangerous, give Acon. Bell. Camp. Coff. or Nux V.—dash cold water on the head. In the advanced stage, to relieve the secondary effects and stupor of intoxication, give

Baryt. Coff. Kreoso. Lach. Nux V. Opi. or Stramo. or Wine. See also Delirium Tremens.

To cure a propensity to drink liquor, the remedies recommended are to put four or five drops of Laudanum in a cup of coffee, and take this three or four times a day, it is said to produce a disgust for liquors ; or one-eighth of a grain of Tartarized Antimony, mixed with water and a little spirits, taken two or three times a day, in many instances produces a loathing of liquor, and cures the morbid appetite for it.

This was essentially the preparation which was extensively sold here a few years ago, by the name of Chambers' *Antidote for Intemperance.* It was reported that a great many were cured by it. To render any of those antidotal articles effectual, the mind and the will requires to be trained and inclined to yield a willing assent to take them to effect a cure, and then a total abstinence condition may be established.

——— To produce a pleasant state of intoxication, take a few drops of the Tincture of Cannabis Indicus of Bengal, repeated several times. This is reported to produce a cheerful and pleasant state similar to intoxication. See this article in the catalogue of Medicine at the latter end of this work. Sabadil given in a similar manner is stated to produce a like effect. These articles are worthy of attention to cure a fit of intoxication, and to destroy a propensity to drink ardent spirits.

——— Reeling sensation is produced by the use of Cann. Ind. Sabad. Silec. or Thuy. When this state takes place as a disease, these medicines will be found useful as curative.

——— Tubercles on the face of drunkards.—Dose them with Ars. or Kreoso.

DYSENTERY.

Dysentery.—In the Allopathic School, the best writers on Dysentery describe it as an inflammatory state of the inner surface of the intestines, attended with more or less fever, and those who have been most successful in treating it have used and recommended the remedies best adapted to the cure of such a condition of disease. Therefore, in Homœopathic practice the remedies should first be used which are known to be most efficient to cure inflammatory states of the villous coat of the alimentary canal.

The proper medicines for this purpose are Acon. Bell. Ipe. Millefo. Merc. Puls. Tart. Anti. or Sulp. In a more advanced stage, when the urgent and febrile symptoms are checked, the following remedies will be useful: Cham. Colocy. Muri. ac. Nitr. ac. Nux V. Sulp. ac. or Plumb. ac.

In the North American Journal of Homœopathy, Petroleum alternated with Ipecac. or Iris. Versic. is highly recommended for this disease.

The remedies should be used in this manner:

If there is fever and pain in the bowels, give Acon. If blood is passed with griping, let the Acon. be followed by Bell. Ipe. or Millefo, or alternated with Acon. If the disease continues with pain, griping, and frequent evacuations, give Cham. Puls. Nux V. or Sulp. If the pain is of a griping, colic nature, give Colocy. or Merc.

If the above named remedies do not control or cure the case, others should be selected and tried according to the symptoms and properties of the drugs, as determined by examining a pure Materia Medica.

If the disease takes on a protracted form, Muriatic acid or Nitr. acid may be used with great benefit. If the discharges are green, give Ars. In most stages, Merc. will be a useful remedy, alternated with the other medicine. When there are crampy, griping pains, or bloody stools in the advanced stage, give Colocy. or Nux V. If there takes place, severe Tenesmus and pressing down at the lower end] of the rectum, give injections of Starch and Laudanum; these frequently are very soothing. In using this remedy, it may be useful to say, their quantity should be very small; two table spoonfuls of Starch and 10 or 15 drops of Laudanum will be about a proper quantity; these may be often repeated.

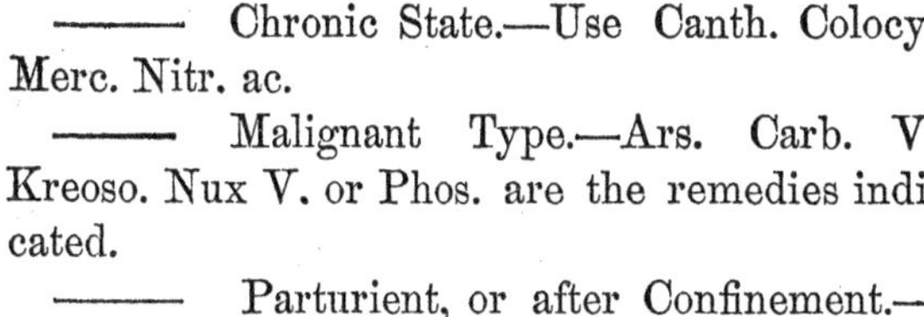

——— Chronic State.—Use Canth. Colocy. Merc. Nitr. ac.

——— Malignant Type.—Ars. Carb. V. Kreoso. Nux V. or Phos. are the remedies indicated.

——— Parturient, or after Confinement.—Give Aloe and such of the other remedies as may be indicated.

——— Tenesmus in.—Use Arnic. Colocy. Lact. Viro. Lobel. Nux V. Sol. Nig. or Sulp.

DYSPNŒA.

Dyspnœa.—The best remedies for this disease are Ambr. Anacard. Ars. Camp. Ignat. Ipe. Lach. Lauroc. Mosch. Phos. Prun. Sp. Puls. Rus. T. Samb. Sep. Sol. Nig. Spong. Staphy. or Sulp. ac.

——— Rattling state.—Use Bromi. Calc. Camp. Kali. Bic. Kalmi. Lat. Lauroc. Lobel. See Asthma.

DYSPEPSIA.

Dyspepsia.—Writers pretty generally agree in describing this disease to be an imperfect and irregular action of the stomach and digestive organs, by which the food is not properly digested and assimilated to the nutrition of the body. This affection is brought on from a variety of causes, and it appears in a great many forms. The immediate exciting cause, when that can be learned, should be avoided or corrected. The remedy may sometimes be used to advantage, directed to what appears to be the cause. In some cases the symptoms present will indicate the remedy. There are but few cases but what will require some studying, and comparing the symptoms with the Pathogenesis of Drugs in the Materia Medica, which course it will be well to pursue.

The remedies proved most useful for this troublesome disease are Arnic. Ars. Auru. Baryt. M. Bell. Bryo. Calc. Caust. Chin. Carb. V. Carb. A. Ferr. Hep. Hyosc. Ignat. Ipe. Kali. Iod. Kali. Bic. Lobel. Lyc. Merc. Nux V. Phos. ac. Podophylin, Prus. ac. Silec. Sulp. or Verat.

If it seems to be the effect of sedentary habits, or the free use of wine or spirits, use Nux V. or Puls. If it is attended with headache or wandering of the mind, or insipid taste, or flatulence or nausea, or burning at the stomach, give Bryo. Calca. Carb. V. Caust. or Ferr. For semilateral headache, giddiness, vertigo, a dullness of the sight, great thirst, or acidity of the stomach, use Cham. Ferr. Nux V. or Sulp. or Sulp. ac. If there are cramps across the stomach and burning pain, and inclined to Diarrhœa, give Carb. V. Ignat. Nux V. Lobel. Podoph. or Prus. ac. When there is great aversion to food, particularly to fat meat, vomiting after a meal, a sinking feeling at the stomach, or headache, use Ipe. Puls. Ferr. or Merc. Phos. ac. or Silec. or Verat. If it is attended with extreme passion or irritability of disposition, or grief, or hysterical excitement, give Asa. F. Ignat. Hyosc. Lach, Nicc. Nux V. or Stramo.

If the case is attended with great weakness and foul taste, burning at the throat, and offensive breath, use Sulp. ac. or Nux V. or Carb. V. Ferr. or Ars. Auru. or Baryt. When there is frequent vomiting, the skin hot or dry, the countenance pale, and a feeble state of the patient, give Ars. Lach. Lyc. Phos. or Coni. or Ferr. When there is a feeble state, an acid stomach, or flatulence, Ferr. is one of the best remedies. Examine Constipation, Flatulence, Eructations, and Stomach, for valuable indications on this subject.

EAR.

This organ is subject to a large number of ailments, which render the department worthy a particular care, and extended enumeration of symptoms, and careful selection of remedies for them, which are detailed as follows:

Air sensation of its whistling in the ear, give Sep. or Str amo.

——— Bells sound in, like the ringing of bells, Silec. Spig. Staphy. Sulp. ac. or Valeri.

——— Boreing sensation in, Stramo. Thuy. are useful.

——— Burning pain in, Sabad. Spong. Spig. Silec. Stann. Staph. or Thuy.

——— Burning in, Nux V. Ol. Anima. Opi. Phos. Selen. Silec. Sulp. Verat. or Zinc.

——— Cramps in, Chin. Silec. Sang. Stann. Staphy. Thuy. Verba. or Zinc.

——— Creeping and painful sensation in—Ranan. Bulb. or Caust.

——— Cracking sensation, Sulp.

——— Deafness.—The most useful remedies are, Anacard. Arnic. Ars. Bell. Calc. Caust. Chin. Graph. Hep. Iodi. Kreoso. Lach. Lyc. Lauroc. Merc. Muri. ac. Nicc. Nux V. Nitr. ac. Phos. ac. Petrol. Puls. Sabi. Sep. Sulp. ac. Zinc. or Caust.

——— Glands under swelled—use Merc. Sarss. Silec. Spong. Sulp. or Thuy.

——— Glass breaking sensation in—Zinc.

——— Grass-hoppers chirping sensation in—Tarax. Thuy.

——— Hammering and singing sensation in, give Coni. Sang. Spong. Stann. Sabad. Sulp. ac. or Thuy.

——— Hearing rendered acute by—Phos. Phytoll. Seneg. Scill. or Sulp.

——— Herpes in, Arg. N. Graph. Kreoso. Lach. Merc Mosch. Nitr. ac. Phos. Petrol. or Sep.

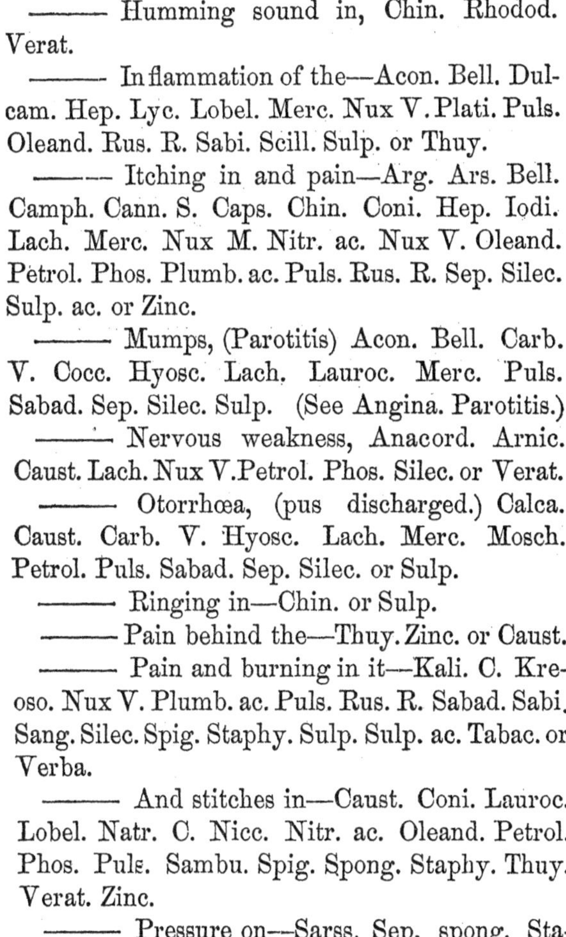

——— Humming sound in, Chin. Rhodod. Verat.

——— Inflammation of the—Acon. Bell. Dulcam. Hep. Lyc. Lobel. Merc. Nux V. Plati. Puls. Oleand. Rus. R. Sabi. Scill. Sulp. or Thuy.

——— Itching in and pain—Arg. Ars. Bell. Camph. Cann. S. Caps. Chin. Coni. Hep. Iodi. Lach. Merc. Nux M. Nitr. ac. Nux V. Oleand. Petrol. Phos. Plumb. ac. Puls. Rus. R. Sep. Silec. Sulp. ac. or Zinc.

——— Mumps, (Parotitis) Acon. Bell. Carb. V. Cocc. Hyosc. Lach. Lauroc. Merc. Puls. Sabad. Sep. Silec. Sulp. (See Angina. Parotitis.)

——— Nervous weakness, Anacord. Arnic. Caust. Lach. Nux V. Petrol. Phos. Silec. or Verat.

——— Otorrhœa, (pus discharged.) Calca. Caust. Carb. V. Hyosc. Lach. Merc. Mosch. Petrol. Puls. Sabad. Sep. Silec. or Sulp.

——— Ringing in—Chin. or Sulp.

——— Pain behind the—Thuy. Zinc. or Caust.

——— Pain and burning in it—Kali. C. Kreoso. Nux V. Plumb. ac. Puls. Rus. R. Sabad. Sabi. Sang. Silec. Spig. Staphy. Sulp. Sulp. ac. Tabac. or Verba.

——— And stitches in—Caust. Coni. Lauroc. Lobel. Natr. C. Nicc. Nitr. ac. Oleand. Petrol. Phos. Puls. Sambu. Spig. Spong. Staphy. Thuy. Verat. Zinc.

——— Pressure on—Sarss. Sep. spong. Staphy. Sulp.

——— Polypus in—Calc. Chin. Lyc. Staphy. Thuy.

——— Roaring in like water falling—Coni. Rus. R. Rhodod. Selen. Silec. Staphy. Sulp. ac. Tabac. or Verat.

——— Tingling in—Arg. Bromi. Calc. Mosch. Muri. ac. Natr. C. Nicc. Nitr. ac. Nux V. Opi. Ol. Anima. Petrol. Phos. ac. Puls. Rus. T. Sep. or Thuy.

——— Sore behind them—Oleand. Petrol. Selen. Silec. Scill. Staphy. Sulp. or Tabac.

——— Throbbing in—Phos. Puls. Sabad. Sang. Seneg. Thuy.

——— Tonsils enlarged.—In the first or inflammatory stage, give Acon. Bell. Cham. Coni. Ignat. In the advanced chronic state, use Baryt. Calc. Coni. Hep. Iodi. Lyc. Nux V. Sulp. Thuy. (See Angina Tonsilitis.)

——— Vermicular motion in them, use Rhodod. Stann. Spig.

——— Whizzing sensation in them, use Sep. Sulp. ac. Tabac. Tart. A. or Zinc.

——— Ecchymosis—Arnic. Ars. Coni. Iodi. Sulp.

EMOTIONS.

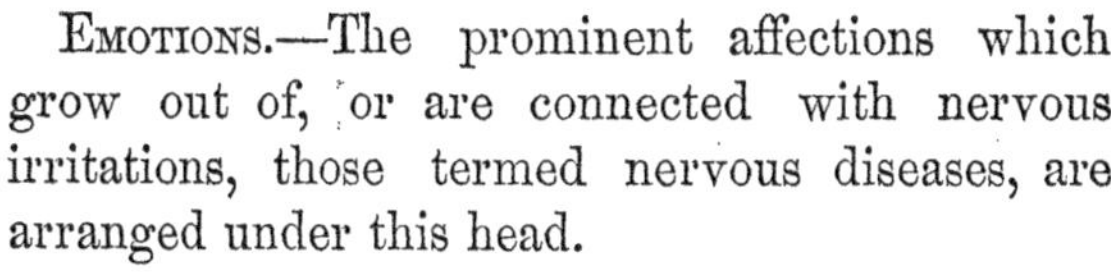

Emotions.—The prominent affections which grow out of, or are connected with nervous irritations, those termed nervous diseases, are arranged under this head.

——— Of anguish—give Puls. Rus. Tox. Sec. C. Sep. Silec. Spong. Stann. Staph. Sulph. ac. Tart. Anti. Thuy. Verat. or Zinc.

——— Of anxiety—use Caust. Mosch. Nicc. Nitr. ac. Nux V. Oleand. Opi. Petrol. Phos. ac. Puls. Ranan. Bulb. Rhodod. Rus. Tox. Sabad. Silec. Spong. Staph. Sulph. Tabac. Tart. Anti. Thuy. Verat. or Zinc.

——— Of cheerfulness to produce—use Lach. Plumb. ac. Sabad. Seneg. Silec. Spig. Staph. Thuy. Verat. or Valer.

——— Of consciousness, loss of—give Oleand. Plati. Rus. Rad. or Verat.

——— Of craziness—give Nitr. ac. Sec. C. Stramo. Sulp. Tart. Anti. or Verat. (See Delirium.)

———Of dancing to excess—Thuy.

——— Of death, great fear of—give Mosch. Nux V. Plati. Puls. Rhodod. Rus. Tox. Sec. C. Spig. Scill. Stann. or Stramo.

——— Of despair and despondency—give Phos. Plumb. Acct. Sarss. Sep. Silec. Stann. Staph. Tabac. Verat. Verba. or Zinc.

——— Ennui, Plum. Aret. or Thuy.

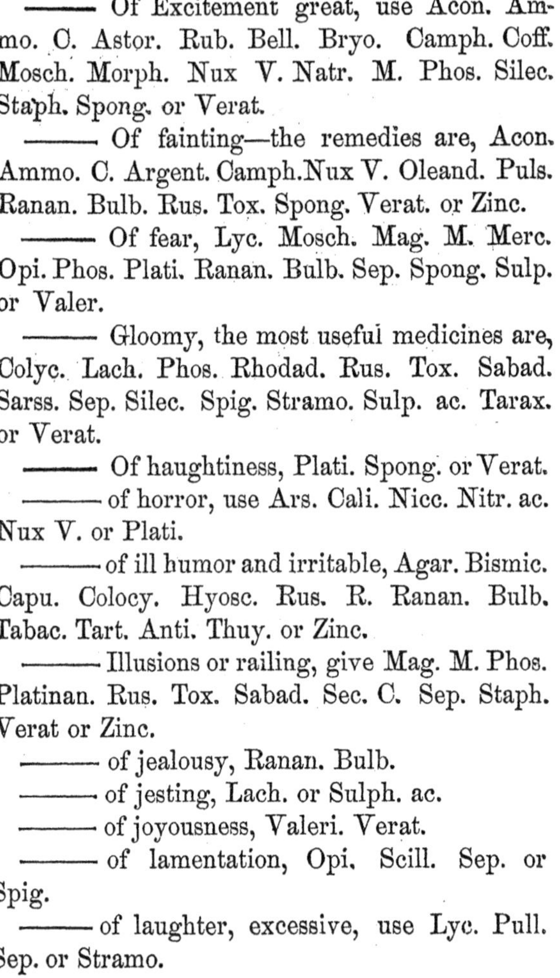

——— Of Excitement great, use Acon. Ammo. C. Astor. Rub. Bell. Bryo. Camph. Coff. Mosch. Morph. Nux V. Natr. M. Phos. Silec. Staph. Spong. or Verat.

——— Of fainting—the remedies are, Acon. Ammo. C. Argent. Camph. Nux V. Oleand. Puls. Ranan. Bulb. Rus. Tox. Spong. Verat. or Zinc.

——— Of fear, Lyc. Mosch. Mag. M. Merc. Opi. Phos. Plati. Ranan. Bulb. Sep. Spong. Sulp. or Valer.

——— Gloomy, the most useful medicines are, Colyc. Lach. Phos. Rhodad. Rus. Tox. Sabad. Sarss. Sep. Silec. Spig. Stramo. Sulp. ac. Tarax. or Verat.

——— Of haughtiness, Plati. Spong. or Verat.

——— of horror, use Ars. Cali. Nicc. Nitr. ac. Nux V. or Plati.

——— of ill humor and irritable, Agar. Bismic. Capu. Colocy. Hyosc. Rus. R. Ranan. Bulb. Tabac. Tart. Anti. Thuy. or Zinc.

——— Illusions or railing, give Mag. M. Phos. Platinan. Rus. Tox. Sabad. Sec. C. Sep. Staph. Verat or Zinc.

——— of jealousy, Ranan. Bulb.

——— of jesting, Lach. or Sulph. ac.

——— of joyousness, Valeri. Verat.

——— of lamentation, Opi. Scill. Sep. or Spig.

——— of laughter, excessive, use Lyc. Pull. Sep. or Stramo.

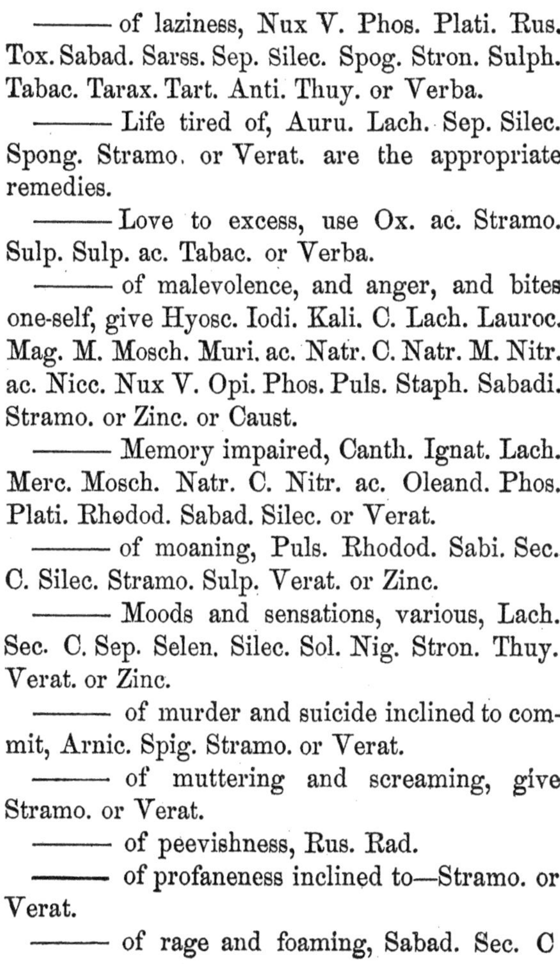

——— of laziness, Nux V. Phos. Plati. Rus. Tox. Sabad. Sarss. Sep. Silec. Spog. Stron. Sulph. Tabac. Tarax. Tart. Anti. Thuy. or Verba.

——— Life tired of, Auru. Lach. Sep. Silec. Spong. Stramo. or Verat. are the appropriate remedies.

——— Love to excess, use Ox. ac. Stramo. Sulp. Sulp. ac. Tabac. or Verba.

——— of malevolence, and anger, and bites one-self, give Hyosc. Iodi. Kali. C. Lach. Lauroc. Mag. M. Mosch. Muri. ac. Natr. C. Natr. M. Nitr. ac. Nicc. Nux V. Opi. Phos. Puls. Staph. Sabadi. Stramo. or Zinc. or Caust.

——— Memory impaired, Canth. Ignat. Lach. Merc. Mosch. Natr. C. Nitr. ac. Oleand. Phos. Plati. Rhodod. Sabad. Silec. or Verat.

——— of moaning, Puls. Rhodod. Sabi. Sec. C. Silec. Stramo. Sulp. Verat. or Zinc.

——— Moods and sensations, various, Lach. Sec. C. Sep. Selen. Silec. Sol. Nig. Stron. Thuy. Verat. or Zinc.

——— of murder and suicide inclined to commit, Arnic. Spig. Stramo. or Verat.

——— of muttering and screaming, give Stramo. or Verat.

——— of peevishness, Rus. Rad.

——— of profaneness inclined to—Stramo. or Verat.

——— of rage and foaming, Sabad. Sec. C

Scill: Selen. Sep. Silec. Sol. Nig. Stramo. Sulp. Verat. or Zinc.

——— Reeling sensation, use Rhodod. Stron. Thuy. or Verat.

——— Religious frenzy, Lach. Verat. Stramo. or Puls.

——— Sadness, Kali. C. Kreoso. Lach. Lact. Viro. Lauroc. Lyc. Mag. C. Mag. S. Mosch. Muri. ac. Natr. C. Natr. M. Nicc. Nitr. ac. Ol. Anima. Opi. Phos. Phos. ac. Plati. Plumb. Rus. Tox. Sabad. Sec. C. Sep. Stramo. or Sulp. ac.

——— Sensibility increased by—Mosch. Muri. ac. Natr. C. Nitr. ac. Petrol. Phos. Puls. Rhodod. Selen. Silec. Staph. or Verat.

——— of singing to excesss, Spong. Stann. Stramo. Tabac. or Verat.

——— Starting, Sambu. Seneg. Sep. Silec. Spong. Stramo. Sulp. Tart. Anti. Verat. or Zinc.

——— of stupor, Morph. Opi. Sep. Silec. Spig. or Verba.

——— of sullenness, give Bell. Ipe. Iodi. Kreoso. Lach. Lact. Viro. Lyc. Mangan. Merc. Nux V. Phos. ac.

——— Taciturn, Lach. Ol. Anima. Opi. Petrol. Plati. Plumb. A. Spig. Spong. Staphy. Sulp. or Verat.

——— Talkative to excess, Stann. or Staphy.

——— Timorous, Puls.

——— of tired feeling, Phytol. Rhodod. Sec. C. Selen. or Spong.

——— Tranquil state of mind to produce, Opi. or Plati.

——— Vexed easily, Verat. or Sabad.

——— Of weeping, much inclined to—Staphy. Stramo. Sulph. Sulph. ac. or Verat.

——— Wildness, Bell. Nux V. Spig. or Verat.

ERUCTATIONS.

Eructations. A disordered raising of unpleasant matter from the stomach, of gas, acrid, sour, or oily material, or small portions of undigested food, the remedies are to be in a measure used according to the nature of the affection. If it comes on soon after a meal, Coffe. or Caust. will be useful; or use Arnic. or Ipec. If there is acidity, use Kali. C. Caust. or Ferr.; if the matter is bitter with nausea, use Ars. Nux. or Carbo. Veg.; should it be attended with fever, give Acon. Bryo. or Ipe. If it is composed of fatty or oily matter, use Puls. or Calca. or Caust.; the other remedies are, Anise. Hep. S. Lach. Carbo. V. China. Consult the articles Flatulence and Nausea, for further directions.

ERYSIPELAS.

ERYSIPELAS, OR ST. ANTHONY'S FIRE.—This disease is considered a cutaneous affection, and somewhat allied to some varieties of Herpes and other diseases of the skin. It is more generally attended with fever and symptoms of constitutional excitement than many other affections of the skin. In addition to the general febrile excitement, there are local symptoms of heat and redness of the skin—a flushed red color, a very fine red eruption—there is a tingling, smarting, or itching; the parts swell and are tumefied. As the case advances, the skin is sometimes affected with larger eruptions or vesicles. In the progress, the skin has a yellowish tinge. If the head is considerably affected, delirium takes place, and stupor may ensue, and even death follow.

The remedies for this disease are Acon. Ars. Bell. [Camphor, in Homœopathic doses, is stated to be almost specific; we have used it with great benefit.]—*N. Y. Jour. of Homœo.* Or give Graph. Hep. Lach. Nitr. ac. Opi. Oleand. Hyosc. Phos. Puls. Rus. T. Stramo. Sulp. or Tart. Anti.

Outward applications generally ought to be avoided as dangerous. But moistening the parts with a weak dilution of Tincture of Arnica or Iodine or Rus. Tox. are admissible, and are found to be very useful; they allay the itching and painful burning.

When the head is affected with eruption, care ought to be taken not to apply cold applications or astringent stimulant lotions to the skin; we have known death to have been produced by such injudicious remedies.

If there is fever, give Acon. Bell. or Bryo.

If these do not check it, give Lach. or Kalmi. L.

If there is spreading red, fine eruptions, particularly if the head is affected, use Bell. Rus. T. or Nitr. ac. or Camp. We have used Camphor, as above named, with good success.

If a drowsiness or dullness of mind takes place, give Coff. Opi. or Stramo.

Should these symptoms continue, use Hyosc. or Rus. T.

If the joints are affected, give Bryo. Puls. Rus. T.

If the skin is of a blueish cast or the eruption runs from one part to another, use Graph. Puls. or Rus. T.

If the knees or feet are swelled or painful, Nux V. or Rus. T.

If the vesicles are of a purple or black color, give Ars. Carb. V. or Sec. C.

If the mind becomes impaired with delirium or stupor, Opi. Stramo. or Hyosc. are proper.

Should there be in the advanced stage a torpid swelling of the skin, Sulph. or Ars. is called for.

When it terminates in ulceration, give Ars. Nitr. ac. or Hep. or Silec. or Sulp.

If the scrotum or genitals are affected, like Chimney Sweeps' Cancer, the remedies are Ars. Clemat. or Rus. T.

When the hands or feet are affected, Arnic. Ars. Bryo. Lach. Puls. or Stramo. are the proper remedies.

If there occur small hard swellings, Hep. or Ars. or Apis. Mellefo.

EXTREMITIES.

Extremities, Diseases of.—The extremities are subject to a great variety of affections; the greater part of them are included in the following list, with the proper remedy connected with the disease.

Arms, hands, and fingers, drawing, numb, or contracted, give Rhodod. Rus. T. Silec. Spig. Spong. Tabac. Tareb. Thuy. Verat. or Zinc.

——— Jerking in, use Valer. Verat, or Zinc.

——— Axilla pain, burning, or sore, use Sambu. Scill. Sep. Silec. Spong. Stann. Staph. Sulph. ac. Valer. Verat. or Zinc.

——— Swelling and ulceration in, Scill. Sep. Silec. Spig. or Sulp. ac. are proper medicines.

——— Burning and itching in feet, legs or hands, give Canth. Caps. Caust. Gum. Gtt. Iodi. Kali. Iod. Kreoso. Lach. Lauroc. Mag. C. Mag. M. Merc. Nicc. Nitr. ac. Nux V. Oleand. Opi. Petrol. Phos. Plati. Puls. Rus. Rad. Rus. Tox.

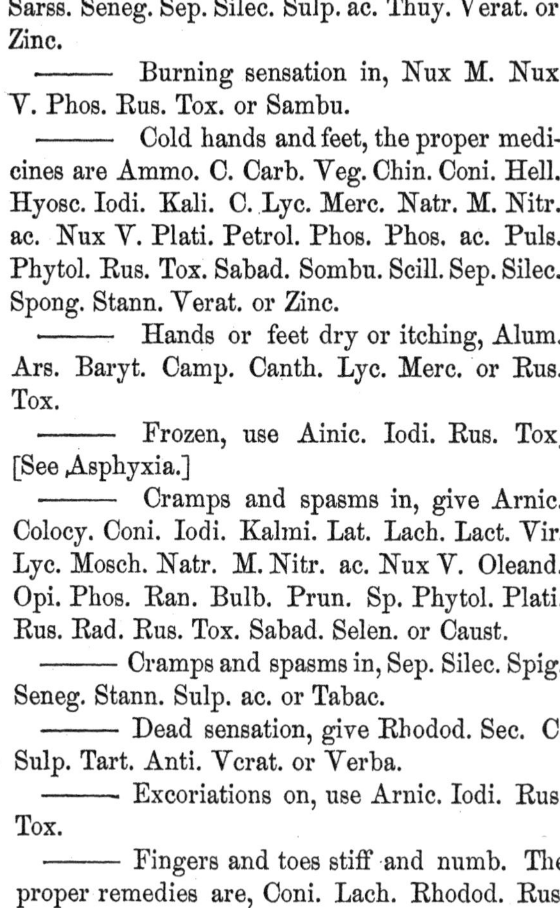

Sarss. Seneg. Sep. Silec. Sulp. ac. Thuy. Verat. or Zinc.

——— Burning sensation in, Nux M. Nux V. Phos. Rus. Tox. or Sambu.

——— Cold hands and feet, the proper medicines are Ammo. C. Carb. Veg. Chin. Coni. Hell. Hyosc. Iodi. Kali. C. Lyc. Merc. Natr. M. Nitr. ac. Nux V. Plati. Petrol. Phos. Phos. ac. Puls. Phytol. Rus. Tox. Sabad. Sombu. Scill. Sep. Silec. Spong. Stann. Verat. or Zinc.

——— Hands or feet dry or itching, Alum. Ars. Baryt. Camp. Canth. Lyc. Merc. or Rus. Tox.

——— Frozen, use Ainic. Iodi. Rus. Tox. [See Asphyxia.]

——— Cramps and spasms in, give Arnic. Colocy. Coni. Iodi. Kalmi. Lat. Lach. Lact. Vir. Lyc. Mosch. Natr. M. Nitr. ac. Nux V. Oleand. Opi. Phos. Ran. Bulb. Prun. Sp. Phytol. Plati. Rus. Rad. Rus. Tox. Sabad. Selen. or Caust.

——— Cramps and spasms in, Sep. Silec. Spig. Seneg. Stann. Sulp. ac. or Tabac.

——— Dead sensation, give Rhodod. Sec. C. Sulp. Tart. Anti. Verat. or Verba.

——— Excoriations on, use Arnic. Iodi. Rus. Tox.

——— Fingers and toes stiff and numb. The proper remedies are, Coni. Lach. Rhodod. Rus. Rad. Sabi. Sambu. Sang. Sars. Sec. C. Sulp. ac. Tereb. Thuy. or Valer. or Caust.

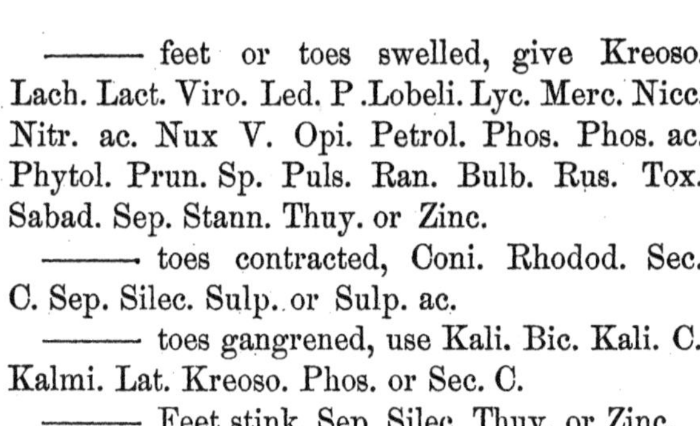

——— feet or toes swelled, give Kreoso. Lach. Lact. Viro. Led. P .Lobeli. Lyc. Merc. Nicc. Nitr. ac. Nux V. Opi. Petrol. Phos. Phos. ac. Phytol. Prun. Sp. Puls. Ran. Bulb. Rus. Tox. Sabad. Sep. Stann. Thuy. or Zinc.

——— toes contracted, Coni. Rhodod. Sec. C. Sep. Silec. Sulp. or Sulp. ac.

——— toes gangrened, use Kali. Bic. Kali. C. Kalmi. Lat. Kreoso. Phos. or Sec. C.

——— Feet stink, Sep. Silec. Thuy. or Zinc.

——— Feet or soles, burning or pain in—give Caust. Colocy. Coni. Scill. Sep. Stann. Stramo. Sulp. or Zinc.

———Feet swelled, Scill. Sep. Stann. Sulp. ac.

———Feet or hands, soles, or palms painful, use Sarss. Sec. C. Seneg. Sulp. Sulp. ac. or Zinc. or Caust.

——— Feet or hands burning in—give Rhodod. Rus. Rad. Sabad. Silec. Sec. C. Seneg. Selen. Sep. Silec. Sulp. or Sulp. ac.

——— Feet or toes, or fingers swelled, or numb, give Caust. Kreoso. Lach. Lactu Viro. Led. P. Lobel. Lyc. Mag. S. Merc. Nicc. Nitr. ac. Nux V. Opi. Petrol. Phos. Phos. ac. Phytol. Prun. Sp. Puls. Rus. Tox. Sabad. Sep. Stann. Thuy. or Zinc.

——— Feet or toes, or fingers cramps in—use Colocy. Oleand. Ol. Anima. Opi. Phos. Phytol. Plati. Prun. Sp. Ran. Bulb. Sec. C. Sep. Silec. Spig. Verat. or Zinc.

——— Fornication, or crawling sensation in —Scill. Sec. C. Sulp. ac. Thuy. or Zinc.

——— Gluteous itching or pain in—give Colocy. Oleand. Phos. ac. Rus. Rad. Rus. Tox. Stann. Staph. Sulp. Sulp. ac. Thuy. or Zinc.

——— Hands chapped, Petrol. Sulp. or Zinc. (See Rhagades.)

Extremities—hip-joint diseases of—these are of several kinds. It may be acute inflammation, or it may be of a rheumatic affection, either acute or chonic, or the disease may be a chronic inflammation or a scrofulous affection; or it may be a sciatic, of a neuralgic character, which is described under the term sciatica.

In treating the diseases of this important part, all those affections ought to be examined into, and the case treated according to the peculiarity of the symptoms.

If there is simple inflammation of the parts about the joint, the usual remedies for such a disease ought to be used, as Acon. Arnic. Bell. Canth. Colocy. &c.

If it is a rheumatic affection, the remedies for this disease detailed in their proper place, will be requisite.

If there is chronic inflammation, use Colocy. Hep. Iodi. Kali. Bic. Lach. Led. P. Merc. Phos. Ran. Bulb. Sabad. Sepi. or Rhodod.

Should it be considered of a scrofulous nature, the general remedies will be, Iodi. Bell. Rus. T.

or Calca. Colocy. Sulp. Silec. phosphate of lime, or phosphate of iron.

If it seems to be sciatica, reference should be made to that head for the remedies there laid down.

——— Fingers and toes jerking or cramps in, give Caust.

——— Hip-joint—sprain bruising or drawing pain or trembling, Caust. Colocy.

——— Paralysed, Nux V. Petrol. Rus. Tox. or Verat. or Caust.

——— Painful, the remedies will be similar to the preceding, Acon. Colocy. Rus. Rad. Sabi. Sang. Sarss. Seneg. Sep. Silec. Spig. Stramo. Staph. Sulp. ac. Tereb. Verat. or Valer.

——— Cramps or stitches in—the suitable remedies are, Acon. Bell. Colocy. Coni. Iodi. Lach. Mosch. Nicc. Nux V. Oleand. Petrol. Phos. Plati. Podoph. P. Ran. Bulb. Rus. Tox. Sabad. Sambu. Stann. Staph. Sulp. ac. Tereb. Thuy. Valer. or Verat.

——— Hot and cold sensation alternating, Opi. Morph. Phos. Phos. ac. Ran. Bulb. or Rus. Rad.

——— Joint bubbling sensation—jerking and stitches in—use Ran. Bulb. Scill. Rhodod. Spong. Stann. Staph. or Sulp.

——— Luxated sensation spontaneous—Rus. Tox. or Thuy.

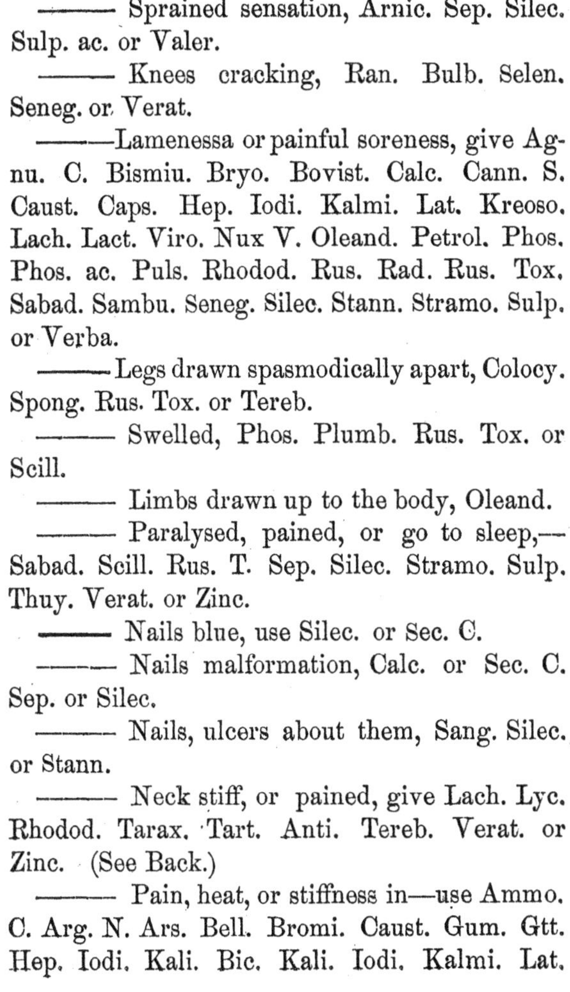

——— Sprained sensation, Arnic. Sep. Silec. Sulp. ac. or Valer.

——— Knees cracking, Ran. Bulb. Selen. Seneg. or Verat.

———Lamenessa or painful soreness, give Agnu. C. Bismiu. Bryo. Bovist. Calc. Cann. S. Caust. Caps. Hep. Iodi. Kalmi. Lat. Kreoso. Lach. Lact. Viro. Nux V. Oleand. Petrol. Phos. Phos. ac. Puls. Rhodod. Rus. Rad. Rus. Tox. Sabad. Sambu. Seneg. Silec. Stann. Stramo. Sulp. or Verba.

———Legs drawn spasmodically apart, Colocy. Spong. Rus. Tox. or Tereb.

——— Swelled, Phos. Plumb. Rus. Tox. or Scill.

——— Limbs drawn up to the body, Oleand.

——— Paralysed, pained, or go to sleep,—Sabad. Scill. Rus. T. Sep. Silec. Stramo. Sulp. Thuy. Verat. or Zinc.

——— Nails blue, use Silec. or Sec. C.

——— Nails malformation, Calc. or Sec. C. Sep. or Silec.

——— Nails, ulcers about them, Sang. Silec. or Stann.

——— Neck stiff, or pained, give Lach. Lyc. Rhodod. Tarax. Tart. Anti. Tereb. Verat. or Zinc. (See Back.)

——— Pain, heat, or stiffness in—use Ammo. C. Arg. N. Ars. Bell. Bromi. Caust. Gum. Gtt. Hep. Iodi. Kali. Bic. Kali. Iodi. Kalmi. Lat.

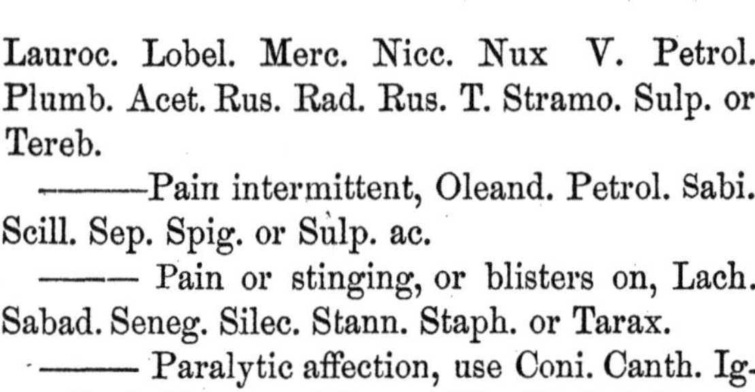

Lauroc. Lobel. Merc. Nicc. Nux V. Petrol. Plumb. Acet. Rus. Rad. Rus. T. Stramo. Sulp. or Tereb.

———Pain intermittent, Oleand. Petrol. Sabi. Scill. Sep. Spig. or Sulp. ac.

——— Pain or stinging, or blisters on, Lach. Sabad. Seneg. Silec. Stann. Staph. or Tarax.

——— Paralytic affection, use Coni. Canth. Ignat. Lach. Mangan. Nitr. ac. Nux V. Opi. Petrol. Phos. ac. Plati. Plumb. Podoph. P. Rus. Tox. Sabad. Sambu. Silec. Stann Sulp. Thuy. or Verat. or Colocy.

——— do. or numbness, or beating in—Coni. Lauroc. Lyc. Merc. Mosch. Muri. ac. Nux V. Oleand. Opi. Petrol. Phos. Phos. ac. Plati. Plumb. Acet. Puls. Rus. Rad. Rus. Tox. Sabad. Sang. Sarss Silec. Staph. Sulp. ac. or Zinc.

——— do. and numbness of hands or feet, Agnu. C. Bell. Bovist. Calc. Caust. Coni. Hyosc. Kali. C. Kreoso. Lach. Sep. Silec. Verat. or Rus. Rad.

——— Rheumatism. (See this article.)

——— SCIATICA is described a pain of the hip-joint, very severe. It partakes of a rheumatic, neuralgic character. The pain frequently runs down to the knee or foot—the remedies are, Acon. Bell. Colocy. NuxV.; or in the progress of the disease, Ars. Cham. Ignat. Rus. Tox.

——— Sensitive, Tereb. Verat.

——— Shoulders pain or stitches in, Lach. Lauroc. Led. P. Lobel. Lyc. Mag. M. Mag. P.

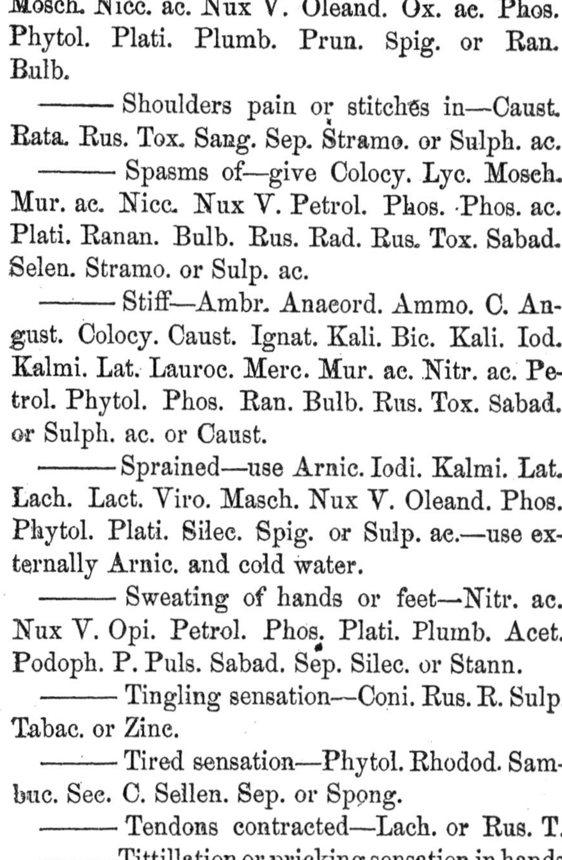

Mosch. Nicc. ac. Nux V. Oleand. Ox. ac. Phos. Phytol. Plati. Plumb. Prun. Spig. or Ran. Bulb.

——— Shoulders pain or stitches in—Caust. Rata. Rus. Tox. Sang. Sep. Stramo. or Sulph. ac.

——— Spasms of—give Colocy. Lyc. Mosch. Mur. ac. Nicc. Nux V. Petrol. Phos. Phos. ac. Plati. Ranan. Bulb. Rus. Rad. Rus. Tox. Sabad. Selen. Stramo. or Sulp. ac.

——— Stiff—Ambr. Anacord. Ammo. C. Angust. Colocy. Caust. Ignat. Kali. Bic. Kali. Iod. Kalmi. Lat. Lauroc. Merc. Mur. ac. Nitr. ac. Petrol. Phytol. Phos. Ran. Bulb. Rus. Tox. Sabad. or Sulph. ac. or Caust.

——— Sprained—use Arnic. Iodi. Kalmi. Lat. Lach. Lact. Viro. Masch. Nux V. Oleand. Phos. Phytol. Plati. Silec. Spig. or Sulp. ac.—use externally Arnic. and cold water.

——— Sweating of hands or feet—Nitr. ac. Nux V. Opi. Petrol. Phos. Plati. Plumb. Acet. Podoph. P. Puls. Sabad. Sep. Silec. or Stann.

——— Tingling sensation—Coni. Rus. R. Sulp. Tabac. or Zinc.

——— Tired sensation—Phytol. Rhodod. Sambuc. Sec. C. Sellen. Sep. or Spong.

——— Tendons contracted—Lach. or Rus. T.

———Tittillation or pricking sensation in hands or feet—Seneg. Stann. Staph. or Sulp.

——— Tremor in—give Caust. Lach. Lauroc. Led. P. Natr. C. Nitr. ac. Nux V. Plati. Phos.

Sabad. Sambuc. Silec. Sec. C. Spong. Stramo. Tabac. Tart. Anti. Thuy. Valer. or Verat.

——— Vesicles on—Lach. Rus. R. Sulp. or Zinc.

——— Warts or excrescenses on feet, Calc. Lach. Spig. or Thuy.

——— Weakness in, Chin. Plati. Prun. Sp. Ranan. Bulb. Rhodod. or Sep.

EYES.

The importance and delicacy of this organ makes it worthy of a careful and extended enumeration of the diseases to which it is subject and the various remedies for them, which are detailed as follows:

EYES.—Amblyopa, impaired vision from nervous affection or weakness of the nerves. The remedies are Anacard. Auru. Bell. Caust. Hyosc. Ignat. Kalmi. Lat. Kreoso. Lach. Lact. Viro. Lauroc. Lyc. Merc. Mosch. Natr. C. Nicc. Nit. ac. Nux V. Oleand. Ol. Anima. Phos. ac. Rus. Rad. Sabad. Sang. Sep. Staph. Stramo. Sulp. Tart. Anti. Thuy. Verat. Verba. or Zinc. or Colocy.

——— Amuroses, paralysed state of the optic nerve, use Lauroc. Opi. Phos. ac. Plati. Plumb. Acet. Rus. Tox. Scill. Sec. C. or Sep. and the above.

——— Balls drawn in or sunken, Seneg. Spong. Staph. or Valeri.

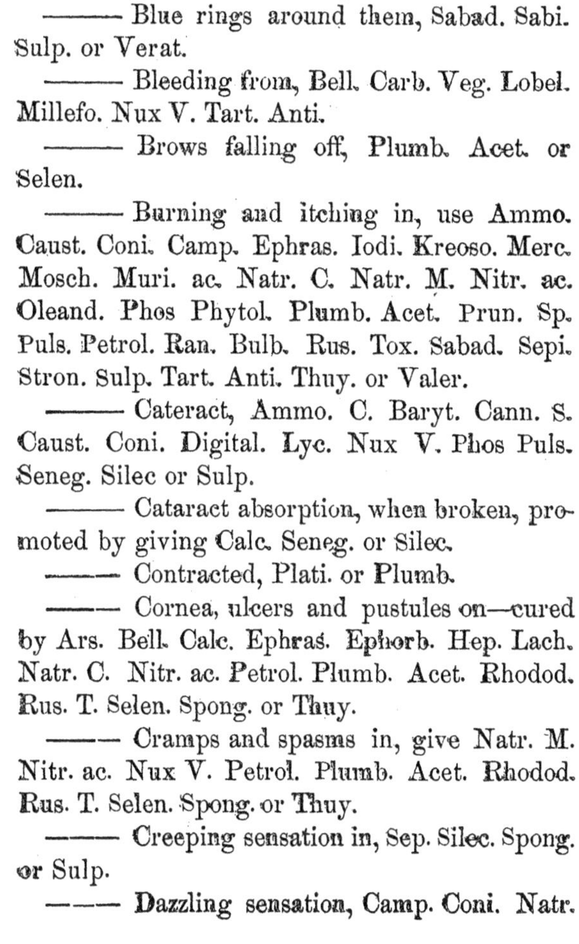

——— Balls pain in, Staph. Stron. or Tabac.

——— Blue rings around them, Sabad. Sabi. Sulp. or Verat.

——— Bleeding from, Bell. Carb. Veg. Lobel. Millefo. Nux V. Tart. Anti.

——— Brows falling off, Plumb. Acet. or Selen.

——— Burning and itching in, use Ammo. Caust. Coni. Camp. Ephras. Iodi. Kreoso. Merc. Mosch. Muri. ac. Natr. C. Natr. M. Nitr. ac. Oleand. Phos Phytol. Plumb. Acet. Prun. Sp. Puls. Petrol. Ran. Bulb. Rus. Tox. Sabad. Sepi. Stron. Sulp. Tart. Anti. Thuy. or Valer.

——— Cateract, Ammo. C. Baryt. Cann. S. Caust. Coni. Digital. Lyc. Nux V. Phos Puls. Seneg. Silec or Sulp.

——— Cataract absorption, when broken, promoted by giving Calc. Seneg. or Silec.

——— Contracted, Plati. or Plumb.

——— Cornea, ulcers and pustules on—cured by Ars. Bell. Calc. Ephras. Ephorb. Hep. Lach. Natr. C. Nitr. ac. Petrol. Plumb. Acet. Rhodod. Rus. T. Selen. Spong. or Thuy.

——— Cramps and spasms in, give Natr. M. Nitr. ac. Nux V. Petrol. Plumb. Acet. Rhodod. Rus. T. Selen. Spong. or Thuy.

——— Creeping sensation in, Sep. Silec. Spong. or Sulp.

——— Dazzling sensation, Camp. Coni. Natr.

M. Nitr. ac. Phos. Phos. ac. Seneg. Sep. or Stramo.

——— Debility of, Anacard. Kali. C. China. Iodi. Lauroc. Natr. C. Nux V. Nicc. Petrol. or Plati.

——— Double vision, Arnic. Baryt. Coni. Muri. ac. Nitr. ac. Petrol.

——— Drawing and stitches in, give Ol. Anima. Sarss. Selen.

——— Dryness, Nitr. ac. Ol. Anima. Plati. Puls. Seneg. Staph. Sulp. Thuy. or Verat.

——— Fire balls sensation of, in—Caust. Camp. Coni. or Zinc.

——— Fistula lacrymalis, the remedies are, Arnic. Calc. Caust. Lyc. Nitr. ac. Petrol. Puls. Silec. Stann. Sulp. or Zinc.

——— Flickering sensation—Coni. Lach. Nitr. ac. Opi. Puls. or Zinc.

——— Gazing sensation, Coni. or Verba.

——— Glands about them diseased, Bell. Coni. Iodi. or Spong.

——— Glistening sensation. Sol. Nig. or Stramo.

——— Hordeolum, (*sty.*) Ammo. C. Baryt. Graph. Lyc. Puls. Seneg. Staph. Sulp. or Thuy.

——— Inflammation of. Use Acon. Ars. Bell. Hell. Kali. Iod. Kalmi. Lat. Kali. Bic. Merc. Mag. M. Muri. ac. Natr. C. Nux V. Plumb. Acet. Seneg. Sep. Spong. Staph. Sulp. Tart. Anti. or Zinc.

——— do. Chronic. Camp. Canth. Chin. Colocy

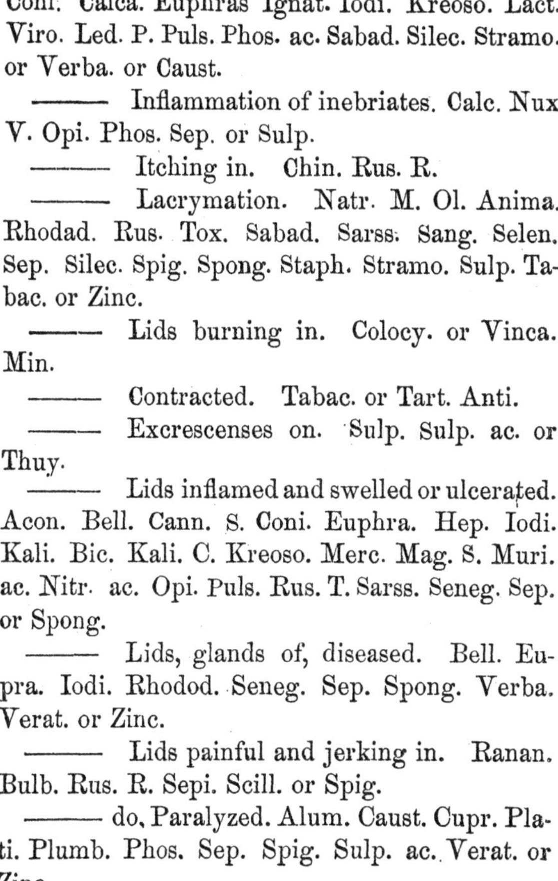

Coni. Calca. Euphras Ignat. Iodi. Kreoso. Lact. Viro. Led. P. Puls. Phos. ac. Sabad. Silec. Stramo. or Verba. or Caust.

——— Inflammation of inebriates. Calc. Nux V. Opi. Phos. Sep. or Sulp.

——— Itching in. Chin. Rus. R.

——— Lacrymation. Natr. M. Ol. Anima. Rhodad. Rus. Tox. Sabad. Sarss. Sang. Selen. Sep. Silec. Spig. Spong. Staph. Stramo. Sulp. Tabac. or Zinc.

——— Lids burning in. Colocy. or Vinca. Min.

——— Contracted. Tabac. or Tart. Anti.

——— Excrescenses on. Sulp. Sulp. ac. or Thuy.

——— Lids inflamed and swelled or ulcerated. Acon. Bell. Cann. S. Coni. Euphra. Hep. Iodi. Kali. Bic. Kali. C. Kreoso. Merc. Mag. S. Muri. ac. Nitr. ac. Opi. Puls. Rus. T. Sarss. Seneg. Sep. or Spong.

——— Lids, glands of, diseased. Bell. Eupra. Iodi. Rhodod. Seneg. Sep. Spong. Verba. Verat. or Zinc.

——— Lids painful and jerking in. Ranan. Bulb. Rus. R. Sepi. Scill. or Spig.

——— do, Paralyzed. Alum. Caust. Cupr. Plati. Plumb. Phos. Sep. Spig. Sulp. ac. Verat. or Zinc.

——— Pressure on. Sulp. Sulp. ac. Tabac. Tart. Anti. Thuy. or Valer.

——— Swelled. Phytol. Plumb. Acet. Puls. Rus. Rad. Rus. Tox. Sabad. Sec. C. Scill. Sep. Stann. or Thuy.

——— Long sighted or seeing at a distance. Petrol. Stramo. Valer. or Verat.

——— Luminous or dazzling illusions. Sec. C. Seneg. Silec. Staph. Stramo. Stron. Sulp. Valer. or Verat.'

——— Mercurial affections. Acon. Arnic. Alum. Calc. Cupr. Hep. Nitr. ac. or Sulp.

——— Mechanical injury. Arni. Bell. Iodi. Rus. Tox.

——— Moats, sensation of, before. Tereb. Thuy. Valer. Verat. Verba. or Zinc.

——— Myope (short sighted.) Ammo. C. Auru. Carb. Veg. Petrol. Phos. Selen. or Sulp. ac.

——— Objects half seen. Mur. ac.

——— Pain in (Photophobia.) Caust. Coni. Colocy. Ephras. Ignat. Lach. Mur. ac. Nux V. Oleand. Puls. Rus. Rad. Seneg. Sep. Spig. Staph. Stann. or Verat.

——— do. and heavy sensation. Nitr. ac. Phytol. or Puls.

——— do. and pressure in. Chin. Coni. Lach. Morph. Petrol. Phos. ac. Phytol. Plati. Puls. Ran. Bulb. Rus. Tox. Sarss. Scill. Sep. Spong. Stann. Stron. Stramo. Tabac. or Thuy.

——— Pupils contracted. Camp. Hyosc. Plati. Plumb. Acet. Puls. Rhodad. Sambu. Sec.

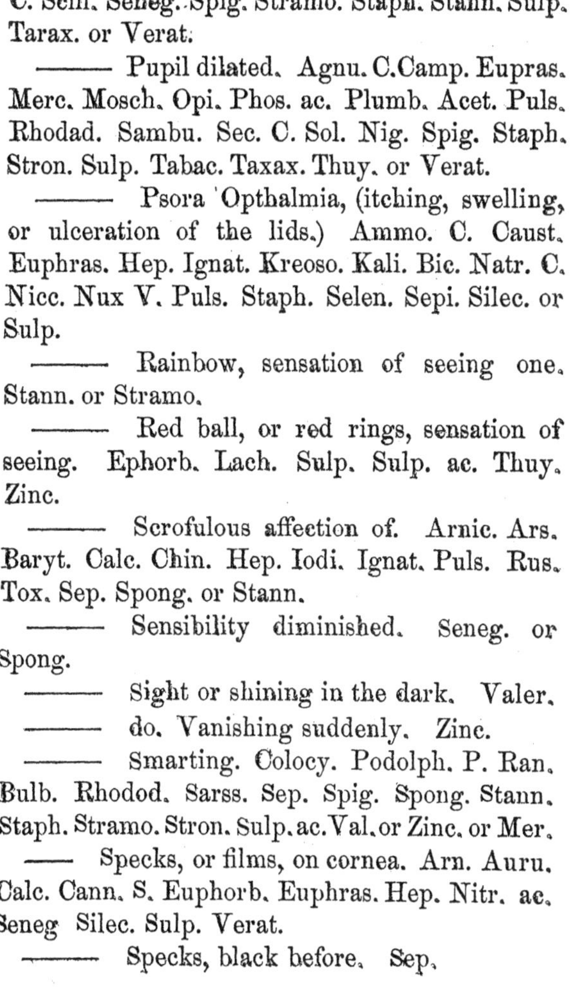

C. Scill. Seneg. Spig. Stramo. Staph. Stann. Sulp. Tarax. or Verat.

——— Pupil dilated. Agnu. C. Camp. Eupras. Merc. Mosch. Opi. Phos. ac. Plumb. Acet. Puls. Rhodad. Sambu. Sec. C. Sol. Nig. Spig. Staph. Stron. Sulp. Tabac. Taxax. Thuy. or Verat.

——— Psora 'Opthalmia, (itching, swelling, or ulceration of the lids.) Ammo. C. Caust. Euphras. Hep. Ignat. Kreoso. Kali. Bic. Natr. C. Nicc. Nux V. Puls. Staph. Selen. Sepi. Silec. or Sulp.

——— Rainbow, sensation of seeing one. Stann. or Stramo.

——— Red ball, or red rings, sensation of seeing. Ephorb. Lach. Sulp. Sulp. ac. Thuy. Zinc.

——— Scrofulous affection of. Arnic. Ars. Baryt. Calc. Chin. Hep. Iodi. Ignat. Puls. Rus. Tox. Sep. Spong. or Stann.

——— Sensibility diminished. Seneg. or Spong.

——— Sight or shining in the dark. Valer.

——— do. Vanishing suddenly. Zinc.

——— Smarting. Colocy. Podolph. P. Ran. Bulb. Rhodod. Sarss. Sep. Spig. Spong. Stann. Staph. Stramo. Stron. Sulp. ac. Val. or Zinc. or Mer.

——— Specks, or films, on cornea. Arn. Auru. Calc. Cann. S. Euphorb. Euphras. Hep. Nitr. ac. Seneg Silec. Sulp. Verat.

——— Specks, black before. Sep.

——— Stareing or contortion. Camp. Caps. Mosch. Scill. Sec. C. Stron. Tabac. or Thuy.

——— Stitches in. Verat. or Zinc.

——— Strabismus, (squinting.) Alum. Bell. Hyosc. Verat.

——— Syphilitic affection. Auru. Merc. Mez. Nitr. ac. or Puls.

——— Trembling sensation. Nitr. ac. Petrol. Phos. Rata. Rus. Tox. or Verat.

——— Twinkling sensation. Anacard. Coni. or Sep.

——— Ulceration of. Ars. Bell. Calc. Euphorb. Hep. Lyc. Mag. M. or Spong. or Sulp.

——— Vesicles on. Seneg. or Thuy.

——— Vibrating sensation. Sabi. Sep. Stramo. Sulp. or Zinc.

——— Vision, blue, green, or yellow shades, Zinc.

——— Web appearance. Tabac. Tereb. or Zinc.

——— Wheels of vision in appearance. Use Caust.

FACE.

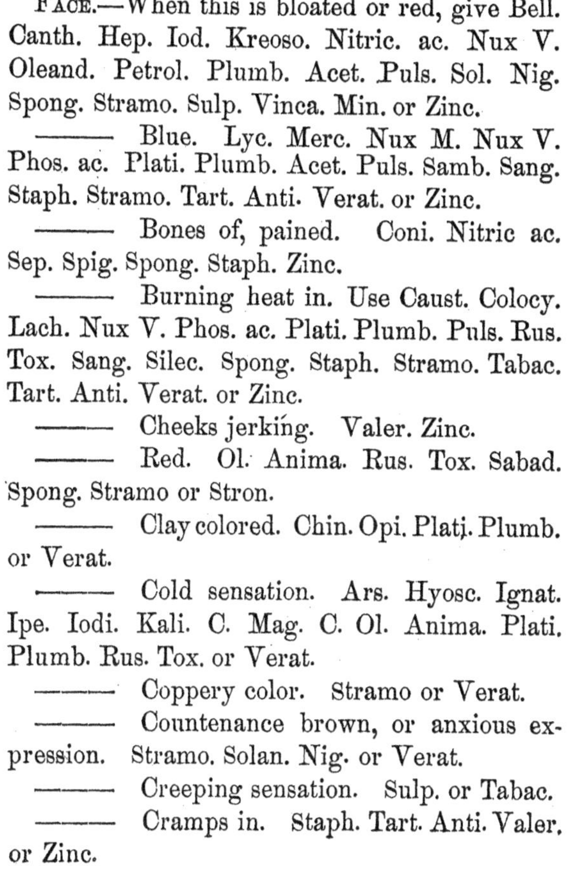

Face.—When this is bloated or red, give Bell. Canth. Hep. Iod. Kreoso. Nitric. ac. Nux V. Oleand. Petrol. Plumb. Acet. Puls. Sol. Nig. Spong. Stramo. Sulp. Vinca. Min. or Zinc.

——— Blue. Lyc. Merc. Nux M. Nux V. Phos. ac. Plati. Plumb. Acet. Puls. Samb. Sang. Staph. Stramo. Tart. Anti. Verat. or Zinc.

——— Bones of, pained. Coni. Nitric ac. Sep. Spig. Spong. Staph. Zinc.

——— Burning heat in. Use Caust. Colocy. Lach. Nux V. Phos. ac. Plati. Plumb. Puls. Rus. Tox. Sang. Silec. Spong. Staph. Stramo. Tabac. Tart. Anti. Verat. or Zinc.

——— Cheeks jerking. Valer. Zinc.

——— Red. Ol. Anima. Rus. Tox. Sabad. Spong. Stramo or Stron.

——— Clay colored. Chin. Opi. Plati. Plumb. or Verat.

——— Cold sensation. Ars. Hyosc. Ignat. Ipe. Iodi. Kali. C. Mag. C. Ol. Anima. Plati. Plumb. Rus. Tox. or Verat.

——— Coppery color. Stramo or Verat.

——— Countenance brown, or anxious expression. Stramo. Solan. Nig. or Verat.

——— Creeping sensation. Sulp. or Tabac.

——— Cramps in. Staph. Tart. Anti. Valer. or Zinc.

——— Deathly look. Plumb. Acet. Sec. C. Staph. or Verat.

——— Distortion. Lach.

——— Dry, sticky feeling. Sulp. ac.

——— Eruptions or vesicles on. Canth. Calc. Coni. Lach. Lauroc. Led. P. Nitr. ac. Nux V. Oleand. Ol. Anima. Petrol. Phos. Phytol. Rhodod. Sabi. Sambu. Sarss. Scill. Silec. Stann. or Sulp.

——— Freckles on. Calc. Carb. Anim. Hep. Kreoso. Lauroc. Led. P. Lyc. Natr. C. Oleand. Sep. or Sulp.

——— Hot sensation. Rus. Tox. Sabad. Sang. Sarss. Sep. Stann. Tabac. or Thuy.

——— Itching. Coni. Lach. Merc. Natr. C. Nicc. Nitr. ac. Nux V. Ol. Anima. Petrol. Plumb. Acet. Prun. Sp. Rheum. Rus. Rad. Sabad. Sabi. Sarss. Sep. Silec. or Zinc.

——— Lips dry or sore. Nitr. ac. Nux V. Phos. Scill. Stann. Sulp. ac. Tarx. Tart. Anti. or Thuy.

——— do. Chapped or sore. Hep. Silec. Tabac. Verat. or Zinc.

——— or mouth distorted or swelled. Lach. Opi. Verat. or Zinc.

——— Pain or drawing, or bruised sensation. Give Caust. Colocy. Sulp. Sulp. ac. Tart. Anti. Tereb. Valer. or Zinc.

——— do. or twinging sensation. Ambr. Arnic. Bromi. Bismu. Hep. Kalmi. Lat. Kreoso. Lach

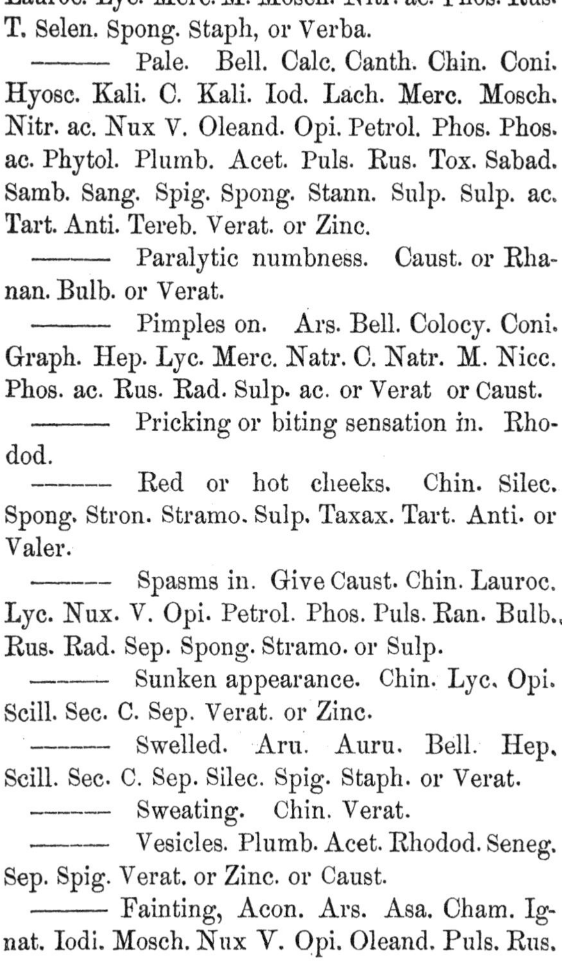

Lauroc. Lyc. Merc. M. Mosch. Nitr. ac. Phos. Rus. T. Selen. Spong. Staph, or Verba.

——— Pale. Bell. Calc. Canth. Chin. Coni. Hyosc. Kali. C. Kali. Iod. Lach. Merc. Mosch. Nitr. ac. Nux V. Oleand. Opi. Petrol. Phos. Phos. ac. Phytol. Plumb. Acet. Puls. Rus. Tox. Sabad. Samb. Sang. Spig. Spong. Stann. Sulp. Sulp. ac. Tart. Anti. Tereb. Verat. or Zinc.

——— Paralytic numbness. Caust. or Rhanan. Bulb. or Verat.

——— Pimples on. Ars. Bell. Colocy. Coni. Graph. Hep. Lyc. Merc. Natr. C. Natr. M. Nicc. Phos. ac. Rus. Rad. Sulp. ac. or Verat or Caust.

——— Pricking or biting sensation in. Rhodod.

——— Red or hot cheeks. Chin. Silec. Spong. Stron. Stramo. Sulp. Taxax. Tart. Anti. or Valer.

——— Spasms in. Give Caust. Chin. Lauroc. Lyc. Nux. V. Opi. Petrol. Phos. Puls. Ran. Bulb.. Rus. Rad. Sep. Spong. Stramo. or Sulp.

——— Sunken appearance. Chin. Lyc. Opi. Scill. Sec. C. Sep. Verat. or Zinc.

——— Swelled. Aru. Auru. Bell. Hep. Scill. Sec. C. Sep. Silec. Spig. Staph. or Verat.

——— Sweating. Chin. Verat.

——— Vesicles. Plumb. Acet. Rhodod. Seneg. Sep. Spig. Verat. or Zinc. or Caust.

——— Fainting, Acon. Ars. Asa. Cham. Ignat. Iodi. Mosch. Nux V. Opi. Oleand. Puls. Rus.

Tox. Sep. Stann. Stramo. Tart. Anti. Tereb. or Verat.

——— Fatigue appearance, Acon. Arnic. Bell. Bryo. Coff. Iodi. Lyc. Morph. or Nux V. (See extremities tired.

FELON OR WHITLOW.

Felon or Whitlow. This a very painful disease which locates on the fingers or hands, of an inflammatory nature; the inflammation or germ of the disease is deep seated at the bone; if matter forms there, it is attended with difficulty to work its way out to the surface, by which it produces great pain and swelling, this affection is generally rendered tedious and serious by injudicious treatment, by the use of hot poultices and hot irritating articles; the proper remedies for it are the internal use of Acon. Bell. Bryo. Ipe. or Silecia. and very low diet; as local applications, use cold water or ice; solutions of acetate of lead applied cold, or usc this in the form of a cold poultice; if these means do not check the disease, it is sometimes arrested or cured by holding the part in lye as hot as it can be borne.

But the best, shortest, and surest remedy is, as soon as the disease is formed, to make a free incision into the tumefied part with a lancet, down to the bone or seat of the disease; this lets out the acrid generating matter and blood, and puts an end to the disease at once Then it is converted into a simple incised wound, which will heal up in two or three days; one half minute's suffering in this way, will save the patient weeks and months of painful anguish, and perhaps, the loss of a joint. If however, the disease does progress, towards suppuration, give Hep. Silec. or Sulp. and apply warm emmolient poultices; as soon as the matter is formed, a free opening should be made to let it out. This may prevent sinuses forming, and afford a chance to apply dressings, when the ulcer must be healed in the common way.

FEVER.

Fever. In most all morbid affections of the body fever is produced. It may be merely symptomatic of an injury, or of a local affection; or it may be a primary disease, brought into action by a genesal disturbance or deranged condition of the system. Or it may be produced as symptoms of specific morbific virus, producing contagious disease. There have been a great many definitions of fever or its proximate cause. It would extend this article to an extreme length to describe them, which would not be very useful. Most authors consider fever an increased degree of heat, an accelerated pulse, a furred tongue, and the functions of the body considerably deranged. It will suffice to enumerate the various kinds of fever, and the appropriate Homœopathic remedies for them as here detailed.

The general remedies for it are, Acon. Bell. Bryo. Cocc. Ipe. Ignat. Lach. Lauroc. Merc. Nitr. ac. Phos. Puls. Rus. T. Sepi. Silec. Spong. or Tart. Anti.

——— Catarrhal, common cold, the remedies most useful are, Acon. Arnic. Nux V. Puls. Phos. Rus. T. Sulp. or Tart. A. (See Angina. Catarrhalis.)

At the commencement when the head and nose are stopped, and affected with a snuffling, use Dulcam. Nux V. or Puls.

If there is fever and slight sore throat, use Acon. Bryo. or Ipe.

If the throat is inflamed and sore, use Bell. Bryo. or Puls.

In children, who have a dry cough and are restless, use Acon. Cham. Dulcam. Sulp. or Nux V.

If there is a painful, bruised feeling, give Drosera. or Arnic.

If there is a raw apthous state of the throat, give Coni. Merc. Borax. or Ipe.

When the joints are swelled and painful, use Bryo. Sulp. ac. or Rus. T.

If there is inveterate cough, with pain in the front part of the head, Bell. Lyc. Puls. or Nux V.

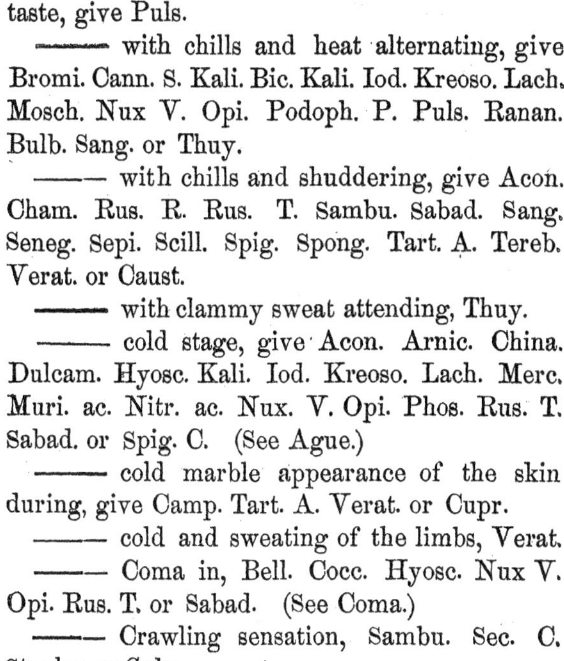

If there is a distress of the head, and loss of taste, give Puls.

—— with chills and heat alternating, give Bromi. Cann. S. Kali. Bic. Kali. Iod. Kreoso. Lach. Mosch. Nux V. Opi. Podoph. P. Puls. Ranan. Bulb. Sang. or Thuy.

—— with chills and shuddering, give Acon. Cham. Rus. R. Rus. T. Sambu. Sabad. Sang. Seneg. Sepi. Scill. Spig. Spong. Tart. A. Tereb. Verat. or Caust.

—— with clammy sweat attending, Thuy.

—— cold stage, give Acon. Arnic. China. Dulcam. Hyosc. Kali. Iod. Kreoso. Lach. Merc. Muri. ac. Nitr. ac. Nux. V. Opi. Phos. Rus. T. Sabad. or Spig. C. (See Ague.)

—— cold marble appearance of the skin during, give Camp. Tart. A. Verat. or Cupr.

—— cold and sweating of the limbs, Verat.

—— Coma in, Bell. Cocc. Hyosc. Nux V. Opi. Rus. T. or Sabad. (See Coma.)

—— Crawling sensation, Sambu. Sec. C. Staphy. or Sulp.

—— Delirium in, Bell. Cocc. Hell. Opi. Phos. ac. Phodoph. P. Rus. T. Sabad. or Sulp.

—— Heat or burning great, give Acon Sambu. Sang. Scill. Silec. Spong. Staphy. Sulp. ac. Thuy. or Verat.

—— Pulse small, or imperceptible, use Camp. Sec. C. Scill. Sol. Nig. Stramo. Sulp. ac. Tabac. Tart. A. Thuy. or Verat.

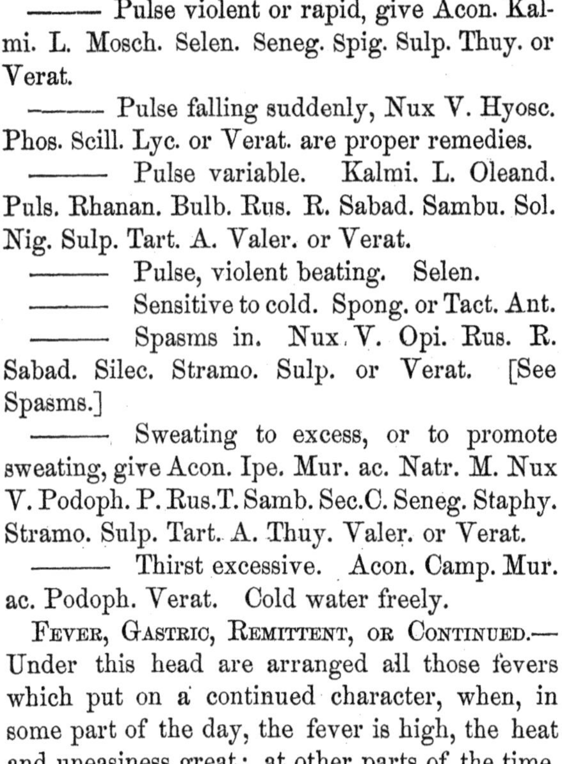

——— Pulse intermittent, Sec. C. Stramo. Tabac. Tart. A. Verat. or Cupr.

——— Pulse slow, use Plumb. Acet. Podoph. P. Rus. T. Sabad. Sec. C. or Thuy.

——— Pulse violent or rapid, give Acon. Kalmi. L. Mosch. Selen. Seneg. Spig. Sulp. Thuy. or Verat.

——— Pulse falling suddenly, Nux V. Hyosc. Phos. Scill. Lyc. or Verat. are proper remedies.

——— Pulse variable. Kalmi. L. Oleand. Puls. Rhanan. Bulb. Rus. R. Sabad. Sambu. Sol. Nig. Sulp. Tart. A. Valer. or Verat.

——— Pulse, violent beating. Selen.

——— Sensitive to cold. Spong. or Tact. Ant.

——— Spasms in. Nux. V. Opi. Rus. R. Sabad. Silec. Stramo. Sulp. or Verat. [See Spasms.]

——— Sweating to excess, or to promote sweating, give Acon. Ipe. Mur. ac. Natr. M. Nux V. Podoph. P. Rus.T. Samb. Sec.C. Seneg. Staphy. Stramo. Sulp. Tart. A. Thuy. Valer. or Verat.

——— Thirst excessive. Acon. Camp. Mur. ac. Podoph. Verat. Cold water freely.

Fever, Gastric, Remittent, or Continued.—Under this head are arranged all those fevers which put on a continued character, when, in some part of the day, the fever is high, the heat and uneasiness great; at other parts of the time, the fever is less; the patient is more calm and quiet; perhaps some moisture of the skin or sweating takes place, but an intermission or entire suspension of the fever does not ensue, The fevers which more generally prevail in the autumnal season, in temperate and northern latitudes are termed Remittent, Bilious, or Gastric Fevers, and those which run into a form of a Typhus character, are all Remittent Fevers, and present one general set of symptoms in the beginning. The fevers connected with inflammatory affections, when the inflammation is seated on some local part, are also somewhat remittent or continued, but they take on the name of Inflammatory fevers, as will be seen by referring to the article headed Inflammations.

The Remittent Fever is ushered in with chills, rigors, or ague, or shuddering; the stomach is often deranged by pain or a sinking sensation, nausea, or vomiting. There is frequently severe pain in the head and in the limbs generally, attended with a loss of strength. As the chill abates or subsides, fever sets in more or less severe, the bowels are generally disordered, sometimes they are costive, and at others a diarrhœa is attending. The tongue has a whitish fur on it, which soon becomes yellowish or brown; the pulse is generally pretty full and firm, though it is sometimes depressed, small, and compressible. A train of other symptoms succeed, and these are very much influenced by the condition of the patient and mode of treatment.

For this form of fever the most advisable remedies at first are those to check the ague, which may be found under the head Ague. If there is nausea or vomiting, give Ipe. or Tart. Anti. in high attenuations, perhaps the twenty or thirty would be preferable; or it may be best to give Acon. in alternation with one of the above named medicines. This course may be pursued with great benefit. As soon as the ague is over and the stomach quieted, give Acon. steadily until the febrile symptoms are moderated; or Bryo. may be used to succeed the Acon. If there is considerable headache and red flushed face, give Bell. In the more advanced state, when the active type has abated, the most useful remedies are Ipe. Merc. Nux V. Podopylin. This last remedy will be very useful to procure evacuations from the] bowels, which may be important. Other remedies, which will be useful in the progress, are Puls. Rus. T. Sabad. Sulp. or Verat.

If the mind gets to be impaired, Cham. Colocy. or Phos. ac.

If there are cramps or spasms, Ignat. or NuxV.

If there is colic or heat or burning in the abdomen, Ars. or Colocy.

If the tongue has a yellow or brown coat, Merc.

If nausea continue, Ipe. Colocy. or Ars. or Nux V.

If there is a sinking faintness and cold skin, Verat.

If there is a fœtid taste of eructations, Carbo V.

If debility and great weakness ensue, Chin. Quini. or Ars. or Wine.

If delirium or nervous irritation take place, consult the articles Delirium and Spasms.

FEVER, HECTIC.

Fever, Hectic. This disease may be brought on from various causes. It is a febrile state, dependent on or connected with a diseased condition of an internal part, and most generally connected with a disease of the lungs. It commonly comes on insidiously and slowly, attended with pain in the chest, short, dry cough, uneasy and irregular sleep, sore throat, dryness of the palms of the hands, flushed cheeks in the afternoon, with slight fever; and as it advances there are night sweats, a small quickened pulse; and as the case progresses there are more numerous and aggravated symptoms. The best remedies in the early stage are Acon. Arnic. Bell. Calc. C. Hep. Kali. Iodi. Ipe, Iodi. Lach. Lyc. Merc. Iodi. Puls. Sulph. or Ars.

For further information of the treatment, see Consumption and Chest Diseases and Cough.

——— Hectic, in the Inflammatory stage, give

Acon. Bell. Bryo. Hyosc. Ipe. Nux V. Puls. Rus. T. or Sulph. See Inflammation.

——— Lethargy in. Give Bell. Cham. Cocci. Opi. See Coma.

FEVER, NERVOUS.

Fever, Nervous Affection. Give Ambr. Ars. Bell. Camp. Canth. China, Hyosc Lach. Lyc. Merc. Mosch. Nux V. Opi. Phos. Rus. T. Selen. Stram. or Verat. See Typhus.

FEVER, INTERMITTENT.

Fever, Intermittent. This form of fever and the manner of attack is so well known, as ague and fever, chills and fever, &c., that in a work of this kind, it seems unnecessary to enter into a detailed description of it. In many instances it is very tedious and troublesome, and difficult to cure.

The remedies most useful are, Acon. Arnic. Ars. Bell. Bryo. Calcara. Chin. Cedron. (cotton seed) Euphorb. Eupatorium. Ferr. Ipe. Puls. Petrol. Rus. T. Stann. Sulp. Verat. or Quinine.

One of the best remedies to use first, to prepare the system for after treatment, is allowed to be Ipe. followed by Nux V.

It is best to give the medicine thus, a dose about every three hours.

The remedies which may with great benefit be

continued through the pyrexia and the apyrexia, or intermission, are, Arnic. Bell. Bryo. Calca. Lach. Nux V. or Ipe. or Puls.; and one of those medicines given in this way often, is capable of effecting a cure.

The plan of treatment which experience has proved to be the most useful, and pursued generally during the cold stage or ague or chills, is to use such remedies as will most readily check the ague, and shorten it as much as possible. The best for this purpose is Agar. Ammo. C. Acon. Ars. Ipe. Nux V. or Puls. (See Ague.)

It will be best to give hot toast, tea, or some other simple hot drink. If the chills continue a long time, warm fomentations or warm water, should be applied to the feet and legs; as soon as the ague or chill abate, and reaction comes on, and fever rises, then those remedies which are well known to be best to allay fever should be used. The most efficacious of these are, Acon. Bryo. Bell. Ipe. Tart. Anti. and cold water, freely used as a drink. If there is pain in the head, or of other parts, or nausea, or distress of the stomach, or abdomen, or nervous irritability or cramps, or other local affections, then give in alternation with one of the medicines above mentioned for fever or a substitute for it, a medicine which will be particularly adapted to those symptoms which is laid down under the heads in the repertory for the peculiar affections which may be present; for instance, if the head is distressed, turn to head, and you will find the proper remedies, and so of the other affections.

The remedies to be used during the intermission, and those generally given, are Calca. China. or Quini. Ferr. or Angust. Eupatori. or Cedron.

——— Intermittent, in the cold stage, give Acon. Agnu. C. Angust. Baryt. Bell. Dulcam. Opi. or Phos.

There is a popular remedy we have known used with so great success, that it seems to be worthy of a place here. In obstinate protracted chills, or ague and fever, take a cup of hot coffee, add to it the juice of one lemon, and drink it hot as soon as the chill comes on; in many cases this has broken up the ague and fever.

——— do. If it is produced from marshy exposure, China. Ars. or Carb. V. Rus. T. Verat. or Ferr.

——— do. In warm weather or hot climate, Bell. Ipe. Caps. Calc. Bryo. Carb. V. Digit. Puls. or Verat.

——— do. When coldness predominates, Ipe. Puls. Sabad. Phos. Carb. V. or Caps.

——— do. When there is excess of heat, Acon. Cocc. Nux V. Ignat. Ars. Bell. Ipe. Sabad. or Valer.

——— do. When there is a regular chill, heat

and sweating, give Ipe. Nux V. Quini. Caps. China. Puls. Rus. T. or Verat.

——— do. If it is attended mostly with heat and sweating, Bell. Bryo. Caps. Cham. Hep. Ignat. or Quini.

——— do. If there is dull headache inclining to stupor, give Opi. Cocc. Bell. Nux V. Hyosc. Stramo.

——— do. Œdematous swelling taking place in the progress, give Bryo. Hell. Ars. Prus. ac. or China.

In places where intermittent fever is prevailing, or when persons are liable to contract it, remedies may be used as preventives to guard against an attack, such as China. Ipe. Nux V.; a dose of one of these taken every day, or one of them on one day, and another the next day, and so on, is said to prevent an attack, and guard the system against it.

PEUERPERAL.

Peuerperal.—The most proper remedy at the first stage is Acon.; after a short time, if there should be a good deal of excitement, or nervous irritation attending, it will be proper to give Nux V. or Ignat. or one of these medicines in alternation with Acon.; after the first or urgent symptoms are over, it will be neecssary to give one of the following medicines according to the symptoms—Ars. Bryo. Canth. Cham. Colocy. Merc. Puls. or Veratrum.

If the pains continue severe, use Bryo. Colocy. or Verat.

If cramps or spasms are attendant, Ignat. or Nux V.

It there is retention of urine, Canth. or Uva. U. or Merc.

For the weakness which may ensue, use Chin. Phos. Calc. or Wine. (See Women, this article.)

PLAGUE.

Plague.—From the best information had, it is thought that the most useful remedies for it in the first stage, are, Acon. Bell. or Ipec. or Ars. As Guaco. is highly useful in the violent fevers of Central America, no doubt it would be useful in the plague. The other remedies enumerated are Nitr. ac. Kreoso. Silec. Carb. V. or Lach.

RAPHANA. ECLAMPSIA TYPHOIDES.

Raphana.—This, fortunately, is a rare disease. It is attended with nausea, vomiting, foul tongue, nauseous taste, headache, giddiness, cramp of the stomach, and throwing up black matter. In the progress, there is a cold clammy skin, great thirst and burning heat, delirium. In a more advanced stage, a putrid state ensues, with delirium and stupor.

For this severe disease, Hahnemann found Solanum Nig. one of the best remedies—almost specific. Others recommended are Acon. Bell. Sec. C. Cupr. Rus. T. Hyosc. Stramo. or Ars. At first, when there is fever, Acon. If burning heat and redness of skin, Bell. Palpitation of the heart or cramps, Ignat. of Hyosc. Brain affected, Stramo. or Hyosc. Cold skin, Cupr. Quick pulse, nervous agitation, and extreme prostration, Ars. or C.

——— Rheumatic—Acon. Bell. Bryo. Caust. Colocy. Cham. Dulcam. Merc. Nux V. Puls. Rus. Ranan. Bulb. are the most useful. (See Rheumatism.)

——— do. Petechial. The remedies are the same as for nervous, typhoid, or putrid fever.

——— do. Putrid. This state takes place in the advanced stage of typhus or malignant fevers. It is a low prostrated condition—the remedies are, Ars. Canth. Carb. V. China. Merc. Phos. Muriatic acid, or Sec. C. and good Wine or Porter.

SCARLET FEVER.

Scarlet Fever. This disease makes its appearance nearly every year, in particular districts, or in different locations. Sometimes it is only sporadic and rather mild, at other times it prevails as an epidemic, and with great severity; it is considered contagious, and when it spreads as a severe epidemic, its contagious character is very manifest.

It comes on with the general symptoms of fever, attended with pain in the head, and limbs, and abdomen, with chills. The throat soon gets sore and somewhat swelled, a dry cough sets in; after a day or two, a fine red eruption appears; sometimes there is a flushed redness without much visible eruption; this generally begins on the face and neck, and then spreads over other parts. At this time the throat and tongue are very red. In severe cases when not checked, swellings and ulceration take place in the throat. If there is considerable fever at the commencement, give Acon. say ten drops of the second or third dilution, or a higher attenuation as the prescriber may prefer: put it into half a gill of water, and give a tea spoonful every two hours, or two or three grains of a trituration of the same attenuation may be mixed in the same quantity of water, and given in a like way. Those who prefer the medicated pellets will use them in preference. As soon as the active fever is moderated and the red eruption appears, give Bell. in the same manner as above directed for using Acon. This is the specific remedy for this form of the disease. With the early and proper use of these medicines, most cases are so checked as to render the disease moderate, or it is cured altogether.

Let the patient drink cold water, and apply a cloth wetted with cold water to the throat and chest; other remedies recommeded and used in some states of the disease, are Baryt. C. Lach. Merc. Nitr. ac. Nux V. Opi. Puls. Phos. Rus. T. or Stramo. If the disease continues obstinately and the throat gets ulcerated, give Merc. alone, or in alternation with Bell. or Rus. T., or such medicine as may be indicated by the symptoms.

If there is prostration, use Ars. or Nux V.

When there is burning of the skin, chillness, or stupor, use Opi. Cocc. or Rus. T.

If the stomach is deranged and face pale, Puls. or Ignat. or Nux V. are the proper medicines.

If the throat and faucies are inflamed or swelled, give Spong. Hep. or Ars. or Merc.

If repercussion, or receding of the eruption takes place, give Bryo. Bell. Cupr. Acet. or Hell. Iodi. Phos. or Rus. T.

In the sinking or typhoid form, give Ammo. C. Muri. ac. Opi. Phos. Phos. ac. or Quinine. In this condition a spoonful of yeast often repeated is advisable, or use wine in the same way.

For the secondary or swelling state, give Ars. Auru. M. Baryt. M. Camph. Hep. Hell. Muri. ac. Nitr. ac. Nux V. Phos. Rus. T. Tart. A. Sulp. or Apis. Mell. When the scarlet fever is prevailing in any place, to prevent an attack, it is found that Belladona is a preventive of the disease; by using it, the disease is so modified, if persons are seized with it, that the case is but a mild one. The proper mode of giving it is, to use three or four drops of the third or fourth dilution once a day, or every other day; or a grain of the second or third trituration may be used in the same manner; or the medicated pellets may be used instead of either of the above named preparations.

SHIP.

Ship, or jail, or nervous.—In this affection, it will be advisable to bear in mind the observations made in the succeeding article on typhus. The mode of treatment generally detailed for the treatment of typhus will be suitable for this disease. If the case is attended with nervous sensibility and continued fever, the remedies are, Acon. Bell. Bryo. or Hyosc. or Stramo. Should there be an inclination to stupor, slow fever, or nervous affection, use Bell. Rus. T.

——— Tertian—Acon. Bryo. Ipe. or Ars. Angust. China. Verat. (See intermittent fever, for a detail of the remedies.

TYPHUS FEVER.

Typhus Fever. That kind of disease termed typhus, or that which runs into a typhus state.

NOTE ON SCARLET FEVER.—In the first stage, when there is nausea or vomiting as there often is, give Ipec. in a high attenuation, say 3d, 6th, or higher, in very minute doses, this allays the vomiting in a short time; if there is much fever as there generally is, give Acon. in alternation with the Ipecac. or when the nausea subsides, omit the Ipecac. and continue the Acon.

When the eruption or flushy redness appears, give Bell. and this may be given alone every two or three hours, or if there is a good deal of fever, give Acon. in alternation with it—the Bell. ought to be continued until the flushy redness abates or subsides, but it had better not be used over 30 or 50 hours, for there is danger of its producing a Belladona aggravation, which, if continued, will cause injurious effects. The best application to the neck at the early stage is cloths wet in cold water, and if there is a good deal of inflammation and heat, ice had better be added to the water. The best and only drink required, or that a child will take is cold water or ice water; small drinks of it should be often given. After this stage has passed, if the fever and swelling at the neck continue, give Bryo. Ipec. and occasionally Bell. or Canth., or if there is a stinging sore pain in the throat, Doloch. will be a good remedy. In the more advanced stage, when the glands of the throat are enlarged, give Merc. and Ipec. in alternation.

With this treatment at this stage of the case, the disease is generally arrested, and the patient recovers. But sometimes as the case advances, the swelling of the glands of the throat and neck become large inside as well as outwardly, and excoriations, apthea or ulcers form on the tonsils and fauces, and there takes place a fullness and stuffing up of the nose or throat, or both ; sometimes a tough ropy corrosive mucus forms and is discharged. In this condition and stage, the best remedies are Carbo. of Ammonia or Bichromate of Potash, given in small repeated doses, and Merc. should be given in alternation with one of these medicines, which will be very useful. In this condition, an excellent application to the neck, (it is rather a domestic remedy, and one I have often used,) apply a slice of salt pork taken from the brine, and let it be kept applied to the neck. By this course, I have carried some severe cases of this kind safely through.

My observation and experience is against the use of blisters or mustard plasters and volatile liniments applied to the throat and neck. With this treatment, there are objections to them, and more decidedly against the use of gargles of cayenne pepper, and such like stimulating and irritating applications to the mouth and throat internally ; if any thing of this kind is used, it had better be some mild fluid, and rather to dilute and wash out the mucus, than to corrode or astringe the part.

A plan of treatment of which this is an outline, has almost uniformly succeeded for years in carrying these cases and the little sufferers safely through to health.

In the progress of the case which appears in the country hereabout, and in the City, we have reason to infer and believe, that there has been some erroneous opinions held respecting it, and sometimes an equally erroneous mode of treatment pursued, and that those opinions so influence the management of cases as to be a means of producing a typhus state, a protracted course of disease, and an increased state of danger. As far as we have been able to investigate this subject for a series of years, we have observed that fevers of this description, or the remittents which runs into typhus, as they appear in this climate or latitude, in the first stage, or at the attack, are of a phlegmasial or compound inflammatory or congestive nature; hence the weakness and debility which is often apparent at this stage is a prostrated condition, and proceeds from an obstructed circulation of the blood, and an interruption of the vital and muscular powers. This character of disease, no doubt, is a different condition of the system from the low typhoid fevers which take place in jails, ships, and among a dense crowded population.

Should the prescriber consider the case before him of a typhoid tendency in the begining, and prone to direct debility, so as to induce him to avoid the use of remedies to relieve phlegmasial action, or to remove congestion, and he directly has recourse to exciting or stimulating sudorific re medies, or opiates, or mercurials, as sometimes is done, they bid fair to have a protracted typhoid case; sometimes prescribers are inclined to give cordial stimulant articles, and even wine, early, to guard against typhus, and to prevent the patient from *running down*, as it has been termed; they also resort to the use of calomel and opium early, reasoning that if the system can be brought under a mercurial action, the disease may be controlled and broken up. Most practitioners may be aware that these remedies used at the first stage of phlegmasial disease, tend to aggravate the affection, and may convert a simple case into an obstinate protracted one. In making these remarks, we do not mean to be understood as objecting to the use of cordial stimulant articles in the advanced stage; after the action or acute febrile symptoms are removed, a very great error practised in the cure of the sick, seems to have been the use of cordial stimulant remedies, in the beginning of febrile phlegmasial diseases, as the history of the severe violent diseases of our country amply shows. (See appendix A.)

When fevers of this character in the first stage are treated with remedies best calculated to remove a compound inflammatory condition, and regulate the action of the blood vessels and the system, the disease may generally be interrupted, and an intermission obtained in about five to seven days; there will seldom be a case which runs on to or beyond nine days; then very slight or no typhoid symptoms appear. Such has been the result of our observation for many years.

Several years ago, Dr. Maygel delivered an address before the New York State Medical Society on the typhus fever of this country, in which it was argued that those fevers were in the first stage of a compound inflammatory nature, and that the advisable and proper remedies at first, were those best calculated to relieve that condition of the system. In Armstrong's treatise on typhus, a similar doctrine is advocated, and a recommendation of a similar treatment.

When the system is laboring under a severe attack of such a disease, by giving freely spicy stimulating or opiate articles, in the first or early stage, tends to overload or depress it still more, or increase the phlegmasial congestive condition; and the more violent the action or depression is at first—if not restrained or relieved or aggravated by remedies, the sooner it runs its course, and the disease changes its type to a typhoid or gangrenous state.

In attempting to treat this kind of disease, disposed to become typhoid, with Homœpathic remedies, which have been pretty well proved to be preferable to those generally used by Allopathic practitioners, the general maxims above detailed had better be borne in mind. The remedies to be selected for the first stage should be those best adapted to cure compound inflammatory or congestive states of disease; at first, use Acon. This should be steadily continued until the chills are over. If there should be nausea or vomiting, it wtll be advisable to give some globules of a high attenuation of Ipec. or Anti. either before the Acon. or in alternation with it, and to continue this course until the urgent symptoms are allayed. If there is severe headache and a red face, give Bell. or Iris. Versic. Or should there take place crampy symptoms, give Nux V. alone, or in alternation with Acon. If there exist marked symptoms of phlegmasial action, use the remedy best adapted to relieve and subdue this state of disease.

If the fever continues high, it will be advisable to continue the Acon. alone, or in alternation with other remedies, which may be indicated. It will be important to procure free evacuations from the bowels, by the use of some of the medicine named under Constipation, or if these do not succeed, a very useful and efficient one may be found in the podophyllin.

It appears some Homœopathic practitioners as we are well informed, suffer cases of disease of this kind to pass along five, six, or more days, without procuring an evacuation from the bowels; this is a very unsafe and injudicious course to pursue. In remittent fevers, and particularly those inclined to become typhoid, there is an accumulation of material in the alimentary canal which ought to be evacuated, and this effect aids much in producing a favorable termination of the case.

The mode recommended by Hamilton of using agents to act on the bowels, is one of the best means in Allopathic practice to cure this kind of disease; and it is doubtful, whether such agents would loose all their efficacy combined with Homœopathic remedies.

When by the course above detailed, the active state of fever and the compound inflammatory symptoms are removed early, much of the subsequent difficulty will be obviated.

If the disease with fever continues, use Bryo. Cham. Puls. or Tart. Anti.

If there is a dullness of the head or stupor, give Cocc. Hyosc. or Opi.

If there is uneasiness or irregularity of the bowels, use Merc. or Cham. or Nux V.

Should there be colic pains, give Colocy. Ignat. or Nux V.

If there is difficulty or irregularity in the uriary organs or functions, use Canth. Uva. Urs. or Petrol.

If there come on cramps of the bowels, or tenesmus, give Ignat. Nux V. or Sulp.

Should the skin become cold or a watery diarrhœa set in, then use Veratrum. or Arsen.

If prostration or typhoid symptoms occur, give Carb. Veg. Silec. or Ars.

For the debility which succeeds the fever, use China. Quinine, Cham. Wine, &c.

If delirium or coma comes on, examine the articles under these heads for a suitable remedy. Should there be a disposition to an affection of the brain, give Acon. Cocc. Bell. or Lach. Stramo. Phos. or Cupr. If there is a pressure on the lungs, with distress of the chest and heavy respiration, give Bryo. Ammo. C. Rus. T. Nux V. Phos. or Ars. or Verat. Should there be distress, pressure, and derangement of the stomach, use Puls. Ignat. Nux V. or Bryo. or Chin. If the case shows a disposition to gangrene, give Merc. Carb. V. or Ars. Chin. Canth. Sulp. ac. Nux V. or Mosch. and some good yeast, Porter, or Wine. (See appendix B.)

Some one hundred and eighty cases of fever, which assumed the typhoid form, are reported to have been cured by Hahnemann, by Bryona. and Rus. Tox. given alternately.

TYPHUS ABDOMINALIS.

———Typhus abdominalis. The remedies useful in this disease, are such as are recommended above. When the diseased action locates on the stomach and bowels, as the term implies, the remedies should be directed to this part. In the first stage, use Bryo. Cham. or Nux V. it will be important to procure evacutions from the bowels.

In the advanced stage, when there is low fever and nervous derangement, use Ars. Mur. ac. or Carb. V. Canth. Rus. T. Phos. ac. or Mosch. (See nervous fever.)

TYPHUS CEREBRALIS.

——— Typhus Cerebralis. Acon. Bryo. Cocc. Rus. T.; the other remedies are the same as those for typhus generally.

YELLOW OR TYPHUS ICTEOROIDES.

Yellow or Typhus Icteoroides. In the first stage, give Acon. Arnic. Bell. Bryo. Canth. or Ipe. If the disease advances, and the symptoms are severe, the remedies most approved are Crotal. Lach. Merc. Nux V. Rus. R. Rus. T. Verat. or Guaco. or Puls. China. or Ars.

FISTULA.

Fistula is an ulcer of a protracted kind. They often form deep holes or cavities in the adjacent parts, or they run along under the skin; these are called Sinuses. Sometimes the sides of these cavities become covered or lined with a hard callous substance; then they are termed Callous or Fistulus Ulcers, meaning a pipe; from their likeness to a tube or pipe, they have attained this name.

By the use of Homœopathic remedies, internally used, this disease is said frequently to be cured. The remedies proper are Calca. Caust. Coni. Lyc. Mur. ac. Nitr. ac. Phytol. Silec. or Sulp.

——— In Ano. This disease is produced by an abscess forming at the extreme lower end of the bowel on the outside of it and directly above the anus. The matter works its way out and discharges by the outer side of the anus and near to it; though in some cases the opening is made through the bowel (gut) and the matter is discharged into the rectum, and so passes off in the usual way with the excrements. The latter mentioned opening may be one, two, or three inches up from the sphincter ani. When the abscess breaks into the bowel, it is called an incomplete fistula; when the opening forms by the side of the anus, it is termed a complete sinus or fistula in ano.

This disease appears to have improperly obtained the name of Fistula in Ano, when it is generally only a sinus; but in progress of time fistulous or callous edges may form in it, and then the term pipe or fistula would be proper enough. This disease is often connected with prolapsus ani, or slipping down of the bowel or some variety of PILES. The internal remedies proper for its cure are Calc. C. Caust. Carbo. Ani., and some one of those above mentioned remedies. Also, local treatment for the ulceration and diseased state of the parts will be requisite. This, however, we leave to the judgment of the medical attendant.

Cases of Fistula in Ano are reported to have been cured by the use of Homœopathic treatment. We have known caustic and sulphur used—a dose of each given in a day, and continued several months, with occasionally Nux V., succeed in curing a fistula, attended with prolapsus ani and bloody purulent discharge.

There are cases of Fistula, however, which cannot be cured by any means short of a surgical operation for this disease, and this course, in many cases, is entirely safe, and the shortest and surest to pursue.

It has fallen to our lot in a number of cases to perform this operation. We have adopted a mode of doing it considerably different in some respects from that described by surgical writers or pursued by practitioners. It appears to be of importance enough to render a description of it worthy of a place here.

Instead of using a probe pointed bistory, take a long, slender sharp-pointed one, and guard the point with a small piece of beeswax as large as a pea. Introduce this instrument into the sinus or fistula; pass the point up to the upper end of the sinus; if the fistula is on the right side of the rectum, the left hand should be used; if on the left side of the rectum, use the right hand. The index finger of the other hand should be guarded with a smooth pine splint, about half an inch wide, a little hollowed on the side next to the finger, and rounded on the opposite side. This splint should extend from the point of the finger into the hand, so as to keep it steady; the finger, thus guarded, introduce into the anus, carry it up as far as the sinus extends and opposite to the point of the bistory; then press the point of the instrument forward toward the splint, and it cuts through the wax, and the rectum and the point settles into the guard; then draw both hands together out and away, keeping the point of the instrument pressed into the splint. The parts are now smoothly and freely divided all the way out, and the sinus fully laid open. Then stuff the cavity with lint, and treat the patient in the usual way.

A number of cases of Fistula in Ano have been operated on in this manner, which has uniformly been successful, and a radical cure has been the result.

FLATULENCE.

Flatulence.—For this affection, which is well known, give Cham. Carbo. Veg. Kali. Iod. Kali. Bic. Nux V. Phos. Silec. or Verat.

FROZEN FEET.

See Asphyxia, Frost Affection, Chillblains.

FUNGUS.

Fungus.—An unnatural growth of spongy flesh or granulations, which form in ulcers, called *proud flesh.* The internal remedies most useful for it are Graph. Iodi. Petrol. Sep. or Tart. Anti. or Sulp.

This affection will also be benefitted by a local application of gentle astringents or exciting or caustic remedies, though severe caustic remedies are often injurious.

——— Hæmatoides.—A species of fungus excrescence. The remedies for it are Phos. Silec. Staphy. and the preceding articles.

GANGLION.

Ganglion.—This is a small hard tumor, unattended with pain, seated on a tendon. They are somewhat movable, and contain a fluid resembling the white of an egg, which is enclosed in a sac; the growth is slow; they seldom become larger than a nutmeg; the limb generally is weaker than the other. If they ulcerate, a painful and foul ulcer is produced. (These are popularly called *Weeping Sinews.*) The remedies for them are Ammo. C. Arnic. Rus. T. Silec. or Zinc. Compression to the part may be used with very good effect.

GANGRENE OR MORTIFICATION.

Gangrene or Mortification.—In the first stage of mortification, it is termed Gangrene. This disease takes place under a variety of conditions of the body; it affects a part locally, or becomes the effect of a general disordered state of the system. The treatment will depend somewhat on the nature of the disease with which it may be united.

The remedies generally most useful are Ammo. C. Ars. Bell. Chin. Ephorbi. Iodi. Kreoso. Silec. or Sec. C. In some stages, wine or porter may be proper. But when gangrene is the effect of acute inflammation from local or mechanical injury, it is better to be cautious in using wine or alcoholic stimulants. Serious injury may result from a free use of these remedies. Cases are sometimes rendered more fatal by a free use of those remedies.

GASTRALGIA.

Gastralgia.—This is a painful affection of the stomach. The remedies for it are Ars. Bell. Baryt. M. Bismuth. Carb. V. Colocy. Ignat. Iodi. Lach. Lobel. Merc. Nux V. Sabad. Silec. or Verat.—[See Stomach.

GASTRITIS.

See Inflammation of the Stomach.

GASTROSES.

See Dyspepsia.

GENITALS.

Genitals.—These organs are subject to a large variety of diseases. Some of the prominent ones affecting the male organs, will be treated of under this head. The affections of the female organs are considered in the section for diseases of Women; the diseases of the Bladder are placed under that head; that of Gonorrhœa under that head, &c.

——— cold and swelled situation. The remedies are Argent. Agnu. C. Baryt. Cann. S. Natr. C. or Sulp.

——— epididymis swelled or enlarged.—Sulp. Thuy. or Zinc.

——— impotence. This is a loss of the virile

powers of erection.—The remedies for it are Anacard. Ignat. Iodi. Merc. Nicc. Nitr. ac. Nux V. Petrol. Phos. Rus. T. Silec. or Sulp.

ONANISM.

Onanism.—This is one of the causes of impotence, the effect of a depraved, libidinous mind, and a deranged state of the body, and of those organs in particular.

——— Onanism is derived from the cognomen of a man named Onan, Genesis, ch. xxxviii. ver. 9: as the term is used, it is incorrect. Onan's crime was not self-pollution—see the verse quoted. A great many persons of both sexes are not aware that a practice does prevail to a considerable extent, by means of which, friction made on the genital organs, a pleasureable sensation is experienced, somewhat similar to that produced by sexual connection; which act, when done *per se*, or by one's self, is termed self pollution or Onanism. The practice is often followed by a train of disease or debility, such as nervous affections, impaired state of the mind, loss of memory, dementia, weak back, emaciation, a loss of the use and the powers of the sexual organs; this latter state is called Impotence. We have witnessed some serious cases of this kind.

To show the correctness of our statements, we

make the following abstract from among a variety of cases.

A gentleman from the south, aged 34, unmarried, came under our observation in 1845. He had for a long time practised Onanism, (as termed.) Although intelligent, and had held a prominent office in the Texan army, he was not aware of the injurious effect of the practice. At last, he experienced the evils, by his health giving way, he was entirely impotent, the testicles were diminished in size, soft and flabby, had dyspepsia badly, was very costive, pain through the chest, severe pain in the back and hips, intense headache and vertigo, sight impaired and flickering, was languid and weak, mind wandering and indifferent, retiring, and avoided female company, depressed in spirits, skin cold and torpid involuntary nocturnal emissions.

By continuing under our care, in the persevering use of Homœopathic remedies, about eight months, he entirely recovered.

The remedies which are recommended and most useful to cure the propensity to such a practice, are Cod liver oil, Iodine, and the medicine mentioned above for impotence. Also, advice and moral restraint ought to be impressed upon the mind, so as to induce the person to abstain from and abandon so injurious a practice.

——— Itching of. Arnic. Anacard. Auru. Ignat. Iodi. Merc. Nicc. Natr. C. Nux V. Petrol.

Phos. ac. Puls. Rus. Tox. Selec. Stann. Staph. or Sulp.

——— Lasciviousness. Canth. Baryt. M. Iodi. Stramo.

——— Pain or burning in. Podoph. P. Raph. R. Rhodod. Spong. Stann. Staph. Sulp. Thuy. Verat. or Zinc.

——— Penis blue. Arg. Nit. Agnu. C. Bromi. Sulp.

——— Cordee. Give Canth. Cann. I. Silec. Tereb. or Bromi.

——— Penis emissions, involuntary. Use Calc. Canth. Caust. Merc. Mosch. Nux M. Petrol. Phos. Plumb. Acet. Ran. Bulb. Rus. Tox. Sabad. Selen. Sepi. Stann. Staph. or Sulp.

——— Penis-erections frequent. Canth. Baryt. M. Spig. Rhodod. Tarax. or Thuy. are the proper remedies.

——— do. eruptions on. Silec. &c.

——— do. excrescences or condolymata on. Sabi. Thuy. (to be used internally and externally.)

——— do. fig warts on. Sabi. Staph. or Thuy.

——— do. glans itching or swelled. Colocy. Sarss. Rhodod. Sep. Spig. Spong. Stramo. Sulp. Sulp. ac. or Thuy.

——— do. inflamed and pain on tip of the glans. Give Acon. Cann. S. Colocy. Coni. Lyc. Merc. Mangan. Nitr. ac. Nux V. Sep. or Zinc.

Penis, erections, jerking sensation in. Stann. Zinc.

——— do. pain and beating in. Sabad. Sabi. Spong. or Thuy.

PHIMOSIS.

——— PHIMOSIS. This is a contraction of the Prepuse or fore-skin, so that it cannot be drawn back over the glands penis, the part is generally inflamed and swelled. The treatment should be adapted to the nature of the affection. If it is produced by friction or chafing, use Anica. internally, and apply it externally. If there is much pain and swelling, fomentation may be very useful; the other proper remedies are, Calend. Rus. T. or Puls.

If the disease is owing to Gonorrhœa, the remedies for that will be proper.

If to Syphilis, use Merc. Nitr. acid, or Thuy. with same local treatment as above stated.

If Pus forms under the fore-skin, and is confined there, it may be necessary to divide the skin to let it out, it is then better to apply dressings. Other useful remedies are Cann. S. Nux V. or Sulp.

PARAPHIMOSIS.

PARAPHIMOSIS. When the fore-skin is drawn back of the glands penis, and retained there, it is known by this term. The remedies for it are warm water or fomentation to the part; aided by giving Acon. Merc. and remedies suitable to those for Phimosis. If the stricture is considerable, and does not give way, it should be divided. If gangrene of the part is threatened, give Ars. or Sec. C.

——— Penis, itching and sore. Colocy. Natr. C. Puls. Silec. Spong. Sulp. ac. or Verat.

——— do. Priapism. Use Canth. Caps. Colocy. Graph. Kali. C. Lach. Lact. Viro. Lyc. Merc. Muri. ac. Natr. M. Nux V. Nitr. ac. Phos. Seneg. Sepi. Spong. Thuy. or Zinc. See Cordee.

——— do. Swelled. Plumb. Acet. Rus. Rad. Spong. Sulp. or Thuy.

——— do. Tittillation of glans. Phot. Feet. Sabad. Spong. Sulp. Tarax. Tart. Anti. Thuy. or Zinc.

——— do. Twitching in. Natr. M. Ol. Anima. Phos.

——— Pubes, hair falling off. Calc. Zinc.

——— Scrotum swelled. Rhodod. Rus. Rad. Rus. Tox. Samb. Silec. Spong. Sulp. or Thuy.

——— do. Itching and twinging in. Nicc. Nux V. Petrol. Plumb. Puls. Rhodod. Selen. Silec. Spig. Spong. Staph. or Sulp.

——— Spermatic cord pained. Coni. or Zinc.

——— do. do. enlarged. Coni. Phos. ac.

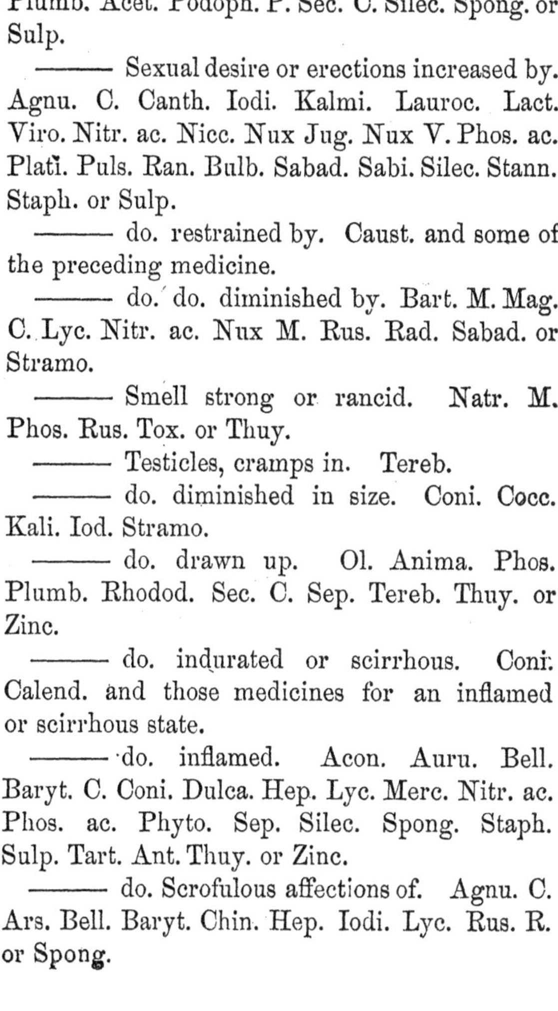

Plumb. Acet. Podoph. P. Sec. C. Silec. Spong. or Sulp.

——— Sexual desire or erections increased by. Agnu. C. Canth. Iodi. Kalmi. Lauroc. Lact. Viro. Nitr. ac. Nicc. Nux Jug. Nux V. Phos. ac. Plati. Puls. Ran. Bulb. Sabad. Sabi. Silec. Stann. Staph. or Sulp.

——— do. restrained by. Caust. and some of the preceding medicine.

——— do. do. diminished by. Bart. M. Mag. C. Lyc. Nitr. ac. Nux M. Rus. Rad. Sabad. or Stramo.

——— Smell strong or rancid. Natr. M. Phos. Rus. Tox. or Thuy.

——— Testicles, cramps in. Tereb.

——— do. diminished in size. Coni. Cocc. Kali. Iod. Stramo.

——— do. drawn up. Ol. Anima. Phos. Plumb. Rhodod. Sec. C. Sep. Tereb. Thuy. or Zinc.

——— do. indurated or scirrhous. Coni. Calend. and those medicines for an inflamed or scirrhous state.

——— do. inflamed. Acon. Auru. Bell. Baryt. C. Coni. Dulca. Hep. Lyc. Merc. Nitr. ac. Phos. ac. Phyto. Sep. Silec. Spong. Staph. Sulp. Tart. Ant. Thuy. or Zinc.

——— do. Scrofulous affections of. Agnu. C. Ars. Bell. Baryt. Chin. Hep. Iodi. Lyc. Rus. R. or Spong.

——— do. Syphilitic affection. Aura. Merc. Nitr. ac.—[See Syphilis.

——— do. Ulcers on. Coni. Thuy. or Sulp.

——— do. Cancerous. Thuy. and those medicines for scirrhous.

——— Urethra, burning and itching in. Arg. N. Auru. Baryt. Bell. Cann. S. Camp. Colocy. [See Bladder, this article.

——— do. Bleeding from. Arnic. Auru. Bell. Coni.—[See Bladder.

——— do. Smarting or itching. Canth. Colocy. Lyc. Merc. Mosch. Nux V. Phos. ac. Prun. Sp. Sabad. Silec. Sulp. ac. Thuy. or Zinc.

——— do. Stricture in. Coni. Petrol. Silec. Sulp. or Thuy.

GLANDS.

Glands.—That part of the body termed the Glandular System is subject to diseases somewhat peculiar to these organs. The remedies for the various forms of diseased glands will now be detailed.

——— Cervicle or axilla, diseased, inflamed, or indurated, the remedies are Coni. Iodi. Lyc. Lach. Natr. M. Nitr. ac. Rus. Tox. Sabad. Sep. Silec. Spong. Staph. or Sulp.

——— enlarged. Give Bovista. Coni. Dulcam. Iodi. Rus. Rad. Sep. Spong. or Thuy.

——— Indurated. Use Ammo. C. Ars. Auru.

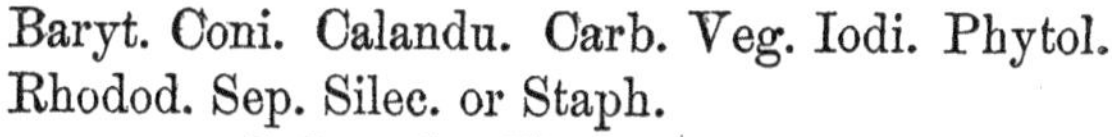

Baryt. Coni. Calandu. Carb. Veg. Iodi. Phytol. Rhodod. Sep. Silec. or Staph.

——— Inflamed. The general remedies are Acon. Arnic. Baryt. Brimi. Hep. Iodi. Lach. Merc. Nitr. ac. Petrol. Rus. Rad. Rus. Tox. Sep. Spong. Staph. or Sulp. ac.

——— Inguinal, inflamed, and enlarged. Give Hep. Iodi. Kalmi. Lat. Lach. Merc. Natr. C. Nitr. ac. Rus. Tox. Sep. Silec. Spong. Staph. Stron. Thuy. or Terb.

——— Lymphatics diseased. Ars. Coni. Iodi. Sep. Silec. Stramo. or Sulp.

——— Prostate, enlarged. Auru. Coni. Kali. Iod. Puls. Spong. Thuy. or Uva. Urs.

——— Scirrhous. Give Ars. Auru.. Bovist. Bryo. Coni. Calind. Carb. Anima. Dulca. Hep. Merc. Nux V. Phos. ac. Plumb. Acet. Rhodod. Sep. Silec. Staph. or Thuy. [See Cancer.

——— Sublingual, diseased. Plumb. Acet. Rus. Tox. Sabad. or Staph.

——— Tonsils enlarged. Bell. Baryt. Calca. Ignat. Iodi. Merc. Mosch. Phos. or Silec. [See Angina, Tonsilitis.

GOITRE.

Goitre.—This disease is similar to Bronchocele, which see.

GONORRHŒA.

GONORRHŒA.—This disease is generally communicated by impure sexual intercourse. It is attended with a discharge from the urethra of males and the vagina of females, of a muco-purulent matter. At first, the parts are affected with smarting and pain of the parts, particularly so on passing the urine.

The proper remedies for this disease in the first stage are those adapted to the cure of inflammation of those parts; such as Acon. Cann. S. Kali. Nitr. Avoid the use of exciting stimulating articles; the diet should be low and mild. It is better for the patient to keep quiet and cool. This course, followed up early, in a few days will frequently succeed in checking or curing the case.

If the symptoms are moderated, or the disease continues, the following medicines will be proper and are recommended: Bals.Cop. Can. Ind. Canth. Lact. Viro. Merc. Natr. C. Puls. Petrol. Petroselinum Sepi. Tussilago Petasites. This last is highly recommended in this disease. It frequently requires great care in selecting and using the remedies.

When there is smarting in passing the urine, use Bals. Cop. or Petroselinum, one or two drops of the first or second dilution.

If the gonorrhœa continues with phimosis, use Merc. and Nux in alternation.

When there is a muco-purulent discharge, Hep. Silec. or Merc.

When the inflammation is relieved, and the discharge is serous, with some pain, use Sulp.

If there is but little pain or swelling, and the running continues, give Merc. Sulp. or Silec; a few globules two or three times a day.

In severe or protracted cases, some of the other named medicines will be useful and worthy a trial.

GLEET.

Gleet.—This is a secondary or chronic stage of the preceding disease. It is often produced by, or is the result of improper or injudicious use of remedies for the first stage of gonorrhœa. The acrid and irritating remedies and injections of this sort, used at first, may check the running, but are frequently followed by a troublesome gleet. It is attended with a discharge of whitish mucous matter. This generally is not very painful, though sometimes it is so, and becomes very tedious and troublesome. The remedies are Ammo. M. Canth. Clemat. Cubeb. Cann. Ind. Kreoso. Merc. Nitr. ac. Nux V. Petrol. Sepi. Silec. Sulp. or Thuy.

This affection is often very obstinate, particularly in females, where it is generally blended with leucorrhœa (whites.) In the treatment, it will be required to change the remedies, and try to adapt them to the peculiar symptoms.

GUM BILES.

Gum Biles.—The remedies for this affection are Ammo. C. Bell. Kreoso. Nux V. Phos. or Sulp. [See Jaws.

GOUT—AITHRITIS.

Gout—Aithritis.—This disease affects the joints very similar to rheumatism. It is considered to be somewhat of a hereditary nature, though not particularly so, for it takes place in persons who have not been contaminated by any hereditary taint. It often attacks severely, continues a length of time, gets relieved by medical treatment, or by an effort of nature, it passes off, and the patient may be well. Some persons are liable to have periodical attacks; in others it takes on a chronic form, and requires a long and careful course of treatment to cure it. The remedies which have proved most useful in it are Acon. Arnic. Ars. Auru. Bell. Bryo. Benzo. ac. Colocy. Caust. Colchi. Iodi. Nux V. Puls. Phos. Sulp. Tart. Anti. or Chloride of Lime: the latter is said to be very efficacious.

In robust, full habits, give Acon. or Bryo.

If the pains shift from one part to another, or are worse at evening, give Puls.

If there are dyspeptic symptoms, use Nux V. or Puls.

If the pain is increased by the part being exposed to the air, give Ars.

If the pain is severe at night, the countenance pale and haggard, give Ferr. or Rus. T. or Chin.

When the pains increase towards morning, and there are cramps or paralytic symptoms, give Nux V.

If the pain is increased by motion, Bryo. is proper.

If the joints are swelled and painful, give Sanguinaria.

——— CHRONIC CASES.—There are a great number of remedies recommended for this stage. Those enumerated at the head of this article are the leading ones. Also, compare this with rheumatism, for which the remedies are very similar.

HÆMORRHAGE.

Hæmorrhage.—This term means a discharge of blood from some part of the body. It may be the product of a full plethoric habit—then it is termed active or acute Hæmorrhage—or it may be connected with a state of weakness and debility; this is called passive bleeding. The remedies most useful for the first or acute variety are Acon. Bell. Ipe. Kali. Iod. Millefo. Nux V. Nitr. ac. Scill. Tart. Anti. or Hamamelis. Mill. and Hamali may be esteemed the most efficacious.

The remedies for the passive or protracted state of bleeding are Ars. Chin. Coni. Kreoso. Nitr. ac. Petrol. Plati. Sabi. Sec. C. Scill. or Cupr. or Terebinth.

The states of the excitement of the system vary and run into each other, so that it is difficult to draw a line of distinction between the active and passive conditions. The remedy, however, may in a measure be learned by observation and some experience, and by examining the Pathoganesis of the drugs.

——— From the Anus, *Hæmorrhoids.* Give Ignat. Lobeli. Lyc. Millefo. Nux V. Sec. C. or Sulp. [See Hæmorrhoids.

——— From the Lungs, *Hæmoptesis.* The lungs are very liable to have blood discharged from them. When it does not often occur, and then only in small quantities, it gives but little inconvenience; but when the bleeding is free or returns often, it becomes a serious matter, and requires attention.

The remedies most beneficial for it—if it is a case of active bleeding—are Acon. Bell. Ipe. Millefo. or Hamamelis and other medicines mentioned above for the active condition of this affection.

If it is attended with weakness, or if the case becomes protracted, the following remedies will be proper: Ars. Chin. Coni. Kreoso. Nitr. ac. Plati. Sabi. Cupr., &c.

If it occurs in females who have a suppression of the catamenia, use Puls. or Sepi. or Hyosc. or Hamamelis.

If the attack is caused by mechanical injury, Arnic.

If there is crampy symptoms or an irritable temper, Nux V.

Those who are liable to attacks of this kind of a disease may do much towards preventing them by daily taking a dose of the 2d or 3d attenuations of Calca. C. or the second or third trituration of Ferr.

——— From the Nose, (*Epistaxis.*) The remedies for this disease are the same as those above mentioned, and the same indications should be observed respecting the active and passive states of the system.

If the hæmorrhage seems to be from congestion of the head, Acon. Bell. Coni. or Cham. or Alum or Rus. T. or Millefo. or Hamam.

In females who have a diminished catamenia or a suppression of it, Puls. or Sepi. or Sabi.

In weakened patients, Chin. Ferr. or Nitr. ac.

If from worms, Merc. or Cina.

If those remedies named do not answer, it will be advisable to try some of the others named.

——— From the stomach, (*Hematemesis.*) Blood discharged from the stomach is generally by vomiting or eructations; it is supposed to come off from the veins instead of the arteries.

If there is a full habit, attended with fever, use Acon. or Ipe.

If there is venous fullness at the stomach, torpid state of the bowels, or hæmorrhoids, Nux V.

If there is moderate pain and bringing up small quantities of blood, Ars.

If it occurs in females when there is suppression of the cataminia, Puls. or Sabi.

When there has been considerable blood thrown up and debility ensues, Carbo. V. or Chin. or Ferr.

Caution should be observed about the diet; it should be light, of a mild kind, and easy of digestion.

HÆMORRHOIDS. (PILES.)

HÆMORRHOIDS.—This disease affects the anus in a painful and troublesome manner; sometimes little lumps or tumors form on the margin of the anus, or just within it. In other cases, there are discharges of blood from the vessels of this part, called hæmorrhoidal bleeding; and another form in which this part is affected is by a thickening or enlargement of the inner surface of the rectum, so that a portion of it protrudes, forming prolapsus ani. This protrusion more particularly takes place when there is an evacuation from the bowels, and then it gives great pain; sometimes it is very difficult to return it.

For this disease the following medicines are the most useful. To effect a cure or permanent relief they should be used a long time, and in this manner cases may generally be cured or relieved. Acon. Aloe. Ambr. Ars. Calca. C. Carb. Ani. Carb. Veg. Chin. Colocy. Graph. Ignat. Iodi. Lach. Merc. Muri. ac. Nux V. Seneg. Stramo. Sulp. or Thuy.

Experience shows that external applications are not to be relied upon for a permanent relief of this or those diseases, though considerable may be done by them to palliate the symptoms. For this purpose some astringent, soothing applications are useful. As some preparations of Lead

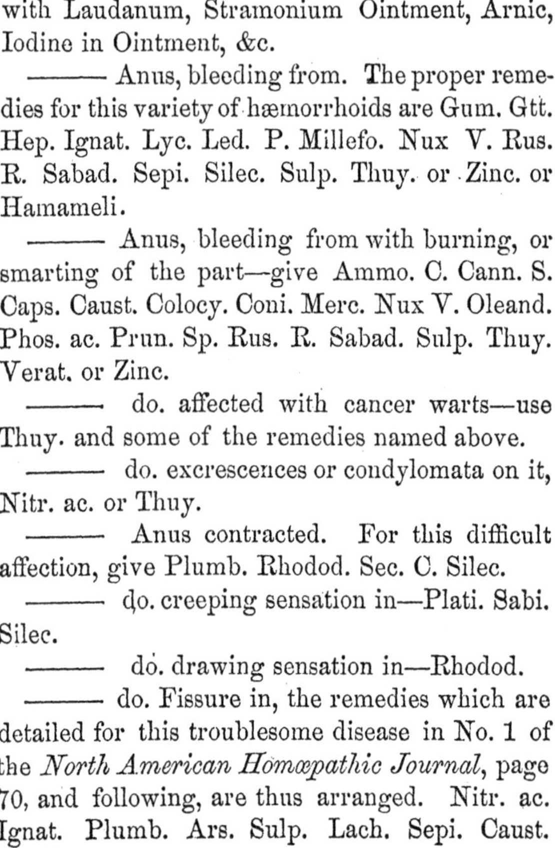

with Laudanum, Stramonium Ointment, Arnic, Iodine in Ointment, &c.

——— Anus, bleeding from. The proper remedies for this variety of hæmorrhoids are Gum. Gtt. Hep. Ignat. Lyc. Led. P. Millefo. Nux V. Rus. R. Sabad. Sepi. Silec. Sulp. Thuy. or Zinc. or Hamameli.

——— Anus, bleeding from with burning, or smarting of the part—give Ammo. C. Cann. S. Caps. Caust. Colocy. Coni. Merc. Nux V. Oleand. Phos. ac. Prun. Sp. Rus. R. Sabad. Sulp. Thuy. Verat. or Zinc.

——— do. affected with cancer warts—use Thuy. and some of the remedies named above.

——— do. excrescences or condylomata on it, Nitr. ac. or Thuy.

——— Anus contracted. For this difficult affection, give Plumb. Rhodod. Sec. C. Silec.

——— do. creeping sensation in—Plati. Sabi. Silec.

——— do. drawing sensation in—Rhodod.

——— do. Fissure in, the remedies which are detailed for this troublesome disease in No. 1 of the *North American Homœpathic Journal*, page 70, and following, are thus arranged. Nitr. ac. Ignat. Plumb. Ars. Sulp. Lach. Sepi. Caust. or Silec.

In 1850, we had a case of fissure and contracted anus in a lady. It was very painful in passing a stool, which was produced only by cathartic articles; the stricture was very rigid. She was extremely costive. On examination, the pain was so exquisite, and the anus so contracted, that the finger could not be introduced into the anus.

We put her upon the alternate use of Nux V. and Sulp.; about the second attenuation of each. She gradually improved so that in six months, she was perfectly cured, and continued so over two years; after that we did not hear from her.

——— Anus, herpes on—Lyc. Natr. M. Petrol. Sabad. Staphy. Sulp. Thuy. or Zinc.

——— Anus, itching in—Acon. Anacard. Arg. Borax. Baryt. Bromi. Caust. Coni. Colocy. Ignat. Iodi. Kali. Bic. Lyc. Mur. ac. Nitr. ac. Nux V. Ing. Petrol. Plati. Phos. Rus. T. Sabad. Silec. Sulp. Tereb. or Zinc.

——— do. Pain in—Nux V. Spong. Scill. Sulp. Tabac. Thuy. or Verat.

——— do. paralyzed—Nux V. Nit. ac. Sabi. Silec.

Hæmorrhoids, anus prolapsus. This troublesome and painful disease is connected with what is termed piles; it is a passing down, or slipping out of the inner lining or diseased portion of the lower part of the rectum, more so when there takes place an evacuation from the bowels. The proper remedies to relieve or cure it are, Aloe. Calc. Carb. V. Caust. Gum. Gtt. Hyosc. Ignat. Muri. ac. Nux V. Phos. Plumb. ac. Podophy. Rus. T. Silec. Staphy. or Sulp.

There are cases in which the quantity of the morbid enlargement comes out in a considerable mass, sometimes as large as a black walnut, a hen's egg, or larger; they become inflamed and are very painful, if this condition continues long and the diseased portion cannot be returned into its place, gangrene may take place; when the excrescence is large and troublesome, and does not yield, or the part is frequently slipping down, it may be advisable to pass a ligature around it at the base, so as to remove it. This generally relieves the patient from all further difficulty by a cure of the disease. There is no particular risk in removing the morbid part in this manner. Such has been the result of our experience in several cases operated on in this way. We refer to two patients among many others who had been affected very painfully and annoyed a long time; there were two clusters of this spongy diseased mass from each removed by a ligature applied around their base; the mass soon digested off. This happened twenty years ago: they have had no inconvenience from this disease since, and are now enjoying good health.

——— do. tumors or varicess on—Lach. Phos. Phos. ac. Plumb. Rata. Sabi. Sep. Silec. or Thuy.

——— do. Ulcer on—Sarss. Sulp.

——— do. Warts, Fig. Thuy.

HAIR.

Hair falling out. The remedies to prevent this are, Ammo. C. Arg. Calc. Carb. Veg. Hep. Hell. Ignat. Iodi. Kali. Iod. Merc. Natr. C. Nitr. ac. Phos. Petrol. Silec. Staph. or Sulp. (See Scalp.)

HEADACHE.

Headache and affections of the head. The general remedies are Acon. Arnic. Ammo. C. Ars. Auru. Agnu. C. Anacard. Bell. Bryo. Bromi. Camp. Caps. Canth. Carb. Ammo. Carb. V. Cocc. Colocy. Coni. Glionine. or Dulcam. Hep. Hell. Hyosc. Ignat. Iodi. Iris. Versic. Kreoso. Kalmi. L. Lauroc. Mosch. Morph. Nux V. Opi. Petrol. Phos. Puls. Rus. R. Rus. T. Ranan. Bulb. Sabad. Staphy. Sulp. Vinca. Min. Thuy. Verat. or Zinc. The remedies should be used in this order.

——— Beating or throbbing in the head, or hot sensation, give Canth. Colocy. Rus. R. Sang. Sepi. Spig. Spong. Sulp. Verat. or Vinc. Min.

——— Burning sensation in—Bell. or Valer.

——— Congestion in—Acon. Bell. Cocc. Hyosc. Millefo. Morph. Nitr. ac. Oleand. Opi. Petrol. Phos. Rus. R. Sabi. Sang. Silec. Stramo. or Tart. Anti.

——— Creeping or itching feeling in—Scill. Spig.

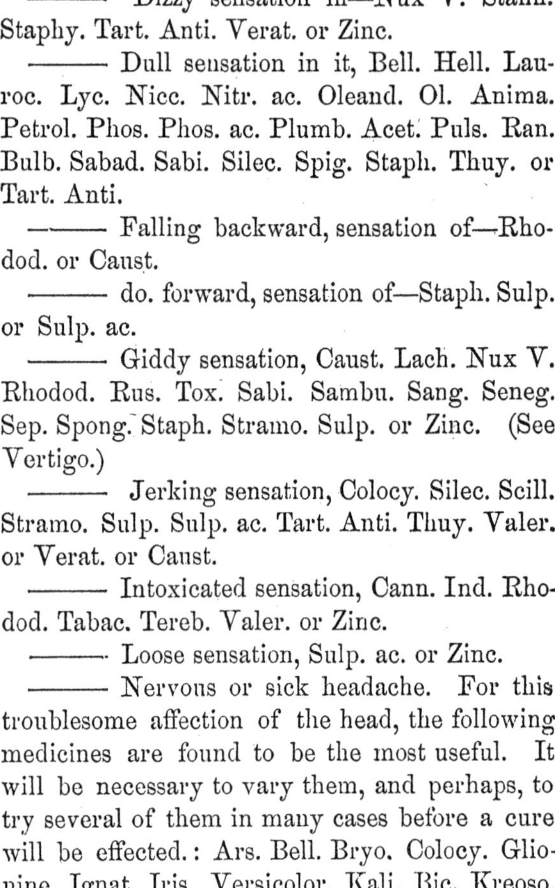

——— Dizzy sensation in—Nux V. Stann. Staphy. Tart. Anti. Verat. or Zinc.

——— Dull sensation in it, Bell. Hell. Lauroc. Lyc. Nicc. Nitr. ac. Oleand. Ol. Anima. Petrol. Phos. Phos. ac. Plumb. Acet. Puls. Ran. Bulb. Sabad. Sabi. Silec. Spig. Staph. Thuy. or Tart. Anti.

——— Falling backward, sensation of—Rhodod. or Caust.

——— do. forward, sensation of—Staph. Sulp. or Sulp. ac.

——— Giddy sensation, Caust. Lach. Nux V. Rhodod. Rus. Tox. Sabi. Sambu. Sang. Seneg. Sep. Spong. Staph. Stramo. Sulp. or Zinc. (See Vertigo.)

——— Jerking sensation, Colocy. Silec. Scill. Stramo. Sulp. Sulp. ac. Tart. Anti. Thuy. Valer. or Verat. or Caust.

——— Intoxicated sensation, Cann. Ind. Rhodod. Tabac. Tereb. Valer. or Zinc.

——— Loose sensation, Sulp. ac. or Zinc.

——— Nervous or sick headache. For this troublesome affection of the head, the following medicines are found to be the most useful. It will be necessary to vary them, and perhaps, to try several of them in many cases before a cure will be effected.: Ars. Bell. Bryo. Colocy. Glionine. Ignat. Iris. Versicolor. Kali. Bic. Kreoso. Kali. Iod. Lach. Mosch. Nux V. Puls. Petrol. Phos. Prun. Sp. Rus. T. Stron. Tabac. Sulp. ac.

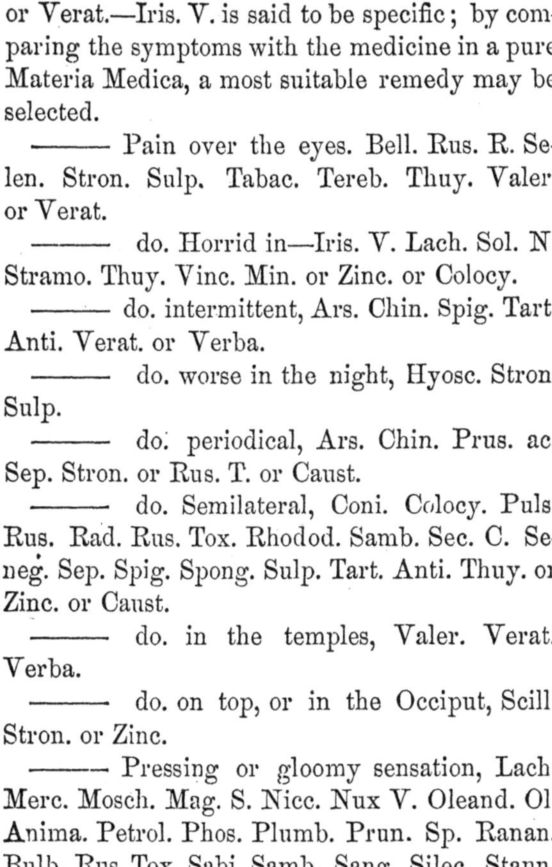

or Verat.—Iris. V. is said to be specific; by comparing the symptoms with the medicine in a pure Materia Medica, a most suitable remedy may be selected.

——— Pain over the eyes. Bell. Rus. R. Selen. Stron. Sulp. Tabac. Tereb. Thuy. Valer. or Verat.

——— do. Horrid in—Iris. V. Lach. Sol. N. Stramo. Thuy. Vinc. Min. or Zinc. or Colocy.

——— do. intermittent, Ars. Chin. Spig. Tart. Anti. Verat. or Verba.

——— do. worse in the night, Hyosc. Stron. Sulp.

——— do. periodical, Ars. Chin. Prus. ac. Sep. Stron. or Rus. T. or Caust.

——— do. Semilateral, Coni. Colocy. Puls. Rus. Rad. Rus. Tox. Rhodod. Samb. Sec. C. Seneg. Sep. Spig. Spong. Sulp. Tart. Anti. Thuy. or Zinc. or Caust.

——— do. in the temples, Valer. Verat. Verba.

——— do. on top, or in the Occiput, Scill. Stron. or Zinc.

——— Pressing or gloomy sensation, Lach. Merc. Mosch. Mag. S. Nicc. Nux V. Oleand. Ol. Anima. Petrol. Phos. Plumb. Prun. Sp. Ranan. Bulb. Rus. Tox. Sabi. Samb. Sang. Silec. Stann. Sulp. or Tart. Anti.

——— Pain pressing outward, Spig. Stann. Sulp. Tabac. Tarax. Thuy. or Zinc.

——— Shaking sensation, Sep. Silec. Spig. or Tart. Anti.

——— Staggering sensation, Rhodod. Sabad. Seneg. Silec. Stramo. Stron. Sulp. Thuy. or Verat.

——— Stitches in, give Caust. Natr. C. Natr. M. Nitr. ac. Oleand. Ol. Anima. Phos. Ran. Bulb. Rhodod. Rus. Tox. Rata. Sarss. Sep. Scill. Silec. Spig. Spong. Stann. Valer. or Chin.

——— Stupifying sensation, Bell. Ol. Anima. Opi. Rus. T. Sabad. Sepi. Spong. Staphy. Stramo. Sulp. ac. Tabac. Tart. A. Tereb. Thuy. or Verat.

——— Vertigo, Lach. Morph. Nitr. ac. Nux M. Nux V. Opi. Petrol. Phos. Plumb. ac. Prun. Sp. Puls. Ranan. Bulb. Sabad. Sabi. Sambu. Sang. Seneg. Sepi. Spong. Stann. Staphy. Sulp. Tarax. Tart. A. Tereb. or Zinc.

——— Violent pain in the back of the head, running to the neck, Kreoso.

——— If the head feels like bursting, burning and piercing, worse at night, give Merc. or Sabad.

——— If the pain is owing to masturbation or onanism, the sight impaired sees luminous objects, has watery eyes.—Agnu. C. Nux V.

——— If the pain is rending or jerking in the temples, Puls.

——— If the pain runs upward from the nape to the top of the head, Silec.

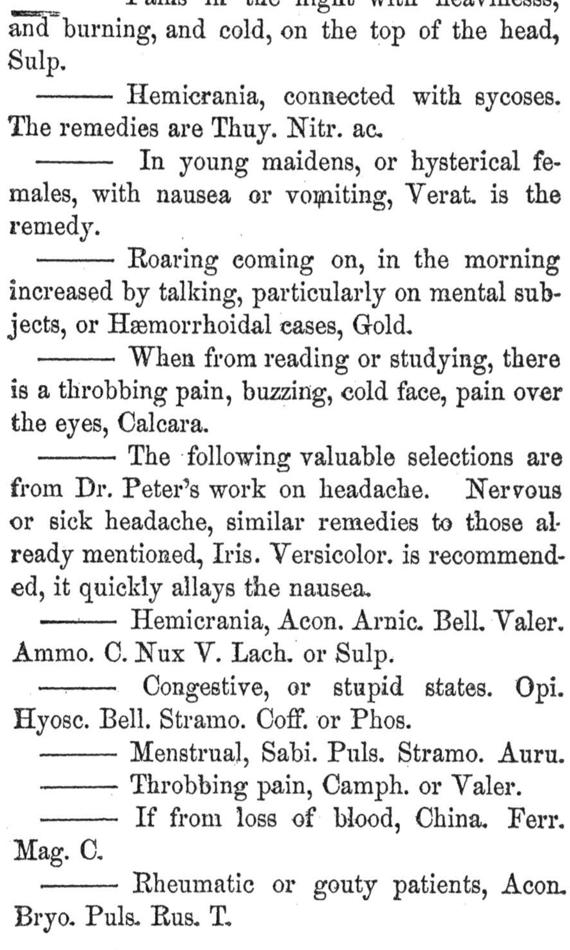

——— Pains in the night with heavinesss, and burning, and cold, on the top of the head, Sulp.

——— Hemicrania, connected with sycoses. The remedies are Thuy. Nitr. ac.

——— In young maidens, or hysterical females, with nausea or vomiting, Verat. is the remedy.

——— Roaring coming on, in the morning increased by talking, particularly on mental subjects, or Hæmorrhoidal cases, Gold.

——— When from reading or studying, there is a throbbing pain, buzzing, cold face, pain over the eyes, Calcara.

——— The following valuable selections are from Dr. Peter's work on headache. Nervous or sick headache, similar remedies to those already mentioned, Iris. Versicolor. is recommended, it quickly allays the nausea.

——— Hemicrania, Acon. Arnic. Bell. Valer. Ammo. C. Nux V. Lach. or Sulp.

——— Congestive, or stupid states. Opi. Hyosc. Bell. Stramo. Coff. or Phos.

——— Menstrual, Sabi. Puls. Stramo. Auru.

——— Throbbing pain, Camph. or Valer.

——— If from loss of blood, China. Ferr. Mag. C.

——— Rheumatic or gouty patients, Acon. Bryo. Puls. Rus. T.

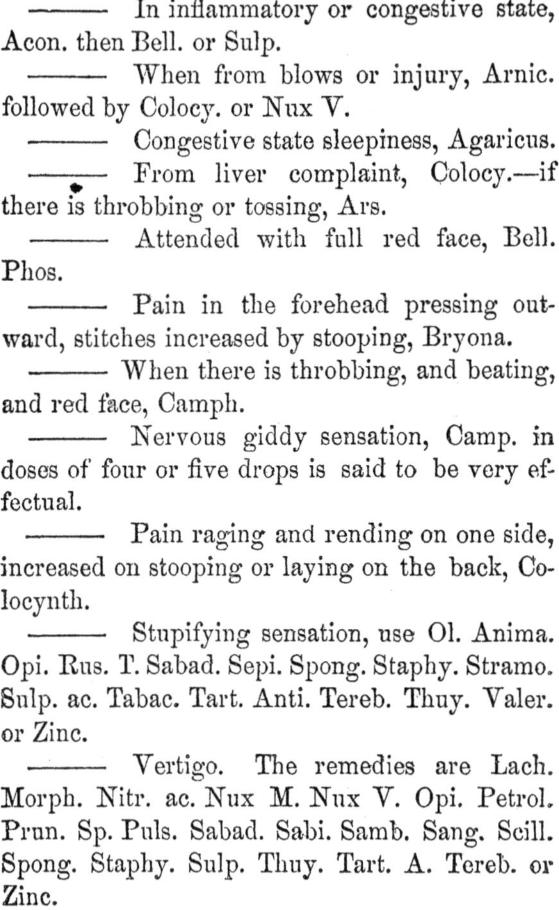

——— In inflammatory or congestive state, Acon. then Bell. or Sulp.

——— When from blows or injury, Arnic. followed by Colocy. or Nux V.

——— Congestive state sleepiness, Agaricus.

——— From liver complaint, Colocy.—if there is throbbing or tossing, Ars.

——— Attended with full red face, Bell. Phos.

——— Pain in the forehead pressing outward, stitches increased by stooping, Bryona.

——— When there is throbbing, and beating, and red face, Camph.

——— Nervous giddy sensation, Camp. in doses of four or five drops is said to be very effectual.

——— Pain raging and rending on one side, increased on stooping or laying on the back, Colocynth.

——— Stupifying sensation, use Ol. Anima. Opi. Rus. T. Sabad. Sepi. Spong. Staphy. Stramo. Sulp. ac. Tabac. Tart. Anti. Tereb. Thuy. Valer. or Zinc.

——— Vertigo. The remedies are Lach. Morph. Nitr. ac. Nux M. Nux V. Opi. Petrol. Prun. Sp. Puls. Sabad. Sabi. Samb. Sang. Scill. Spong. Staphy. Sulp. Thuy. Tart. A. Tereb. or Zinc.

HEART.

Heart. This organ may be considered the most important in the body; it is the active agent in its functions, and on this action the continuance of life immediately depends, while all other organs and functions of the body are at times more or less quiet and at apparent rest, the heart is always in active operation to propel the sanguineous fluid through the arteries, to every part of the body. When this organ ceases to act, the circulation of the blood stops, and the vital principle soon leaves the corporeal tenement.

In some conditions of disease an increased quantity of blood is forced upon the heart, or it accumulates in the lungs, so that its action is curbed or obstructed, and it is unable freely to discharge the quantity of fluid from it in the ordinary and necessary manner, when an increased energy or relief in some way is required to overcome the resistance. [See pages 15 and 16, and the article on Congestion.] As one instance of this kind, congestion of the lungs may be mentioned; in such cases the circulation is slow, the pulse is flaccid, and there is evidence of a diminished quantity of vital air in the system.

The supreme and controlling position of the *heart*, as being the first moving power of life, the steady faithful performer of its office, and its continual efforts to preserve and perpetuate life—would seem to be sufficient to shield it from reproaches frequently cast upon it, such as a depraved heart, an evil heart, a malignant heart, a wicked heart, and a heart continually inclined to evil and vice; it may be suggested whether *will* or *disposition*, would not be a better term. The *heart*, however, is subject to diseases, such as dropsy, inflammation,—the substance of it may be diseased by enlargement, forming organic affection, or as it is termed *hypertrophy*, in the cells and cavities where ossification sometimes takes place. Aneurism of the great artery where it arises from the heart may take place; we have witnessed a case of this kind where the aorta was distended to four times its natural size, yet, singular as it may seem, the patient lived in this state many months. From pressure of the tumor and pulsation against the clavicle, the clavicle was absorbed through it, at length a rupture of the vessel took place over the top of the clavicle, a copious hæmorrhage ensued, and life soon was extinct.

But the most common disease affecting the heart is an increased nervous sensibility, producing palpitations and irregular actions f various kinds.

——— Inflammation of the.—When this takes place, it is very difficult to distinguish it from similar diseases of the adjacent parts; there is fever, severe pain through the part, and a full quickened pulse. The remedy first is Acon. and cloths wet in cold water applied to the side. It would be proper to follow this with Ipe. or Bryo.

If there are crampy symptoms, use Nux V.

The general treatment would be similar to that for inflammation of the lungs or chest.

For organic affection and aneurism, Ars. Coni. and Nux V. or Lyc. would be the best medicine. See also Hyperthrophy.

The remedies for nervous irritability and palpitation, Acon. Arnic. Ambr. Angust. Ars. Auru. Bell. Caust. Coni. Digital. Hep. Lach. Nux V. Oleand. Opi. Phos. Puls. Rus. T. Silec. Spig. Staphy. Sulp. Verat. or Zinc.

——— Cramps in or about it.—Ambr. Kreoso. Lach. Morph. Opi. Oleand. Ol. Anisi. Phos. Rus. T. Sec. C. Thuy. or Zinc.

——— Double beat, or violent or irregular action, Natr. M. Opi. Oxalic. ac. Spig. or Stramo.

——— Dropsy of the. Acon. Arnic. Ars. Colchi. Spong. and the other remedies for heart diseases.

——— Hypertrophy or organic enlargement, Digital. Rus. T. or Ferr. Chin. Ignat. or Ars. Iodi. ox. ac. Phos. Spong. Spig. or Verat.

——— Nervous irritation of. Arg. N. Asa. F. Bismu. Cham. Coni. Lach. Lact. Viro. Lauroc. Nux V. Oleand. Phos. Puls. Plati. or Verat.

——— Palpitation of. Acon. Arnic. Angust.

Arg. N. Ars. Arnic. Bell. Carb. Ani. Calc. Chin. Colocy. Ignat. Ipe. Iodi. Kalmi. L. Kreoso. Lach. Lyc. Merc. Nitr. ac. Nux V. Oleand. Phos. Silec. Podophy. Puls. Rus. R. Sabad. Staphy. Sulp. Sulp. ac. Thuy. Valer. or Verat.

——— Pain in and about it.—Morph. Oleand. Opi. Rus. R. Sang. Sulp. Sulp. ac. Thuy.

——— Spasms in. See Cramps.

——— Tremulous action. Spig. and the remedies for Cramps.

HERNIA OR RUPTURE.

Hernia or Rupture.—From some deficiency in the structure of the parts and fibres composing the surrounding sides of the abdomen, or from a strain or violent action, a yielding or giving way, which sometimes occurs, and a portion of the bowel or contents of the abdomen are pressed through the aperture, forming what is termed a Hernia or Rupture.

Those who have this disease should wear a truss well adapted to keep the bowel up in its place. Unless this precaution is used, the part slipping down is apt to become larger and more troublesome; sometimes by neglect or other causes the protruded part gets to be distended, inflamed, and swelled, so that it cannot be easily returned to its place; then a contraction or stricture is formed at the place where it passes out of the abdomen, and strangulation takes place. In such cases it is often very difficult to return the contents, and the circulation of the blood in the bowel protruded, and the passage of the contents of the canal is cut off and interrupted. If it is not very early removed, gangrene of the part takes place.

The part where the rupture commonly takes place is in the groin, at what is termed the abdominal ring. Though ruptures do occur at other places, such as at the navel, on the sides or under Poupart's ligament in the upper and inner part of the thigh, &c. When a rupture is strangulated, to reduce it, place the patient on the back, and in a position to relax the muscles of the abdomen, then with the hands make a pressure on the tumor according to the rules laid down in the books on surgery.

If there is much resistance and difficulty, the process may be aided by giving the patient a few doses of Acon. Bell. Nux V. Opi. or Rus. T.

If by these means used five or six hours the reduction cannot be effected, surgeons direct taking a large quantity of blood to produce a relaxation of the system, by which also violent inflammation may be prevented and the stricture removed. In some instances we have witnessed happy results from this course.

If the stricture is not relieved by these means, it is recommended to give a large dose of an Opiate; this produces a favorable effect after the loss of blood.

The proper remedies for external use are cloths wet in cold water, or ice applied to the tumefied part.

If by these means the reduction is not effected, and particularly after bleeding, it will be very serviceable to use warm fomentations to the part.

By these means perseveringly used the patient may generally be relieved.

When all these means fail, as sometimes they do, there is great danger in a short time of gangrene and mortification of the protruded part taking place.

To prevent this fatal result, it will be proper and sometimes necessary to perform the operation for strangulated hernia. Surgical writers and teachers have given advice that after strangulation takes place, and proper means are used to relieve it, and if they do not succeed in twenty-four or thirty-hours, there is great danger of gangrene and mortification. Therefore, by this lapse of time, or soon after, the operation for the patient's safety had better be performed.

In the course of our professional experience several cases, as above detailed, have come under our care, and a sense of duty placed us in a situation to attempt a relief of the patient by the operation; fortunately, they have thus been attended with success.

It may be important and worthy of record, particularly to the reader, to state that when the bowels or part of the contents of the abdomen protrude, as above stated, a hernia or rupture is formed; generally, this takes place just over the pubes, in the groin. When the contents of the rupture become inflamed or obstructed, it distends, swells, and is very painful; the part or opening where the bowel passes out, contracts and forms a band like a ligature around the bowel. If this stricture is not removed early, the life of the protruded portion may be destroyed, and the death of the patient is likely to ensue.

The operation for incarcerated hernia consists in cutting through the skin over the tumor, dissecting down through the subcutaneous parts so as to arrive at the ring or place where the stricture is formed; then by a delicate cutting instrument divide the fibres which form the band or ligature; this removes the stricture; then the bowel or contents of the rupture may be safely and readily returned into its place in the abdomen, when the parts should be brought together, and the wound dressed in a surgical manner. By this course, if the operation is well performed, the life of the patient is preserved, and the part where the protrusion took place may likely unite and grow so firmly together that it will not be necessary to wear a truss afterward.

The Homœopathic remedies which will be useful to prevent and cure this disease are Auru. Coni. Ignat. or Nux V.

Some one of these medicines used steadily for a length of time, particularly in infants and young persons, will sometimes cure the complaint or very much lesson the difficulty, though the patient should wear a truss, and it would be advisable to consult a Homœopathic physician.

To illustrate this matter, and to show the importance of prompt and correct action in such cases, we trust it may be a useful admonition to those immediately interested in such diseases to refer to some cases.

Many years ago, (about twenty,) a medical council was called to a case of Mrs. C——, of which we were one. It was about twenty miles from the county-seat, and in the country. It was ascertained that she had a femoral hernia; the part had protruded out under Poupart's ligament. It was now three days since it occurred. Judicious means had been used by the medical attendants for its relief, without success. The council of six members concluded that the only chance of relief was by an operation, and at once that was proceeded with. By a free incision of the skin, and dissecting down to the sac, we opened it, when the intestine appeared. It was purple, and in a gangrenous state. By a slender bistory, we now divided the fibres which formed the stricture, when the bowel was, without difficulty, returned to its place in the abdomen. She became very quiet and comfortable, and continued so two days, when symptoms of mortification of the bowels came on, and, after lingering two or three days, she died. Had the operation been done in twenty-four or thirty hours after the incarceration took place, this patient, no doubt, would have recovered.

About two years after this, a farmer, Mr. Mariott, who lived several miles farther in the country than the former, had an inguinal hernia, which became strangulated. We were informed by the friends that persevering means were used for his relief, but no operation was performed, and the hernia was not reduced. After suffering three or four days he died!

In about two years after this case, a respectable farmer, Mr. Carpenter, residing near the previous case, had an inguinal hernia, which became strangulated. On visiting this patient, we learned that the disease had existed twenty-four hours. The tumor was large, extremely hard and painful. The means for its reduction had been judicious. After some further trials, it was found impossible to reduce it. To obtain further useful surgical advice was equally impossible, the nearest surgeon being 20 miles off, which would delay an operation about 24 hours. The question was then submitted to the patient, and his Quaker friends, who were numerously in attendance, whether the operation should be performed at once or not, knowing as they did the result of the last mentioned case of their neighbor and friend, they soon concluded in favor of the operation, and wished it to be performed, with a single assistant. The operation was commenced, (as was desired in the call we went prepared with instruments.) After a free incision of the skin with a calm mind and steady hand, the dissection was continued until the stricture of the abdominal ring was arrived at. When the contracted fibres were cut, and the protruded contents were returned into their place in the abdomen, the parts were brought together; the wound dressed; the patient was soon calm and quiet, and recovered in a reasonably short time. After this he did not find it necessary to wear a truss. At the time of our writing, he is in the enjoyment of good health.

——— Hydrocele. This disease is often classed with hernia, but properly belongs to dropsy where it is placed.

——— Inguinal rings pressing on them, as if hernia would proturde; in such cases, use Colocy. Kreoso. Lyc. Nitr. ac. Nux V. Petrol. or Silicia.

——— Spasms or crampy pains in it, Mosch. Nux V. or Ptoleum.

Hernia strangulated, or pain in it similar to strangulation, give Acon. Bell. Nux V. Opi. Phos. Silec. Sulp. or the remedies above detailed.

——— Umbilical, similar treatment to that above recommended—apply a compress over the navel with a bandage round the body.

——— Sensation as though a protrusion of hernia was coming out, give Auru. Nux V. or Silec.

HERPES.

HERPES. The skin is subject to a great variety of diseases of an eruptive kind; the general name for them is herpes. Also there are other names used for them according to their variety or peculiarity. Affections of the skin are frequently very obstinate and difficult to cure; but the process of cure is rendered much more certain now, than it was formerly, by the use of specific Homœpathic remedies given internally. In most cases it is thought not advisable to use external applications to those diseases, for as they are the effect of a peculiar impure state of the system or the fluids, local remedies drives the exciting cause or humor back into the system without eradicating it, which may produce other and internal diseases of a serious nature.

The general remedies are Acon. Ammo. C. Ars. Arnic. Baryt. Bryo. Calc. Canth. Clemat. Coni. Graph. Hep. Kreoso. Ipe. Kalmi. L. Kali. Bic. Kali. Iod. Lach. Lyc. Merc. Muriate of Gold. Nux V. Oleand. Petrol. Phos. Psorinum. Ranan. Bulb. Rus. R. Rus.-T. Sepi. Silec. Staphy. Sulp. Tart. Anti. or Zinc.

——— Crusta lacta, a blotchy eruption, Sars. Sep. Silec.

——— Dry scabby variety, Sep. or Sulp.

——— Eccema, Ammo. C. Dulcama. Kali. Iod. Kali. Bic. Merc. Petrol. Phos. or Verat. or Caust.

——— Of the face, Acne. Ars. Arnic. Canth. Dulcam. Graph. Kali. Iod. Kreoso. Lach. Merc. Sol. Muri. ac. Rus. T. Sep. or Verat. or Caust.

——— do. swelled, use Ars. Arnic. Carb. Animi. Merc. Nux V. Sep. or Sulp.

——— Fine eruptions, Mosch. Oleand. Petrol. Phos. ac. Rus. T. Sang. or Sulp.

——— Furfuraceous, or scaly scabby state of the skin, Arnic. Ars. Auru. M. Oleand. Sepi. Sulp.—externally apply Iodine very much diluted.

——— Impetegines, Ambr. Ammo. C. Ars. Carb. V. Coni. Graph. Hell. Kali. Bic. Lyc. Merc. Oleand. Rus. T. Sep. Sulp. or Tart. Ant.

——— Itch—common itch, Arg. Nit. Barbaris. Carb. V. Caust. Crot. Tig. Kreoso. Lach. Lobel. Nitr. ac. Psorinum. or Ranan. Bulb. Rus. T. Sulp. or Tart. Ant. Dr. Hering recommended Psorinum. as the most specific.

——— itching and burning sensation, Arg. N. Ars. Carb. V. Caust. Coni. Iodi. Kreoso. Kali. Iod. Lobel. Merc. Nitr. ac. Oleand. Rus. T. or Sulp. or Sepi.

——— Of the scalp, Graph. Lyc. Oleand. Silec. or Sulp.

——— Lichen or nettle rash, Carb. V. Graph. Iodi. Phos. Rus. T. Tart. Anti. or Sulp. (See skin.)

——— Rash fine eruption, Kali. Bic. Led. P. Puls. Sarss. Sep. or Puls.

——— Small pox like eruption, Stramo. Sulp. Vaccina. or Variolin.

——— Tinea capitis (dow worm) Bell. Hep. Petrol. Phos. Sep. Silee. Stramo. or Sulp. and the other remedies for herpes.

——— Vesicles, Lach. Lyc. Petrol. Ranan. Bulb. Zinc.

HICCOUGH.

HICCOUGH. The remedies for this affection are Ammo. C. Agar. Ambr. Ars. Bell. Carb. V. Caust. Camp. Carb. A. Hyosc. Iodi. Merc. Mur. ac. Nitr. ac. Nicc. Ol. Anisi. Petrol. Sabad. Spong. Stramo. Sulp. Tart. A. Vegetable acid Verat. or Verba. These remedies must be used according to the peculiarity of the case. For a guide in addition to this head, see Dyspepsia, Flatulence, Gastrioses and Stomach.

HOARSENESS OR APHONIA.

HOARSENESS. An imperfect state or loss of the voice—this is a very common affection, as a consequence of colds, or affections of the faucies and throat. The remedies for it are, when there is considerable fever and soreness of the throat, use

Acon. or Bell.; in the more advanced states, or when there is little or no fever, give Ammo. C. Bryo. Coni. Caust. Colocy. Merc. Nitr. ac. or Muri. ac. or Phos.

If there is a smarting sensation in throat, Caps, or Dolico. or Tart. Anti.

In chronic lingering cases, Iodi. Kali. Iod. Rus. T. Sabad. Seneg. Spong. Thuy. or Verat.

HYDROPHOBIA.

Hydrophobia or canine madness, is a disease produced by the bite of an animal in a madened state, from a peculiar animal poison introduced into the system. The remedies found most useful for this disease are Belladona Lach. Hyoseramus, Stramonium, or Cantharides Cuprum, or Hydrophobin, (the matter of infection.)

In the *North American Journal of Homœopathy*, vol. 1, p. 273, Cedron is recommended; it is used in Central America, and stated to be specific for this disease. Dr. C. Hering and others recommend dry radiating heat to be applied to the wound. This should be used in this manner; a red hot iron or live coals, or any other convenient heat must be placed as near the wound as possible without burning the skin, or causing a too sharp pain; keep up the heat steadily a long time, confine it to the wound as much as possible, apply oil or grease to the wound, and this should be repeated whenever it becomes dry. The heat should be continued in this way, until the patient shivers; the process should be continued about an hour, or until the morbid symptoms diminish. Internal remedies should be administered at the same time; a little Brandy or wine will be useful. If the pains shoot towards the heart, give Arsenicum, in doses of three or four globules of the 2d or 3d attenuation, in a spoonful of water; if the suffering continues, the dose should be repeated in half an hour, or if there is an aggravation of the medicine, it will be better to wait two or three hours. In cases where Ars. doesnot afford relief after being given three or four times, it is best to use Bell. in the same way.

Hahnemann states that he considers Belladona, a very small dose given after the bite, every three or four days, to be a certain preventive of the disease.

As soon as convulsions set in, Lach. should be given—two or three globules every one or two hours.

If there comes on drowsiness, or burning of the throat and frothy mucus in the mouth, or an inclination to drink, which is refused, or there is a stricture and suffication of the throat, or a glowing fulness of the face, or inclination to strike or bite with convulsive twitching, give Belladona, place a few globules on the tongue, repeated as directed for Lachesis.

Should the convulsions be severe or of long duration, or there is not much inclination to bite or spit, with moderate spasms in the throat, and shooting or burning pain, a dread of fluids, or severe convulsions, or raving, or dread and fear of people, use Hyosciamus.

When convulsions are produced by looking on a glass or a brilliant object, or mentioning to the patient water, fits of laughter or singing take place, or are attended with great fury, wildness or pupils dilated, give Stramonium, in the same manner as directed for Lach. and Bell.

If there is great dryness and burning in the mouth or great aggravation in attempting to swallow, it is recommended to give Cantharides.

As one of the most effectual remedies, the Hydrophobin is recommended; it is recorded that cases have been cured by it; also, for animal poisons. It is stated in the journal above named that Guaco. is used with great success in South America.

In the North American Journal of Homœopathy, No. 6, page 518, there is an account of several cases of hydrophobia being cured or prevented by Euphorbium.

HYPOCONDRIA.

Hypocondria.—This disease is considered an affection of males somewhat similar to hysterics in females. Persons liable to it are those of nervous temperament, dull or melancholy disposition. They have pain and distress in and about the abdomen, flatulence and eructations; they are subject to erroneous and fanciful ideas; apt to imagine themselves more ailing or sick than they really are.

In the treatment of such cases the fancies of the patient should be indulged and endeavors made to direct the mind to other and agreeable subjects. The remedies proper to use are Acon. Anacard. Arnic. Ars. Auru. Bell. Bromi. Hyosc. Lach. Merc. Mosch. Nux V. Petrol. Phos. Rus. R. Staphy. Sulph. Tereb. or Verat.

If there is fever, with flushed face, give Acon. or Bell.

If there are crampy, nervous symptoms, Nux V. Bromi. or Hyosc. or Staphy.

If there is ill humor, Anacard. Hyosc. or Sulp.

When there is low spirits, Calc. or Auru.

There should be an endeavor to select and use the remedies according to the peculiarity of the case.

HYSTERIC.

See this article, under the head of Women, Diseases of.

IMPOTENCE.

See Genitals.

INFLAMMATION.

INFLAMMATION. There are very few diseased states of a general nature, of a febrile character, which take place, without being attended, more or less, with inflammatory action.

This condition is defined by writers and in Lexicons plogosis, or phlegmasia, a disease characterized by heat, pain, redness of the skin, attended more or less with tumefaction and fever. Inflammation is divided into two species, phlegmonous and erysipelatous; besides these distinctions, inflammation has a great variety of species and forms of appearing, such as acute, chronic, congestive, and passive.

In this article the diseases which, in the early ssage, are attended with features of acute inflammatory symptoms, will be treated on with the suitable remedies for them detailed.

The remedies generally most useful for this class of diseases are, Acon. Bell. Bryo. Ipe. Kalmi. T. Tart. Anti. Nux V. or Phos. and many others will be proper as the condition of the cases may present.

——— Inflammation of the brain, phrenitis,

and encephalitis. We introduce a description of this disease taken from Dr. Pulte's book. "The brain and its two coverings are subject to inflammation separately, and the symptoms show themselves particularly in the beginning of brain fever, the first species called meningitis, when the duramater is inflamed.

The acute meningitis attacks a person suddenly, exhibiting immediately stupor and drowsy symptoms, the patient cannot be raised easily to keep the head erect; he complains of vertigo and dizziness, reels in walking, pupils contracted, cannot bear the light, eyes are not red yet, constipation, scanty red urine, fever with a soft pulse.

——— Second species, or (arachnoides) when the next covering of the brain is inflamed—this commences with pain violent over the whole head, increased by congestion and violent beating of the blood vessels, attended with wakefulness, muttering, pulse quick; if not early relieved, stupor and delirium ensues, and the patient is likely to die.

——— The third species is inflammation of the substance of the brain. It begins with violent symptoms of congestion and pulsation of the arteries of the neck and head; the face is red and bloated, the eyes blood-shot, intense heat in the head and delirium; the patient tosses about, is very sensitive to light, skin dry, violent thirst, hard full pulse, fever high, frequent retchings or vomiting."

In practice it will be extremely difficult to distinguish between the varieties of diseases of the brain above laid down, but fortunately, there are some general remedies which apply pretty well to them all.

For the first species, it is recommended to use Opi. or Hyosc. with other remedies for fever.

In the second variety, use Aconite, Bell. or Hyosc.

For the third variety, Acon. is the remedy to use first; this should be followed by Bell.

When, from the foregoing symptoms, or from there being fever, severe pain in the head, a flushed face, red or blood-shot eyes, it may be pretty satisfactorily ascertained that the patient has an attack of inflammation of the brain, or its appendages; begin by giving Acon. at once; the dose should be repeated every half hour at first; after three or four hours, the period should be lengthened to an hour, and after a few doses are given in this way, the periods may be lengthed to two hours. If the patient is of full or plethoric habit, blood should be taken from the arm. We should have no confidence in a temporising inefficient mode of abstracting blood by leeching or cupping in such cases. A neglect or refusal to bleed may very much jeopardize the life of the patient.

We have had a good deal of experience in this matter. Cold water or ice should be applied to the head, and cold water given freely as a drink; the feet should be put in water as hot as it can be borne, let salt be put in it; keep the feet there a long time; when taken out of the warm water, keep them warm, apply cabbage leaves to them, or some softening article; many useful remedies may be found which will keep them moist and warm, and be useful in the various symptoms which will be presented

After there is a mitigation of the symptoms, the proper remedies to use are Bell. Digital. Hell. or Opi.

After the acute stage of the disease is over, or the violence of it is checked, the most proper remedies are Ars. Hyosc. Merc. Puls. or Sulp.

In this stage of diseased brain, and in congestion, Hahnemann and Teste recommend warm water and spirits applied to the head in preference to cold applications.

The patient should be kept in a dark cool room.

Inflammation of the brain from concussion. From blows on the head, falls and other injuries, the brain may receive such a severe shock or concussion as to produce Inflammation. In such cases the first remedy should be Arnica; also apply it very much diluted externally, on the part injured. If reaction comes on so as to produce fever and pain, give Acon. Digital. or Sulp.

8*

If stupor or darting crampy pain takes place, use Cocc. Camp. Ignat. Nux V. or in a late stage of the case, give Ars. (See Injuries Mechanical.)

INFLAMMATION OF THE BLADDER, (CYSTITIS.)

INFLAMMATION OF THE BLADDER, CYSTITIS. This organ among others is subject to attacks of inflammation, the symptoms attending it are pain, and a burning heat through the part in the bladder; it soon becomes full or distended, the urine is hot and passed with difficulty; fever is attending, the pain extends to the bowels, back, and to the ribs. Acon. will be the proper medicine, but early after it, Canth. Caps. Cann. S. or Uva. Urs. will be required and necessary, in more advanced stages, Arnic. Digital. Iodi. Nux V. Phos. Puls. Rus. T. Scill. or Terebinth will be proper to be used, according to the symptoms presented.

In this manner, if there is a difficulty of urinating, give Cann. S. Canth. or Digital.

If there is pressing down on the neck of the bladder, Canth.

If there are urgent efforts with pain to pass urine, Nux V. Phos. or Scilla.

If Cantharides may have caused the disease, give Camphor.

If there is diminished action in the parts, and inability to pass urine, Terebinth. (Refer to Disease of Bladder.)

INFLAMMATION OF THE BOWELS, (ENTERITIS.)

INFLAMMATION OF THE BOWELS, ENTERITIS. This disease is characterised by pain more or less severe in the bowels; sometimes it is very severe, this is attended with fever. The pulse is small and fine, or hard; in some cases it appears in the form of a colic, attended with cramps or twisting pains—the bowels are costive.

This disease appears in the form of primary acute inflammation; also it is frequently either symptomatic of, or connected with other diseases, such as indigestion, colics, dysentery, &c.

It is the first, or acute nature of the disease which will be directed for in the treatment here, (leaving the other forms to be considered along with the disease with which they may be connected.)

The first remedy should be Acon., and this is to be given often; a dose every half hour or hour at first; it should be continued until the fever moderates. Apply cloths wet with cold water to the abdomen. Dr. Currie recommends a free use of this article in this way, and Dr. Abercrombie directs cold water to be dashed on the abdomen. Let the patient take cold water as a drink in small quantities, repeated often; and after this early period passes, give Bryo, or if there are crampy pains, give Nux V.

If the pains are of a colic kind, give Colocy.

If the symptoms continue obstinate, and the skin becomes cold, use Ars. or Verat.

It is not advisable to attempt to give purgative medicines in the early stage. Let the bowels remain quiet until the inflammation is removed and the stricture passes away; then it will be proper to procure an evacuation.

We have long observed, it is a very common practice among practitioners that in the treatment of such cases, which is generally called *Bilious Colic*, attempts are made at once to force a passage through the bowels by active and sometimes drastic purgative medicines, in which there is very frequently a failure; and we have often learned that cases of this kind, and under such treatment, have terminated fatally.

The better and proper way is to cure the inflamed state of the bowels, and to relieve the stricture which exists at the diseased parts, before harsh attempts are made to produce evacuations by Cathartic medicines.

If there is much pain and colicy symptoms, give Opi. Puls. Rus. T. or Colocy.

Should the fever and sickness continue, give Merc. Nux V. Tart. Anti. or Ipe.

After the first stage, we have observed great benefit to accrue from fomentations with alkaline solutions applied to the abdomen.

——— Of the bowels, *chronic form*. Sometimes the preceding disease as well as in other states, the inflammation assumes a lingering chronic form, attended with pain and soreness of the abdomen, irregularity and griping; a part of the time, fever; the proper remedies are Bell. Bryo. Cham. Merc. Sulp. or Zinc.

INFLAMMATION OF THE KIDNEYS.
(NEPHRITIS.)

INFLAMMATION OF THE KIDNEYS. The indications for the existence of this disease are pain in the lumbar region, of a shooting severe kind; it extends to the bladder, and to the urethra, producing urinary obstructions; the urine is high colored; the testes are drawn up and painful, in the progress, pain and cramps affect the legs, fever sets in with a full tense pulse.

The first remedy is Acon. when the fever or pain is somewhat moderated, give Bell. or Cann. S.

If there is a pressing pain on the bladder or urethra, Cantharides will be useful, or alternate this with Acon.

In the progress of the case, the other useful remedies will be, Bals. Cop. Merc. or Tussilago. When the pain is severe or of a darting form, Ether is a valuable remedy.

When the acute type is somewhat mitigated, and there is pain in urinating, it will be of service to use Canth. or if the use of this drug may have produced the disease, give Camp. For other remedies, see Bladder, Kidneys, Colic and Nephritis.

INFLAMMATION OF THE LIVER.

(HEPALITIS.)

INFLAMMATION OF THE LIVER. This disease is defined a severe pain in the region of the liver, attended with fever and derangement of the bowels; it is often attended with nausea or vomiting. It appears in an acute or chronic form; the latter is called liver complaint, and may be of a very protracted nature.

——— The acute type will be considered here, and the chronic form we refer to the head of Liver and its diseases. The remedies most useful for this affection are, Acon. Bell. Merc. Lach. or Bry. Cham. Nux V. Puls. or Sulp. At the beginning during the fever and pain, give Acon.; continue it until the fever and pain have abated; at this stage it will be best to make cold applications, such as cold water or ice, over the liver. After this course, if there is rather dull pain in the part and fulness of the chest, a pressure to the head or giddiness, or faintness, give Bell. This may be followed to advantage by Merc. or alternated with it. Dr. Beach found Bell. and Bryo. alternated, very useful for this disease.

When the pains are shooting and there is great tenderness at the part, or there is derangement of the stomach, give Nux V.

If in the progress there is burning pain, heat of skin, anxiety, or vomiting of dark matter, give Ars. Puls. or Sulp.; or Cham. or Lach. may be very useful in the latter stage. (See Liver.)

INFLAMMATION OF THE LUNGS.
(Pneumonia.)

Inflammation of the Lungs. This disease is characterised by rigors, chills, pain or stitches in the side or chest; these are soon followed by fever; the respiration is short and hurried, a short dry cough, a scanty tough expectoration; this is generally tinged or mingled with blood; the pain in the chest is generally severe, though at times there is more of a pressing fullness than pain. The pulse is commonly full and tense, but sometimes it is small, slow, and compressible; the face is red and flushed, but in some cases, it is of a dull and purple or dingy color.

For this disease early and active treatment is required; at first use Acon.; this should be often repeated, and continued until there is an abatement of the symptoms; let the patient drink cold water freely, and apply cloths wet in cold water over the chest, or use a bag of ice.

Bryo. should be given next, every one or two

hours, or Tart. Anti. will be a very useful remedy instead of Bryo.

If there is a full flushed face, with some headache, give Bell.

The following medicines are recommended in the progress of the case, Ipe. Merc. Phos. Rus. T. Sambu. or Ammo. C.; it will be better for the patient to be in a cold or cool room.

If the expectoration is streaked with blood, or a sore throat, Bell. or Ipe.

In the progress of the case, Tart. Anti. is highly recommended; also in this condition, Phos. will be very useful, particularly when there are shooting pains in the chest or dry hoarseness.

In the advanced stage, when there is heaviness across the chest and scanty expectoration, Ammo. C. will be very useful.

For the use of other remedies, reference is made to Chest, Cough, &c.

INFLAMMATION OF THE PERITONEUM.
(PERITONITIS.)

INFLAMMATION OF THE PERITONEUM. As this membrane immediately invests the bowels lining the abdomen, it is rather difficult to distinguish this disease form Enteritis. It is attended with pain and tension of the abdomen, tenderness to the touch, constipation, difficulty of urinating—the other symptoms are similar to those of Enteritis.

The remedies are about the same as those pointed out for Enteritis.

Treatment during the acive fever, use Acon.; as soon as the active fever has moderated, Bell.

When the symptoms are considerably moderated, Merc. is a useful medicine.

If there is distension and pain, Nux V.

If symptoms of prostration ensue, Ars.

Other remedies useful are Canth. Lach. Cham. Lyc. Colocy.; the remedies further will be very similar to those for Enteritis.

INFLAMMATION OF THE PLEURA.
(Pluritis, Pleurisy.)

Inflammation of the Pleura. The membrane which lines the ribs on the inside of the chest, is the seat of this disease; the lungs are directly in contact with it, so that when the pleura is inflamed, the portion of the lungs on that side is very likely also to partake of the disease. The symptoms of it are, a pain or stitch in the side, difficulty of breathing, and dry barking cough.

Slight expectoration at first, which is sometimes streaked with blood; the skin is hot and dry, pulse full and tense, great thirst, urine high colored, with active fever

At first give Acon. let it be continued until the fever and pain moderate, then Bryo. will be proper.

When there are cutting pains or burning sensation, or a mucus expectoration, and this streaked with blood, Bryo. or Millefo.

These remedies being used, and there is a mitigation of the disease, use Sulp.

If there is headache and red face, Bell.

When the active fever is checked, and pain and dyspnoea continue, Merc. or Arnica.

If the disease has been produced by contusion or injury, use Arnica.

Other remedies recommended are, Phos. Tart. Anti. or Digital. Ipe. Sabad. Scill.; these should be used as the symptoms are presented, much in the same manner as are stated for inflammation of the lungs: reference is made here for a detail of the remedies.

INFLAMMATION OF THE PSOAS MUSCLES. (Psoitis.)

Inflammation of the Psoas Muscles. The symptoms are pain in the lumbar region, moving the limbs up or down, gives pain; turning, or any exertion increases the pain, the kidneys being placed on this part, and are somewhat connected with this inflammation. The symptoms are similar—inflammation of this part may lay the foundation of that serious disease termed Psoas abscess.

The remedies for Lumbago under Rheumatism, will be useful for this disease; during the active stage, use Acon. This should be succeeded by Bell.

If there is contraction or cramps in the part, Colocy.

If there are symptoms of suppuration, Staphy. Silec. or Hep. (See Nephritis and Psoas abscess.)

INFLAMMATION OF THE SPLEEN.

(Splenitis.)

Inflammation of the Spleen. The symptoms are sharp darting pains through the spleen, with fever; the part is enlarged; it is attended with vomiting of blood, or the passing of bloody stools.

This is a rare disease, and is difficult to be distinguished from other inflammations of the abdomen.

If there is active fever, give Acon. or Bryo.; in the progress Arsen. is well recommended, also Nux V. or Arnic. or China.

If it is complicated with Ague, Ars. or China.

The chronic form, when the spleen is enlarged, is termed *ague cake:* for this state Ars. Baryt. M. Lyc. Carbo. Vig. Ferr. Stann. or Sulp. are the proper remedies.

INFLAMMATION OF THE STOMACH.

(Gastritis.)

Inflammation of the Stomach. There are two forms in which this disease appears, one is an inflammation of the coats of the stomach proper, the other is an inflammation of the internal lining of the stomach or villous coat.

The former is the one to be treated here, the latter or villous inflammation of the stomach and intestines, are to be found under Cholera and Dysentery.

The symptoms are severe pain, burning or pricking in the part, heat, distension of the stomach, retching or vomiting, hiccough, a prostration, or sinking sensation, features sunken in, and cramps, pulse is small and quick, and firm, though sometimes it is compressible—high fever ensues.

The remedies most useful are Acon. Canth. Bell. Ipe. Nux V. Anti. Puls. or Bryo. Hyosc. or Ars.

In the first stage, give Acon. in doses of high attenuation often repeated.

If there is nausea or vomiting, let Ipe. or Camp. be given in alternation with Acon.; apply cloths wet in cold water over the stomach; after the symptoms have somewhat moderated, use Bell.

Should nausea continue, Ipe. or Anti. or a high attenuation of Ars. should be used.

If the patient has indulged in alcoholic drinks, or there are crampy pains in the region of the stomach, use Nux V.

If there is a good deal of retching and a coldness of the skin, give Ars. or Verat.

As the case advances, some of the other remedies named will be useful.

When the first or acute stage has passed, fomentations with hot alkaline solutions, will be very useful.

If the disease does not yield and become considerably moderated in twenty-four or forty-eight hours, it may be advisable and even necessary for the safety of the patient to resort to blood-letting; sometimes by the aid of this remedy, with the continuance of the Homœopathic remedies, the disease will very soon yield, and the patient approach toward a cure. Such has been our observation.

In the milder cases, when it may be caused by suppression of the catamenia or coldness of the stomach, Puls.

If there is burning pain in it, Canth.

If there takes place an apparent sinking, with a fluttering pulse, Ars. or Verat.

In the latter stage, when there remains uneasy soreness, Cham. or Sulp.

INFLAMMATION OF THE TESTICLES.
(Hernia Humoralis.)

Inflammation of the Testicles.—This disease may be produced by external injury or from gonorrhœa. One or both testicles may be affected. The testicle swells, is painful, and tender to the touch; the spermatic cord swells, and is also painful.

The remedies for inflammation generally will be proper for this disease, such as Acon. Bell. Bryo. or Ipe. The patient should lie in bed. For local remedies, a solution of Acetate of Lead or Muriate of Ammonia, applied cold or in the form of cold poultice, will be very useful; or Arnica in the same way, will answer a good purpose.

After the first or acute stage is over, these articles applied warm will be very proper; or if there is a good deal of pain, Laudanum may be added to them with great advantage. Also, at the more advanced stage, give Merc. Ipe. Anti. or Puls. For the induration of the testicle, use Coni. or Iodine.

A popular and very useful remedy is a poultice of white beans. When the patient sits up or walks about, the testicle should be suspended in a truss or bandage.

If there is irritation and pain of the urethra, give Puls.

If the swelling is the effect of external injury, Arnic. should be used internally and externally.

For other remedies, consult Genital Organs and Indurated Glands.

INFLAMMATION OF THE TONGUE.
(GLOSITIS.)

INFLAMMATION OF THE TONGUE.—It is attended with swelling, redness, and heat.

The medicine best adapted to this affection are the following:—

If there is acute inflammation, swelling or fever, give Acon. After this is used, the useful articles will be Arnic. Merc. Bell. Lach; and in the advanced stage, Ars.

INJURIES, MECHANICAL.

INJURIES, MECHANICAL.—There are a great variety of ways by which bruises, cuts, contusions, and lacerations of the body externally, are produced, and from this cause many serious internal diseases are caused. When these occur, in the first place, the patient will need immediate attention for comfort. The wound, if any, should be cleansed and dressed. If there is dislocations or fractures, they should be properly reduced, and the bones put in place. The proper and most useful remedy for internal use is Arnica; give the 2d or 3d dilution, or a higher attenuation; a dose every half hour, or hour or two at first, and after awhile, at longer periods, according to the severity of the injury. For external use, mix a teaspoonful of the Tincture of Arnica in a gill of water or a larger quantity, and use it to bathe

the injured part with; apply it to the part, often changing it. Generally, it will be best to add a little spirits to this lotion. All the external remedies should at first be used cold. In the same manner, instead of Arnica, it will do well to use Calendula, Conium, or Euphorbium. In the progress of the case, instead of Arnica, it will do well to give Hep. Iodi. Nux V. Rus. T. or Sulp.

SPRAINS.

SPRAINS—Wrenches and Injuries of the Knee and other Joints. These frequently occur; they require particular attention to prevent inflammation, which may prove tedious and very serious. Avoid at first using any warm or hot application to the part, or hot stimulating articles.

The plan of treatment above detailed will be preferable to any other.

In severe or extensive cases of injury taking place, particularly if the vital functions or important organs are injured—as soon as the reaction of the arterial system takes place, blood should be taken in small or large quantities, answering to the severity and urgency of the case; so say Laurie and Hull.

INJURY OF THE BRAIN FROM MECHANICAL CAUSES.

INJURY OF THE BRAIN.—This organ is liable to have concussion, compression, lesion, laceration, and inflammation produced from this cause. Generally, the use of Arnica, as above directed, at first it will be proper to use and for other remedies; they may be found under Inflammation of the Brain, Congestion, Coma, and Head Diseases.

Although injuries to so delicate an organ as the brain often leads to serious and fatal results, yet under some circumstances it sustains great and serious diseases, when by prompt and proper means it recovers from their effects. This principle may be illustrated by recording an interesting case.

In June, 1836, P. Butler, a farmer near the city of Poughkeepsie, went out with a large musket to shoot crows that were pulling up his young corn. On firing at them, the birds were unhurt, but the gunner was prostrated and wounded; the explosive power forced out the breech pin of the gun in a reverse direction towards the man; the point entered the cranium near the centre of the forehead, and penetrated two inches into the brain. He was prostrated and insensible, but before I arrived, he had somewhat recovered from the stupor, and the iron had been drawn out. On clearing away the coagulated blood, I ascertained that the bone was fractured, that portions of it were driven in upon the brain, and the brain was seriously wounded. To keep down the inflammation he was freely bled, and preparations were made for trepanning him. As soon as things could be got ready, and with the assistance of some medical friends, I proceeded to the performance of the operation. After perforating the bone at the injured part, the fragments of the fractured bone were removed from the brain, and the depressed portion of bone elevated. An important point now was to guard against inflammation of the brain. Here was impressed upon my mind the principle laid down by Sir Astley Cooper, in such cases to keep down the increased arterial action by abstracting a portion of the blood to prevent inflammation and congestion from taking place on the brain, which would likely prove fatal. As the action of the arterial system came up or was increased, the patient was bled, so that the inflammation was kept down; he had very little severe pain to encounter; in all he lost about 70 ounces of blood. The sanies and matter passed off from the wound; the aperture in the bone closed up in a reasonable short time, and he was restored to health, and resumed his labor. He enjoyed good health for twelve years or more afterwards. A fair inference is, that the copious bleeding kept down the inflammation of the brain, and was the means of saving this man's life.

——— Mechanical, of the Brain. Use the remedies, similar to those mentioned above, at first.

If there comes on a heaviness or dull stupor, give Bell. Cocc. or Hyosc. or Opi.

If considerable fever sets in, give Aconite.

——— do. Concussion of the Brain. Give Acon. Arnic. Coni. Hep. Iodi. Opi. or Rus. Tox. Externally, apply Arni. Iodine or Rus. Tox. in the form and manner above pointed out.

INFLUENZA, OR GRIPPE.

INFLUENZA.—This disease affects very similar to common cold, though it is more severe and more general in the attacks on a great number of persons at a time. Among the symptoms, the following are enumerated:—

The nose and throat are stuffed up; there are chills and fevers; soreness of the throat and upper part of the chest; severe headache, giddiness, red eyes, cough, and hoarseness.

It frequently prevails in an epidemic form, and when it does, it attacks people more uniformly and extensively than any other disease. Instances are stated that in a town where it prevailed, not a single one was known to escape it.

The remedies most useful for this disease are Acon. Anti. Ars. Camph. Coni. Dulcam. Ipe. Merc. Nux V. Sabad. Verat. or Phos. or Puls.

At the commencement, a few doses of Dulcam. or Camp. will frequently prevent or cure it.

Should there be fever, use Acon.

If the throat gets sore with cough, Bell.

If there is shooting pains or crampy feelings in the neck or chest, give Nux V.

If the case continues obstinate, with cough, cramps, &c., use Merc. or Ars. Sabad. or Verat.

If there are secondary symptoms of tumefaction or little lumps on the skin, or hoarseness, &c., use Caust.

ITCH AND ITCHING.

See Herpes.

JAWS AND GUMS.

Jaws and Gums.—These parts are subject to many important diseases, many of which may be relieved by Homœopathic treatment.

——— do. Articulation, pain and stiffness in, give Bell, Colocy. Rus. T. Phos. Silec. or Verat.

——— do. Bleeding. Calc. Iodi. Mag. C. Millefo. Nux V. Phos. Sepi. Silec. or Sulp. ac.

——— do. Painful. Ammo. C. Bell. Cann. S. Colocy. Hep. Iodi. Merc. Nitr. ac. Petrol. Phos. Stramo. Sulp. Sulp. ac. Thuy. or Verat.

——— do. Brown, black, or yellow gums. Plumb. ac.

——— do. Excrescences on. Stann. or Thuy.
——— do. Falls and raises involuntarily. Lach. Sang. Valer.
——— do. Glands on them inflamed. Bell. Sepi. Silec. Spong. Stann. Sulp. or Thuy.
——— do. Soft and swelled. Nitr. C. Nux V. Petrol. Phos. Spong. Sulp. ac. Verat. Zinc.
——— do. Tittillation, easily. Staphy.
——— do. Ulcerated. Iodi. Merc. Nitr. ac. Nux. V.

JEALOUSY AND MADNESS.

Jealousy and Madness.—Lyc. Lach. Nux V. Stramo. See Emotions, this article.

JOINTS.

Joints.—See Extremities and Injuries, Mechanical.

KIDNEYS.

Kidneys.—These parts are subject to inflammation, which has been treated of under that head, and to colic or spasms, to burning sensation, ulceration, morbid secretion of urine, producing diabetes, and to what is termed Bright's disease.

——— For colic and spasms, termed Nephritic Colic, the remedies are Ether. Bell. Canth. Lyc. Nux V. Sulp. Tereb. or Uva. Urs.

If the spasms or pains are severe at first, give Ether or Nux V.

If there is a burning sensation, Canth.

If there is dull pain, with fever, Bell.

In the progress if there is suppression of urine, Uva. Urs. or Canth.

When the acute form has passed over, if there is pain and difficulty in passing urine, Tereb. or some of the other remedies may be useful.

——— Ulcerated condition. Give Iodi. Merc. Nitr. ac. or Nux V. See Psoas Abscess.

BRIGHT'S DISEASE.

Bright's Disease.—In *Copeland's Medical Encyclopædia*, it is stated under the head of Dropsy, that "attention has been called to glandular disease of the kidneys, as described by Bright. It is considered as a primary inflammatory affection, attended with a secretion of albuminous urinaria. Cases have been published, in which Bright's disease existed without albuminous urine; and, on the other hand, albuminous urine was present without Bright's disease. By some, who look upon glandular disease of the kidneys as the result of inflammation, glandular disease has been thus regarded. However, it is owing to an error of the system, which is inexplicable."

The Homœopathic remedies for this disease are found to be Tart. Anti. or Muriate of Mercury.

LASCIVIOUSNESS.

LASCIVIOUSNESS.—A disposition to this practice, or an indulgence in it. The medicines for it are Canth. Chin. Graph. Lyc. Phos. Silec. Stramo. Sulp. or Verat.

LANGUOR, OR A TIRED SENSATION.

LANGUOR.—Give Chin. Nitr. ac. Nux V. Phos. ac. Plati. Seneg. Silec. Stramo. Sulp. ac. or Zinc. See Extremities, this article.

LEPROSY.

LEPROSY.—This loathsome disease, so much noticed in Sacred Writ, which caused great annoyance and suffering, and one which was the means of degradation among the chosen people, has not been much noticed by modern writers, and it appears that no intelligible or successful mode of treating it has been pointed out, until the Homœopathic method was introduced, and determined the properties and powers of drugs, by learning their effects on the healthy person. By this means some remedies have been discovered, which prove very useful in curing this kind of affection. They are Alum. Ars. Carbo. Ani. Carbo. Veg. Caust. Petrol. Rus. T. Silec. and Sulp.

Many cases of disease presenting this character, are reported to have been cured by those medicines, given in minute doses, and long continued.

LETHARGY.

Lethargy.—For this condition of disease, the remedies are Baryt. Cocc. Tart. Anti. See Coma.

LIVER.

Liver.—This organ holds an important place in the body, from its office being to furnish bile to aid in the process of digestion and in the support of life.

It is subject to diseases which interferes with its functions and operations, and may produce affections of a serious kind, though it is very doubtful whether the *bile* proceeding from the *liver* has as much to do with producing disease and causing morbid derangement, as some are in the habit of charging to it; for there cannot be an ailment of the stomach or a febrile attack, nor a derangement of the system, of almost any kind, but what it is by some ascribed to the bile, or it is a bilious affection or bilious interference with the animal economy, when in a great portion of those cases the bile has very little influence in the case or nothing to do with it.

The term *bilious* has a very indefinite meaning, but it is said that this term furnishes an excuse and a reason among Allopathic practitioners for many of the remedies used, frequently to treat a disease that does not exist. The liver is, however, subject to inflammation, which has been treated of under that head.

——— To a burning sensation in it, with painful stitches. For this affection, give Bryo. Calc. Lyc. Nitr. ac. Nux V. Sabad. or Sulp.

——— Gall, Bladder, pains in or through it. The remedies are Sabad. Sabi. or Oleander.

——— Gangrenous symptoms present. Ars. Sec. C. Silec. or Carb. V. and Wine.

——— Heavy, lumpy sensation in it. Sulp.

——— Induration of it. Arg. N. Ars. Auru. Coni. Iodi. Kali. C. Lyc. Lauroc. Merc. Nux V. Silec. or Sulp.

——— Chronic disease or chronic inflammation of it—There is a large number of medicines useful for this affection; the following are the

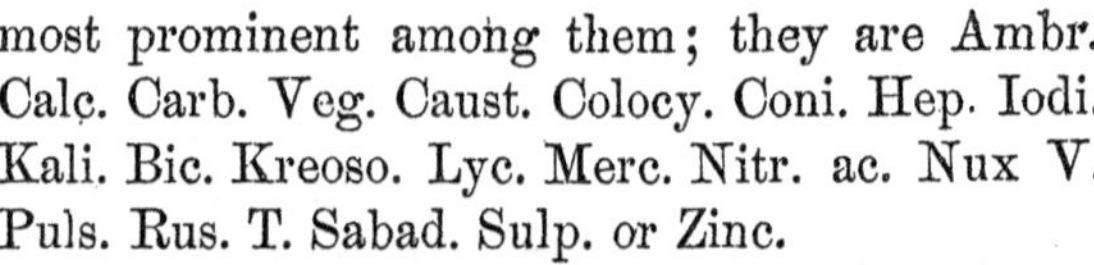

most prominent among them; they are Ambr. Calc. Carb. Veg. Caust. Colocy. Coni. Hep. Iodi. Kali. Bic. Kreoso. Lyc. Merc. Nitr. ac. Nux V. Puls. Rus. T. Sabad. Sulp. or Zinc.

——— Jaundice, this is connected with the preceding affection or produced by it; give Ambr. Berba. Coni. Cham. Lyc. Merc. Nux V. Puls. Rus. T. Sulp. or Sulp. ac.

——— Pain of a cutting nature attended with shuddering—Nux Jug. Nux V. Phos. Prun. Sp. Rus. R. Sabad. Stann. Tabac. or Valer.

——— do. Intermittent in—Ars. or Zinc.

——— Spasms or stitches in—Nux V. Sulp. Tabac. or Zinc.

——— Ulcers in it—Ars. Chin. Lach. Seler. or Silec.

LICE, BODY.

Lice, Body. The remedies are Ars. Chin. Merc. Sabad.; these should be given internally, and a lotion or ointment of the latter applied outwardly.

——— Crab, Sabad. internally and externally to be used.

MANIA AND ALIENATION OF THE MIND.

Mania and Alienation of the Mind.—There are a great number of causes which operate upon the body and mind, which are calculated to produce this state of disease. The peculiar causes from which these diseases arise and their pathological nature, have been very ably examined and explained by medical writers, yet the subject is still enshrouded in much obscurity and darkness. It is the intention here merely to lay down the symptoms presented, and the manner of attack, with appropriate remedies for them.

It will be required to use the remedies in a measure according to and corresponding with the symptoms. Those affected with this disease should have mild indulgent treatment, as far as is consistent with their safety and comfort, and that of their attendants and friends—they should be indulged in their fancies, and have their minds diverted and amused as much as possible.

The remedies which are found to be most useful, are Arn. Anacard. Ars. Auru. Canth. Coni. Lach. Opi. Origani. Plati. Puls. Quini. Sec. C. Sepi. Stramo. or Sulp. Tart. Anti. or Verat.

If the disease is in consequence of a fright, use Opi. or Acon. Bell. Anti. or Verat.

If it seems to be caused by home sickness, Phos. ac. Staphy. or Colocy.

If it is produced by disappointed love, give Hyosc. Ignat. or Phos.

If from jealousy, Lach. Hyosc. or Nux V.

If it is brought on by passionate anger or sense of revenge or insult, Ignat. Plati. or Colocy. or Staphy.

When it seems to have been produced by religious excitement or frenzy, Stramo. Hyosc. or Puls. (See Emotions.)

When it proceeds from intemperance, Nux V. Opi. or Hyosc. (See Drunkenness.)

When it is the effect of a full sanguineous habit, or the patient is of such a temperament, attended with fever, give Acon. Bell. Hell.

If the derangement is on one particular subject, termed MONO MANIA, give Auru. Stramo. or some of the preceding named remedies.

When there is a state of debility and feebleness of the body, givs China. Ferr. or Quinine.

For other indications and remedies, the reader will please examine Emotions, Coma, Delirium, Drunkenness, Onanism, Mind and Memory, and Melancholy.

MARASMUS. (ATROPHIA.)

MARASMUS. This affection is described by writers as a depressed habit of the body, an apparent deficiency in the process of nutrition; there is a wasting away and emaciation of the system, attended with a feeble languid state.

It is divided into marasmus of old age; termed Senelis, or the decay of old age; and marasmus Infantile, or that affecting infants. The remedies for that of old age are Conium. Baryt. Opium. nourishing diet, and whatever may seem to add strength to the patient and vigor to the system. The marasmus of infants will be treated on under the article on Infants.

MEASLES, (Rubeola.)

Measles. This is a contagious disease; it may spread about sporadically or mildly, or it may prevail as an epidemic with great severity; this disease is in itself not a very serious affection, but it is often rendered severe and malignant by injudicious treatment, which is often used by kind friends, and by some others, (allusion is here made to the use of warm heating, and stimulating remedies to drive the eruption out; this increases the fever and makes the case worse.) The case commences with symptoms of common cold; sneezing is one of the common symptoms, watery red eyes, dry cough, and there are generally symptoms of fever. As all these eruptive diseases and common colds are attended with fever, and begin very much alike, the nature of the case cannot be exactly known until the eruption comes out; but as the remedies for inflammatory fever would be very proper in either case, there need be no error about the treatment.

The proper remedies for it are Acon. Bell. Ipe. or Anti. Give cool drinks, and keep the patient in a cool room.

In the first or inflammatory stage, give Acon. or Bell.

When the disease is determined on, give Acon.

If there is a catarrhal affection and a stopping up of the head or nose, use Dulcam. or Puls.

If the throat is sore and inflamed, give Bell.

If the eruption does not come out, give Bryo.

If vomiting and distress at the chest attends, give Tart. Anti. or Ipe.

If there is a belching from the stomach, give Ars. 30th, or in a high attenuation.

In the early period, let the patient drink cold water, and gargle the throat with it.

If delirium comes on, give Bell. Cocc. Opi. Stramo. or Hyosc.

MELANCHOLIA.

Melancholia.—This disease, which affects body and mind, is very difficult fully to understand, and equally in some cases difficult to cure. It appears in various forms and degrees. The patient is gloomy, dejected, and gets discouraged; the mind dwells on unpleasant, discouraging topics; strange and inconsistent fancies pervade the mind. The remedies most generally found useful are the following, from which such may be selected, as on examination of the Materia Medica, if needful, appears best for the case.

Acon. Agar. Anacard. Arnic. Ars. Auru. Bucci. Calc. Caust. Coni. Hyosc. Ignat. Kreoso. Nux V. Nitr. ac. Opi. Petrol. Puls. Plati. Rus. R. Sec. C. Silec. Stramo. Staph. Sulp. Verat. or Zinc.

——— If there is deep melancholy, give Ars. Auru. Lach. Nux V. or Sulp.

——— If the patient is gloomy and silent, use Ignat. Cocc. Lyc. Puls. or Sulp.

——— If it is an impaired state of mind, caused by religious excitement, Auru. Bell. Lach. Puls. or Sulp. are most appropriate.

——— Should there be a disposition to commit suicide, give Ars. Bell. Hyosc. Puls. Scill. or Auru.

——— Should there be an inclination to rove about, Bell. Hyosc. or Stramo.

——— If there is anger and inclination to curse and swear, give Hyosc. or Bell. or Stramo.

If there is rage, give Bell. Hyosc. Verat. or Stramo.

See Emotions, for other peculiarities.

MIND AND MEMORY.

MIND AND MEMORY.—This furnishes another variety of an impaired condition of the mind to those of alienation, melancholy, and those states of the mind mentioned under emotions; they all appear to be more or less connected together in the symptoms exhibited.

——— do. Anxiety, excessive. The remedies for this state are Sepi. Stramo. Sulp. ac. Thuy. or Verat.

——— Cheerfulness. Sabad. Sec. C. Spig. Staph. Stramo. Tarax. or Thuy.

——— Desponding. Sep. Thuy. or Zinc.

——— Fanciful and Visionary. Cann. Ind. Rhodod. Stron. Stramo. Sulp. or Tarax.

——— Imbecility. The remedies are Acon. Arnic. Anacard. Ars. Auru. Camp. Hyosc. Ignat. Kreoso. Nitr. ac. Nux V. Opi. Petrol. Plati. Puls. Phytol. Plumb. Acet. Rus. Rad. Rus. Tox. Sec. C. Seneg. Sep. Silec. Staph. Stramo. Sol. Nig. or Sulp. ac.

——— Gloomy. Sabad. See Emotions and Melancholia.

——— Loss of. Agnu. C. Angust. Ars. Baryt. Hyosc. Kali. C. Lach. Ignat. Opi. Phos. Plati. Rus. Rad. Silec. Stramo. Sulp. ac. Tart. Anti. Thuy. or Verat. or Caust.

——— Sad. Sep. Stann. Staph. Stramo. Sulp. Thuy. or Verat. or Caust.

——— Thinking and talking faculty, loss of. Sec. C. Silec. Staph. Stron. Sulp.

——— Wild and morose. Ran. Bulb. Sang. Verat.

MERCURY—DISEASES FROM IT.

Mercury.—Within the present century this article has been brought into use much more extensively than it was at any former period. It was found to produce very searching and influential operations on the body; it was thought to have a specific power to overcome and eradicate diseases; and as it proved capable of producing a diseased action on the system, peculiar to itself, it was resorted to as a counteracting agent to raise up a new train of action, by which, on the plan of using counteracting agents for the cure of diseases, it would probably suspend the existing diseased action, regulate the secretions, and bring about a favorable state of health. For these or some other reasons, within the last half century, this drug has become very generally and extensively used. However salutary and useful *mercury* may have been when moderately and judiciously used in some cases, the free and excessive manner in which it has been employed, has no doubt produced great injury on the body, and the means of ruining many constitutions. This drug is not used at all by Homœopathic practitioners in *doses to produce a purgative effect, nor to bring about a salivation, neither to effect what is termed a mercurial action on the system.* By the Homœopathists it is only used in an attenuated form, or in infitismal doses. By its effects it is shown that in many instances it leaves a train of diseases on the body, which marks well its contaminating deleterious effects; these furnish a great number of cases for Homœpathic practitioners to detect, prescribe for, and to cure.

It is the morbid consequences of this drug, and the remedies for them, that will be considered here.

There are some medicines which experience has shown to be very salutary to relieve and cure those diseases.

The remedies are Angust. Auru. Ars. Carbo. V. Hep. Lyc. Mezere. Nitr. ac. and Sulp. or Kali. Iod.

——— Its effects on the bones, attended with nodes, pain, tenderness, and caries, give Angust. Kali. Iod. Mezere. Nitr. ac.

——— Mouth and throat sore, and painful from it. Arg. N. Caust. Ignat. Kali. Bic. Mezere. Nitr. ac. or Sulp.

——— Salivation. To check it, use Baryt. Bromi. Calc. C. Ephorb. Nitr. ac. or Sulp.

Hahnemann directs the body to be bathed in warm water and acid.

For chronic lingering cases of disease derived from it, the proper course will be to use some one of the remedies herein named, in small, highly attenuated doses, a long time, by which the patient will be very much relieved or cured.

The reader may consult to advantage the article Mercury, in *Jhar's Symptomen Codex.*

The opinions of two distinguished members of the profession on this subject are introduced here:—

As the injudicious use of mercury has been mentioned in this place, we think proper to refer to some eminent opinions on that subject. For many years before his demise, Dr. Hosack, as he often expressed it, abstained from its use as a common remedy in fevers and diseases. In remarking on the common and rather promiscuous use of mercury in diseases of the liver, he said, that it produced more liver diseases than it cured.

The following remarks are stated as being a part of a lecture, given by Professor Chapman, of Philadelphia, extracted from the *Homœopathic Examiner*, vol. iii. page 124:—

"Gentlemen, if you could see what I see—persons in the very last stage of wretched existence, emaciated to a skeleton—with the skull almost perforated—the nose half gone—rotten jaws—ulcerated throat—breath more pestiferous than the poisonous Upas—limbs racked with pain—mind imbecile—a disgusting spectacle to others—you would exclaim, as I often have done, O! the lamentable want of science, that dictates the abuse of that noxious thing Calomel, in the Southern States—what merit do gentlemen flatter themselves they possess by being able to salivate a patient. Cannot the veriest fool in Christendom salivate; give calomel? But I will ask another question—Who is it that can stop the career of Mercury, after it has taken the reins in its own destructive and ungoverable hands? He who for an ordinary cause, resigns the fate of his patient to Mercury, is a vile enemy to the sick."

MOUTH, DISEASES OF.

MOUTH, DISEASES OF.—Abscess in.—Borax. Merc. Natr. C. Rus. R. Sabi. See Jaws and Gums.

——— Bleeding. Chin. Mag. C. Millefo. Nitr. ac. Nux V. Phos. ac. Staph.

——— Burning or itching in. Colocy. Mag. C. Merc. Merc. Iod. Nitr. ac. Nux V. Phos. ac. Prus. Sp. Rus. Rad. Staph. Sulp. Tart. Anti. Tereb. or Verat.

——— Distorted. Opi. or Verat.

——— Dry or hot. Canth. Nat. M. Plumb. Rus. Rad. Rus. Tox .Sang. Silec. Verba.

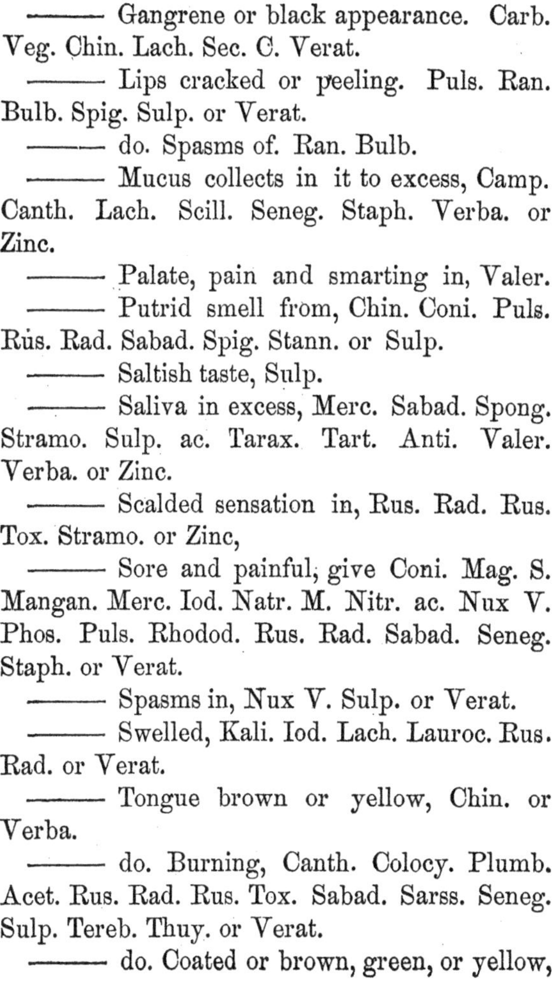

——— Gangrene or black appearance. Carb. Veg. Chin. Lach. Sec. C. Verat.

——— Lips cracked or peeling. Puls. Ran. Bulb. Spig. Sulp. or Verat.

——— do. Spasms of. Ran. Bulb.

——— Mucus collects in it to excess, Camp. Canth. Lach. Scill. Seneg. Staph. Verba. or Zinc.

——— Palate, pain and smarting in, Valer.

——— Putrid smell from, Chin. Coni. Puls. Rus. Rad. Sabad. Spig. Stann. or Sulp.

——— Saltish taste, Sulp.

——— Saliva in excess, Merc. Sabad. Spong. Stramo. Sulp. ac. Tarax. Tart. Anti. Valer. Verba. or Zinc.

——— Scalded sensation in, Rus. Rad. Rus. Tox. Stramo. or Zinc,

——— Sore and painful, give Coni. Mag. S. Mangan. Merc. Iod. Natr. M. Nitr. ac. Nux V. Phos. Puls. Rhodod. Rus. Rad. Sabad. Seneg. Staph. or Verat.

——— Spasms in, Nux V. Sulp. or Verat.

——— Swelled, Kali. Iod. Lach. Lauroc. Rus. Rad. or Verat.

——— Tongue brown or yellow, Chin. or Verba.

——— do. Burning, Canth. Colocy. Plumb. Acet. Rus. Rad. Rus. Tox. Sabad. Sarss. Seneg. Sulp. Tereb. Thuy. or Verat.

——— do. Coated or brown, green, or yellow,

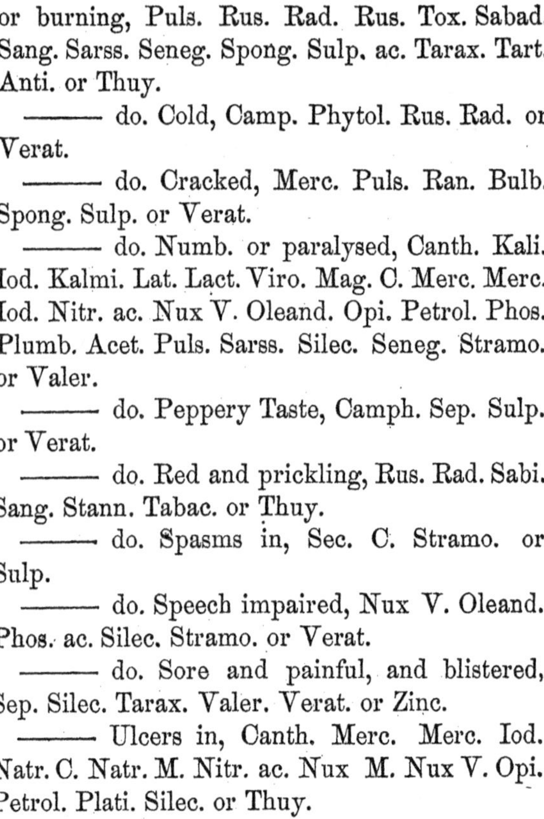

or burning, Puls. Rus. Rad. Rus. Tox. Sabad. Sang. Sarss. Seneg. Spong. Sulp. ac. Tarax. Tart. Anti. or Thuy.

——— do. Cold, Camp. Phytol. Rus. Rad. or Verat.

——— do. Cracked, Merc. Puls. Ran. Bulb. Spong. Sulp. or Verat.

——— do. Numb. or paralysed, Canth. Kali. Iod. Kalmi. Lat. Lact. Viro. Mag. C. Merc. Merc. Iod. Nitr. ac. Nux V. Oleand. Opi. Petrol. Phos. Plumb. Acet. Puls. Sarss. Silec. Seneg. Stramo. or Valer.

——— do. Peppery Taste, Camph. Sep. Sulp. or Verat.

——— do. Red and prickling, Rus. Rad. Sabi. Sang. Stann. Tabac. or Thuy.

——— do. Spasms in, Sec. C. Stramo. or Sulp.

——— do. Speech impaired, Nux V. Oleand. Phos. ac. Silec. Stramo. or Verat.

——— do. Sore and painful, and blistered, Sep. Silec. Tarax. Valer. Verat. or Zinc.

——— Ulcers in, Canth. Merc. Merc. Iod. Natr. C. Natr. M. Nitr. ac. Nux M. Nux V. Opi. Petrol. Plati. Silec. or Thuy.

——— Watery drooling, Natr. M. Plumb. Rus. Tox. Sabad. or Silec.

MUCUS MEMBRANES.

Mucus Membranes. This portion of the body which forms the lining or covering of the internal surface of most or all the cavities and tubes of the system, such as the bronchial tubes of the lungs, the internal surface of the alimentary canal, the urethra of the male and the vagina of females, are subject to diseases, which at first are generally of an inflammatory nature, either acute or chronic; the acute form requires remedies for the cure of this variety of disease generally, such as Acon. Ipe. Tart. Anti. or Cann. S. Nux V. or Spong.

For the chronic kind, Ars. Auru. Baryt. M. Canth. Bals. Cop. Merc. Nitr. ac. Iodide of Merc. Puls. or Sulp.

MORBUS NIGER.

Morbus Niger. A black disease, or black death, as it has been called. This condition of disease sometimes takes place in the progress of violent malignant cases; it is the effect of previous violent inflammatory action, or deep congestion of the system; when it does occur, the remedies for it are, Ars. Carbo. Veg. Carbo. Ani. China., Quinine. or Sec. C. and Wine or Porter.

In the 14th century, there was an epidemic of a malignant type spread over Europe, attended with great fatality, in which the patient turned brown or black during life, and after death putrefaction took place very rapidly ; this was called the *black death epidemic.*

In the description of this disease, it is represented to have been attended with "violent inflammation; the brain was affected and delirium attended—a burning thirst with a hot pestiferous breath; abscesses and diseased glands took place; there was decomposition of the blood, and sudden death." From this short description, it is shown to have been a very highly inflammatory disease, and that the blackness was the result of the blood being deprived of vital air, and a process of decomposition suddenly taking place.

This condition has more or less taken place in more modern epidemics.

NAUSEA AND VOMITING.

Nausea and Vomiting. This disease appears under a variety of forms, either as a primary affection, or connected with other diseases; there is a great number of remedies useful for it; among them may be enumerated, Acon. Anisi. Arg. N. Bell. Calc. C. Camp. Caust. Coni. Hyosc. Ipe. Mosch. Morph. Nitr. ac. Nux V. Phos.

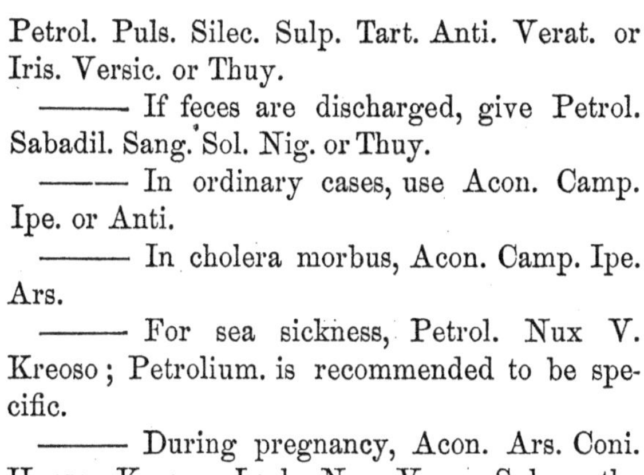

Petrol. Puls. Silec. Sulp. Tart. Anti. Verat. or Iris. Versic. or Thuy.

——— If feces are discharged, give Petrol. Sabadil. Sang. Sol. Nig. or Thuy.

——— In ordinary cases, use Acon. Camp. Ipe. or Anti.

——— In cholera morbus, Acon. Camp. Ipe. Ars.

——— For sea sickness, Petrol. Nux V. Kreoso; Petrolium. is recommended to be specific.

——— During pregnancy, Acon. Ars. Coni. Hyosc. Kreoso. Lach. Nux V. or Sulp.; the other medicine will also be useful in many cases.

NEURALGIA.

Neuralgia. The remedies most useful for this painful disease are, Acon. Agar. Anacard. Asa. F. Caust. Camp. Cham. Colocy. Ferr. Iris. Vers. Guaco. Mosch. Nitr. ac. Nux V. Petrol. Phytol. Plati. Phos. Puls. Rus. R. Rus. T. Stramo. Sulp. Thuy. or Verat.

——— When the face is affected, (as in Tic Doloreux) give Acon. Bell. Caust. Phos. Staphy. or Veratrum. or Nux V.—Cream, mixed with a little Veratrum, and used as a lotion on the affected part, is very efficacious to quiet pain; Colocy has been very effectual in some cases.

——— When the digestive organs are dis-

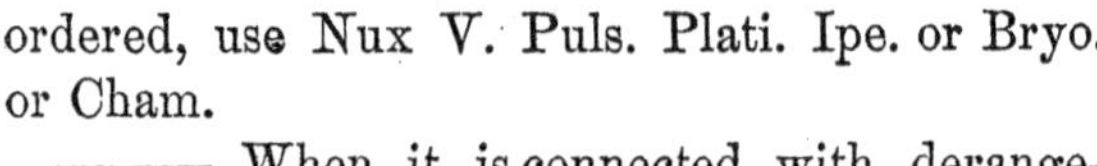

ordered, use Nux V. Puls. Plati. Ipe. or Bryo. or Cham.

——— When it is connected with derangement of the womb, give Nux V. Puls. Plati. China. Ignat. or Sepi.

——— If it is influenced by worms, give Spig. Bell. Cina. Ferr. Graph. or Sulp.

——— If rheumatism accompanies it, use Acon. Bryo. Rus. T. Merc. Phos. Puls. Nux V. Lach. or Rus. T.

——— In gouty subjects, give Nux V. Rus. T. or Caust. Merc. or Colch. or Colocy.

——— When there is an inflammation of the part with fever, give Acon. Bell. Bryo. or Merc. Staphy. or Verat. or Thuy.

——— Should it be from the effects of mercury, give Auru. Hep. Bell. Nitr. ac. or Sulp.

——— If it is connected with Mumps, or disease of the parotid glands, Acon. Bell. Puls. Merc. Mezere. or Silec.

——— In young persons of full habit, use Acon. Bell. Phos. or Lach.

——— In persons of a nervous irritable habit, give Bell. Lach. Spig. Nux V. Ignat. or Verat.

For other nervous affections, consult Spasms.

NECK STIFF, AND WRY NECK.

Neck Stiff, and Wry Neck. The neck is liable to become stiff, so that it is very painful to move it, or to move the head; this is produced by several causes. It is often connected with common colds, when the parts of the throat and the muscles of the neck are inflamed; in such cases, the remedies adapted to the cure of the cold will be proper for the neck.

It may be produced by sprains or wrenches; in such cases, give Arnica. and apply externally a lotion of diluted Tincture of Arnica. to the neck.

It frequently is a rheumatic state of disease; then the remedies pointed out for that complaint will be proper.

WRY NECK.

Wry Neck. This commonly is a sudden stitch or pain of the part, of the nature of nervous cramps; during the attack, the neck is often almost immovable; the head is frequently turned to one side. The remedies for it are Lycopodrium, Nux V. or Ether, or Phosph.

NIGHT-MARE.

Night-mare. This well known disease sometimes takes place in a distressing form, when remedies are required for it; those most useful are Ammo. C. Agar. Ambr. Asa. F. Puls. Sulp. Sulp. ac. or Thuy.

NIGHT SWEATING.

NIGHT SWEATING. To check this excessive and weakening discharge, give Phos. Sambu. Sang. Silec. Sulp. ac. or Ferr.

NOSE.

NOSE. This organ is subject to a variety of diseases, which are here detailed with the appropriate remedies for them.

——— Bleeding, Acon. Bell. Kali. Iodi. Millefo. Merc. Mosch. Muri. ac. Nitr. ac. Phos. Spong. or Thuy. (See Hæmorrhage.)

——— *Bleeding* and burning condition, Petrol. Phos. Plumb. Puls. Rus. R. Sabad. Sang. or Caust.

——— *Bleeding* and mucus discharge, Sepi. Silec. Sulp. or Ammo. M.

——— Cancer on, or in it, Ars. Calend. (See Cancer, in its alphabetical place.)

——— *Caries* of the bones of—Ars. Angust. Arnic. Calc. Merc. Phos. Silec. Sulp. or Verat.

——— *Coryza*, (Catarrh so called.) The remedies most useful are Alum, Ammo. C. Ars. Caust. Coni. Euphorb. Hep. Ignat. Iodi. Kreoso. Kali. Bic. Calc. Iod. of Merc. Mezere. Petrol. Puls. Sabad. Spong. Staph. Sulp. Tart. Anti. Thuy. or Zinc.

——— *Coryza* dry, Ignat. Lyc. Lauroc. Nux

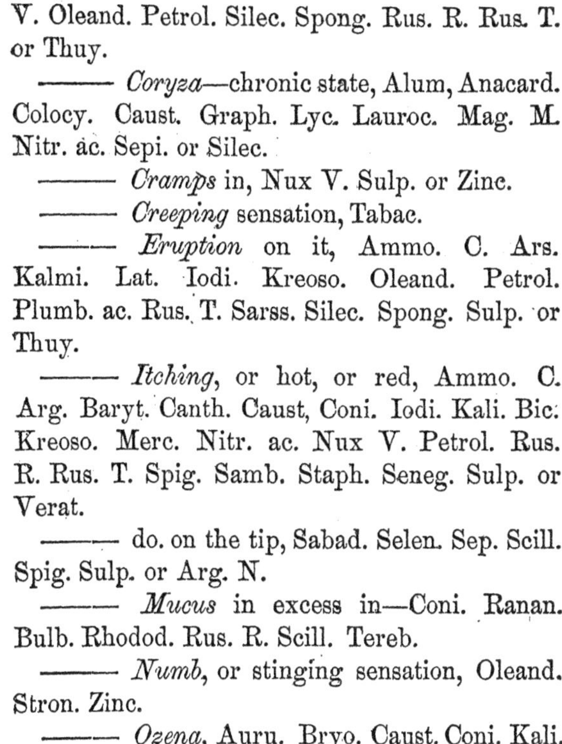

V. Oleand. Petrol. Silec. Spong. Rus. R. Rus. T. or Thuy.

——— *Coryza*—chronic state, Alum, Anacard. Colocy. Caust. Graph. Lyc. Lauroc. Mag. M. Nitr. ac. Sepi. or Silec.

——— *Cramps* in, Nux V. Sulp. or Zinc.

——— *Creeping* sensation, Tabac.

——— *Eruption* on it, Ammo. C. Ars. Kalmi. Lat. Iodi. Kreoso. Oleand. Petrol. Plumb. ac. Rus. T. Sarss. Silec. Spong. Sulp. or Thuy.

——— *Itching*, or hot, or red, Ammo. C. Arg. Baryt. Canth. Caust, Coni. Iodi. Kali. Bic. Kreoso. Merc. Nitr. ac. Nux V. Petrol. Rus. R. Rus. T. Spig. Samb. Staph. Seneg. Sulp. or Verat.

——— do. on the tip, Sabad. Selen. Sep. Scill. Spig. Sulp. or Arg. N.

——— *Mucus* in excess in—Coni. Ranan. Bulb. Rhodod. Rus. R. Scill. Tereb.

——— *Numb*, or stinging sensation, Oleand. Stron. Zinc.

——— *Ozena*, Auru. Bryo. Caust. Coni. Kali. Bic. Kali. C. Kreoso. Lach. Lyc. Muri. ac. Nux V. Phos. ac. Puls. or Rus. T.

NOSE. (Ozena.)

Nose. For ulcers in the nose, or a green discharge from it—give Ars. Auru. Scill. Sep. Silec. Sulp. Tart. An. or Thuy.

——— *Obstructed*, Sabi. Silec. Spig. Staph. or Tereb.

——— *Red* from intemperance, Ars. Carb. Anima. Canth. Caps. Caust. Hep. Kali. Iod. Merc. Mezere. Nux V. or Verat.

——— *Pain* in it, Coni. Nitr. ac. Petrol. Puls. Sang. Selen. Seneg. Silec. Spong. or Zinc.

——— *Polypus* in—Arnic. Calc. Coni. Staph. Nitr. ac. Phos. Sep. Silec. or Seneg.

——— *Scurf* on—Thuy. Sulp. or Caust.

——— *Smell* acute, Sabad.

——— do. *Horrid* sensation in—Coni. Plumb. Acet. Rhodod. Seneg. or Sep.

——— do. Loss of—Arg. Auru. Arnic. Caust. Coni. Kali. Bic. Kali. Iod. Plati. Sep. Sulp. Zinc. or Garlic or Sabad.

——— *Snuffling*, Sep. Sabad. or Dulcam.

——— *Sneezing* to excess, Anacard. Ars. Canth. Mosch. Nitr. ac. Oleand. Phos. Rus. Rad. Rus. Tox. Sabad. Stramo. Sulp. Tabac. Tart. Anti. Thuy. or Zinc.

——— *Sore* or *Smarting* in, Staph. or Rus. T.

——— *Swelling* or itching, Arg. Arnic. Ars. Auru. Bell. Caust. Hep. Kali. Iod. Kreoso. Nux V. Rus. Tox. Scill. Sepi. or Zinc.

——— *Syphilitic* affection, Mezere. Merc. Nitr. ac. (See Syphilis.)

——— *Tingling* sensation in, Nitr. ac. Ol. Anima.

——— *Tittillation*, Seneg. Spig. Sulp.

——— *Tip cold*, or pricking in, Sarss. Silec. Sulp.

——— *Vesicles* on or in, Sec. C. Spig. Tereb. or Zinc.

ŒDEMA.

Œdema.—This affection is noticed under Dropsy, by the term Anasarca.

OSTOITIS. Inflammation of the Bones.

Ostoitis.—The bones or the membranes immediately connected with them, may become inflamed and very painful. This affection may lead to or terminate in caries. The remedies in the early stage are Acon. Bell. Bryo., and cold applications to the part, calculated to check the inflammatory disease. In the progress of the case, it will be beneficial to give Angust. Asa. F. Auru. Colocy. Hep. Merc. Silec. or Nitric. ac. or Sepi.

OVERHEATING. Coup de Soleil, (*termed Sun Struck.*)

Overheating.—When this condition is produced, and prostration or fainting takes place in consequence of sudden or excessive heat of the sun. It is advisable not to drink cold water until sometime has elapsed; then it may be given in small quantities; wet the hands and feet with cold water, also the head. Give Acon. at once, or Bryo. Ipe. or Anti. To counteract congestion of the brain, which is likely to take place, use Bell. Cocc. or Opi.

If nausea or vomiting occurs, Silecia gives relief, or use Ipe. or Anti.

If the patient revives and regains his faculties, he should be kept quiet, placed in a cool place, and some of those remedies to aid reaction of the powers of the system, and to prevent an increase of fever, should be given.

PAIN.

PAIN.—The great variety of pain, its frequent occurrence, and the various parts of the body liable to be affected with it, renders it important to arrange a list of those cases, with the remedies suitable for them, in the following manner:—

——— Of the Anus. Give Aloe. Ignat. Lobelia. Lauroc. Merc. Nux V. Rus. T. Sulp. or Thuy. (See Hæmorrhoids.)

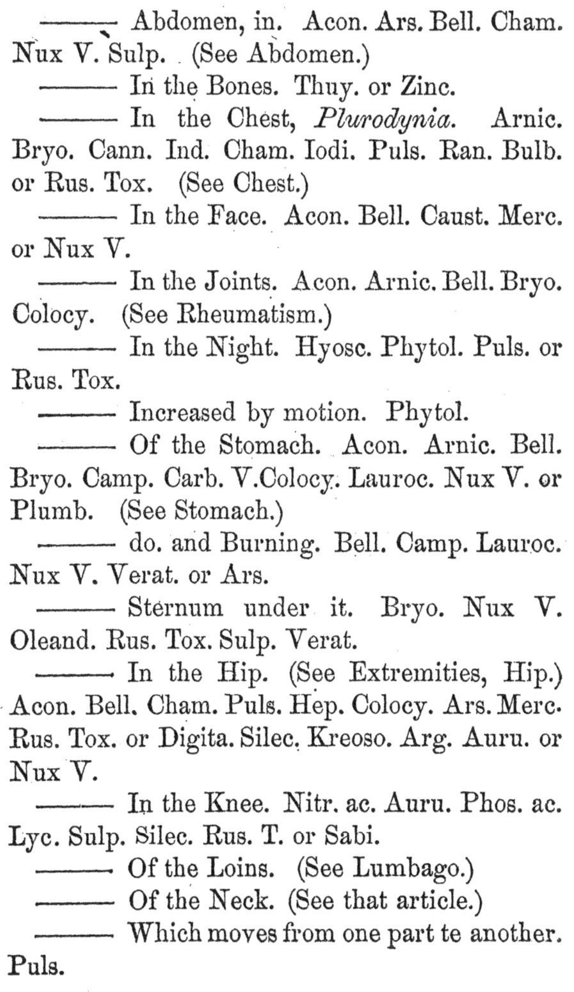

——— Abdomen, in. Acon. Ars. Bell. Cham. Nux V. Sulp. (See Abdomen.)

——— In the Bones. Thuy. or Zinc.

——— In the Chest, *Plurodynia.* Arnic. Bryo. Cann. Ind. Cham. Iodi. Puls. Ran. Bulb. or Rus. Tox. (See Chest.)

——— In the Face. Acon. Bell. Caust. Merc. or Nux V.

——— In the Joints. Acon. Arnic. Bell. Bryo. Colocy. (See Rheumatism.)

——— In the Night. Hyosc. Phytol. Puls. or Rus. Tox.

——— Increased by motion. Phytol.

——— Of the Stomach. Acon. Arnic. Bell. Bryo. Camp. Carb. V. Colocy. Lauroc. Nux V. or Plumb. (See Stomach.)

——— do. and Burning. Bell. Camp. Lauroc. Nux V. Verat. or Ars.

——— Sternum under it. Bryo. Nux V. Oleand. Rus. Tox. Sulp. Verat.

——— In the Hip. (See Extremities, Hip.) Acon. Bell. Cham. Puls. Hep. Colocy. Ars. Merc. Rus. Tox. or Digita. Silec. Kreoso. Arg. Auru. or Nux V.

——— In the Knee. Nitr. ac. Auru. Phos. ac. Lyc. Sulp. Silec. Rus. T. or Sabi.

——— Of the Loins. (See Lumbago.)

——— Of the Neck. (See that article.)

——— Which moves from one part te another. Puls.

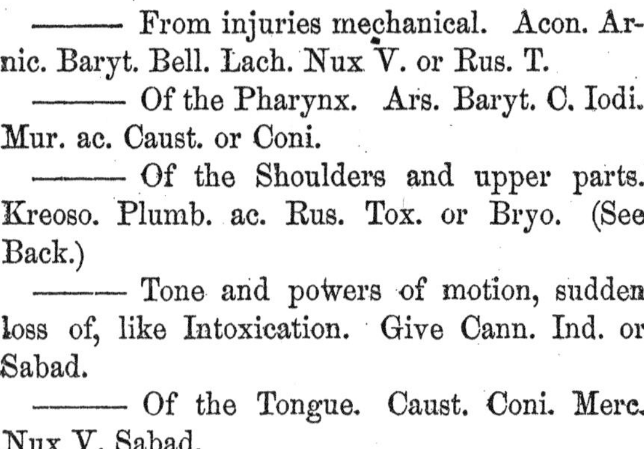

——— From injuries mechanical. Acon. Arnic. Baryt. Bell. Lach. Nux V. or Rus. T.

——— Of the Pharynx. Ars. Baryt. C. Iodi. Mur. ac. Caust. or Coni.

——— Of the Shoulders and upper parts. Kreoso. Plumb. ac. Rus. Tox. or Bryo. (See Back.)

——— Tone and powers of motion, sudden loss of, like Intoxication. Give Cann. Ind. or Sabad.

——— Of the Tongue. Caust. Coni. Merc. Nux V. Sabad.

PALATE.

PALATE.—The palate or uvula frequently becomes inflamed or elongated from colds or some other cause. When this is the case, it produces a tickling or irritation on the tongue, and an unpleasant condition of the parts. It is frequently recommended and practised in such cases to cut off a piece of it, but this is an unadvisable and unnecessary course to pursue.

It may generally be relieved by giving Nux V. or Bell., two or three doses in twenty-four hours. If these do not afford relief, use Merc. or Calca. Sulp. or Dolicho. By these means followed up, the affection will, in short time, be removed, and the patient cured.

PALSY.

PALSY.—This disease is described by authors as a loss of the muscular powers, and an inability to use the limb or part affected. It is frequently attended with numbness of the part or diminished sensation.

The remedies which are most useful for this affection, and generally recommended, are Ambr. Ammo. C. Ammo. M. Arnic. Ars. Bell. Bryo. Caust. Kreoso. Kali. Iod. Hyosc. Lach. Lyc. Merc. Mosch. Nux V. Oleand. Plati. Plumb. Rus. T. Silec. Stram. or Sulp. or Cinebar.

The following is a general mode in which they should be used, according to the conditions of the case.

When the disease is brought on, or is the effect of apoplexy, we refer to this article for a detail of the treatment.

——— If it is connected with, or owing to, Rheumatism, give Arnic. Bryo. Colichi. Rus. T. Lyc. Silec. or Sulp. (See Rheumatism, for further detail.)

——— Should the affection proceed from general debility or succeed any exhausting sickness, give Chin. Ferr. Baryt. C. Nux V. Kali. Iod. Plumb. or Sulp.

——— If it proceeds from, or is caused by suppressed cutaneous eruptions, use Lach. Sulp. or Hep. Kali. Iod. or Rus. Tox. or Puls.

—— If it is produced by the effect of lead, as is sometimes the case in painters, give Opi. Bell. Plati. or Alum. Bell. Puls. Nux V. or Sulp. or Castile Soap. (See Colic, from Lead.)

—— Hemiplegia. A case of this kind of palsy came under our treatment sometime since, which we think of importance enough to relate here.

Mrs. S., aged about fifty years, of spare frame, was suddenly seized, and at once completely paralyzed in the left side, and was nearly speechless. The foot was almost insensible to touch or pinching. We gave her Nux V., by which, in a short time, the speech returned; some other remdies were used without a perceptible benefit, when she took Rus. Tox. Mother Tincture, one drop twice a day, which was increased a drop day until fifty drops were given at a dose. In a few days she began to improve; she felt a prickling sensation, and had twitches in the limbs, and soon began to move the arm; there came feeling and warmth in the foot and leg; the limb was rubbed with a hot solution of salæratus, and cloths wet in it were wrapped around it. This was all that was applied externally, and she gradually improved from day to day till she used the hand, and walked the room at the end of fifty days; then the medicine was diminished one drop a day until it run out, when she had fully recovered and walked the street. (We refer to *Jhar's Symptomen Codex*, article Rus. Tox., for this authority for using Rus.)

——— Of the Anus Sphincter. Aloe. Hyosc. Rus. Tox. or Nux V.

——— Of the Muscles of the Face. Caust. Kali. Iodi. or Nux V.

——— Of the hands or feet. Ars. Bovista. Ferr. Kreoso. Plumb. Rus. T. Sabad. Silec. or Thuy.

There does not seem to be much benefit derived in paralytic cases by the external use of exciting or other remedies; the host of those recommended and used, frequently produces much inconvenience, and may do injury. If it is recollected, that in cases of general palsy, the origin of the disease is in the brain or at some large nerve, it will appear unlikely that irritating the extreme points of the nerves at the skin can be of much use. The remedies which are likely to be useful and effect a cure, must be given internally.

Hahnemann disapproves of the use of external exciting remedies; he also condemns the use of electricity, and says it may give some temporary relief at first, but exhausts the nervous energy, and thus proves injurious in the end. If it is used at all, it should be in a mild manner.

PAMPHIGUS.

Pamphigus.—A kind of fungus excrescence raising up on the skin. The remedies for it are Asa. F. Auru. Bell. Coni. Graph. Hep. Iodi. Merc. Rus. T. or Sulp. or Caust.

PLICA POLONICA.

Plica Polonica.—This is a disease which affects the inhabitants of Poland and some others of the North of Europe; the hair of the head becomes adherent or plaited together, produced by some morbid gummy secretion, which exudes from the scalp.

The remedies found useful for it are such as are used for scald head; to wit, Calc. C. Nitr. ac. Nux V. Petrol. Podoph. P. Rus. T. Sepi. Sulp. or Thuy.

The hair should be cut off close, and the skin washed and cleansed with soap and water, and such dressings applied to it as are used for scald head.

PURPURA RUBRA.

Purpura Rubra.—This affection is considered a modification of cutaneous disease, somewhat similar to scarlatina. The skin is represented to exhibit a brownish or purple appearance. The remedies are Acon. Bell. Dulcam. Iodi.

In the *American Journal of Homœopathy*, No. 3, p. 391, it is stated that Spirits of Turpentine is a specific remedy for it.

PYROSES—Commonly called Heartburn.

Pyroses.—It is an unpleasant and sometimes a painful affection. There is a burning sensation at the stomach, somewhat similar to those of eructation, and the effects are much the same.

The remedies for it are Calc. C. Morph. Nitr. ac. Nux V. Petrol., and the medicine for eructations.

RHEUMATISM.

Rheumatism. This troublesome and painful disease which affects the limbs, the joints, and more or less all parts of the body, is produced by various causes, and appears under different circumstances. It is well known, and its effects are so visible, that a detailed description of it seems to be unnecessary. It is generally divided into acute and chronic rheumatism, but the line of distinction cannot easily be drawn.

The most advisable method of treating the acute form will be here detailed. The remedies are, Acon. Ars. Bell. Bryo. Cann. Ind. Colch. Hyosc. Ipe. Kali. C. Kali. Iod. Kalmi. L. Nitr. ac. Phos. Podoph. P. Puls. Ranan. Bulb. Rus. T. Sang. Stramo. or Tart. Anti.

——— In the first stage, when there is fever, pain, swelling, or inflammation of some parts, Acon. is the best medicine; give three or four drops of the 2d to the 6th dilution, every three to six hours; or give a grain of the 2d or 3d trituration at a dose. If there is shooting pains at night, or the part is red and swelled, give Bell.

In continued pain, with moderate fever increased on motion, if Acon. or Rell. does not check it, give Bryo. Puls. or Hyosc.; when there is a numbness or cramps in the part, use Nux V.

If the pain is deep seated, give Kali. Iod. or Merc.

If the pain is changing from one place to another, use Camp. Puls. or Kalmi. L.

When there is torpor, numbness, or trembling, worse when still, Rus. T.

If the pain is dragging, or burning, or lancinating, Ars. is proper.

When the stomach is deranged, use Colch. or Nux V. The other remedies may be selected if these fail, and they should be used in accordance with the symptoms compared with their properties, as shown in pure Materia Medica.

When the pain seizes a part, and suddenly

leaves it and fixes on another part, give Puls. or Acon. or Tart. Ant. or one of these latter may be used to advantage, alternated with Puls.

In the acute or inflammatory stage, apply cold water freely to the painful part; cloths wet in ice cold water are the most useful; to this may be added to advantage, a little acetate of lead, Muriate of Ammonia, or tincture of Arnica.; leave the pained part to the open air as much as may be convenient.

This course has been pursued in a great number of cases, and for years, with decided advantage; generally in a short time it may be expected that a cure will be effected.

——— *Chronic.* In many cases it will be difficult to distinguish this kind from the preceding; the points of difference mostly relied on, are, that in the acute rheumatism, there is swelling and severe pain in the part; the skin is red, there is fever; and these symptoms are frequently quite severe, though in this variety at times, there is not much fever, pain, or sickness. In the chronic rheumatism, the case is more protracted; it continues worse and better a length of time, without much swelling or fever: the part sometimes is numb, or partially deprived of usefulness.

The same remedies frequently are useful in each form; those most useful in the chronic or protracted kind, are, Ars. Auru. Bryo. Cann.

Ind. Caust. Colch. Colocy. Kali. Iod. Kreoso. Lyc. Merc. Nux V. Phytol. Puls. Sabi. Stramo. Sulp. Thuy. or Verat.

The directions given for selecting a proper remedy on page 10, should be observed here, as well as in other cases.

If the pain runs about and changes from one part to another, or runs upward, give Arg. N. Asa. F. or Caust. Lyc. Puls. Thuy. or Verat.

When the pain is fixed in a joint, give Acon. Bryo. Bell. Rus. T. Tart. Anti. Ars. Lobel. Sulp. or Arg. N.

If the upper extremities are the seat of the pain, use Acon. Bryo. Lyc. Puls. or Rus. T.

If the pain is worse at night than in the day time, give Hyosc. Stron. or Bell.

If gout is connected with it, see Gout.

RHEUMATISM, LUMBAGO.

Rheumatism, Lumbago. The remedies which prove most useful for this painful disease are, if there is fever, use Acon. Bryo. or Ipe.; when there is not fever, use Iodi. Kali. Bic. Kali. Iod. Kreoso. Lach. Merc. Phytol. Prun. Sp. Rus. R. Rus. T. Sabad. Staphy. Sulp. Tabac. Verat. or Zinc.

——— If the skin is inclined to be cold, or has an itching on it, give Ammo. C. Arg. N. Bell. Bryo. Ipe. Iodi. or Prun. Sp.

——— If the parts are stiff and rigid, give

Carb. Ani. Camp. Ipe. Lach. Led. P. Phytol. Silec. or Staphy.

——— If there is numbness with the pain, or it appears to be connected with a syphilitic contamination, give Kalmi. L. Merc. Mezere. Nitr. ac. Petrol. or Podophy.

——— If the pains are increased by a chill, give Acon. Bryo. Dulcam. Merc. or Sulp.

——— Should it be brought on, or increased by stormy weather, use Rus. T. Dulcam. or Lyc. or Verat.

When any change of the weather brings on an attack, guard the system by taking Calcara. Silec. Sulp. or Lach. or Rus. T.; or if the pain sets in at the time, one of these medicines will be the proper remedy to take.

It will be observed that external remedies are not recommended here, except cold water, and articles combined with it to reduce fever and inflammation; but if there should be a rigid stiff state of the affected part in the advanced stage, some mild emollient or softening remedies would be proper and useful. But the multitude of exciting and stimulating articles recommended and used for the cure of this disease are generally of very little use, and experience proves, that they frequently have a tendency to aggravate the pain.

When Homœopathic treatment is pursued, all those articles are inadmissible. In this as well as in other difficult diseases, it will be well to run over the list of medicines named in a Materia Medica, to see which corresponds best with the case, and then fix on that.

RICKETS.

RICKETS. This disease commonly affects young children. The indications of it arė, a large developemeut of the head, a prominent forehead, the breast bone is full and prominent, the ribs flattened, the abdomen is enlarged; there is emaciation, and a state of languor and debility; as the case advances the muscles become flaccid, the skin pale, the bones distorted, curved, and deformed, attended with a slow fever and poor appetite.

The most useful remedies are Asa. F. Bell. Calc. C. Colocy. Iodi. Merc. Sol. Nitr. ac. Silec. or Sulp. (See Cachexia.)

RING-WORM.

RING-WORM. This is a species of Herpes; the remedies for it are Ars. Graph. Merc. Rus. T. Sep. or Sulp. (See Herpes.)

RISUS SARDONICUS. SARDONIAN OR INVOLUNTARY LAUGHTER.

RISUS SARDONI US.—The remedies for it are Ranan. Bulbosa. This affection is nearly allied to Chorea, which is placed under Spasms. (See Spasms.)

SALT RHEUM.

Salt Rheum.—For this inveterate and troublesome disease, the most useful remedies are Ars. Hep. Petrol. Thuy. or Sulp. Hep. is allowed to be the most certain. (See Herpes.)

SCALD HEAD. Tinea Capitis.

Scald Head.—This well known disease is also called *Dow Worm*. Some one of the following medicines will be capable of effecting a cure; they should be continued a long time. Ars. Baryt. Calc. C. Carb. V. Graph. Hep. Kreoso. Lyc. Merc. Oleand. Petrol. Psorinum. Rus. T. or Sulp. (See Herpes.) Apply to the scalp Citron Ointment or solution of Nitrate of Silver, or Muriate of Mercury, and wash and cleanse it every day.

SCIRRHUS.

Scirrhus.—The most appropriate remedies for this disease are Bell. Calendula, Conium. Sep. Silec. or Ars. (See Glands, Cancer, &c.)

SCIATICA.

SCIATICA is defined by surgical and other writers a disease of the sciatic nerve at the hip joints, partaking of an inflammatory, neuralgic nature. The pain is often very severe, sometimes it extends to the knee and foot—it differs from the disease of the *Hip Joint proper*, *so called*, which is an inflammatory affection of the ligaments and parts about the joint. That disease may and does at times partake of a scrofulous or rheumatic character. This is more confined to the nerves. The remedies most suitable for Sciatica, are Acon, Bell. Cham. Ignat. Nux V. or Ars. Colocy. or Rus. T.

When there is considerable fever, give Acon. or Bell.

If there is dragging or burning pain in the joint, Ars. will be a proper remedy.

If the pain is most severe in the night, with irritability of temper, and it is irregular, use Cham. or Ignat.

If the pain is more severe towards morning, with a stiff paralysed feeling, Nux V.

If the pain increases towards evening, or when the patient is still, Puls. or Rus. T.

When the pain is aggravated by anger, or there is an irrascible temper, Colocy. or Hyosc.

If the pain is more severe when the patient is at rest, Rus. Tox. or Puls.

For the other symptoms of the part, examine Rheumatism, Scrofula, and Hip Joint disease, for other remedies which may useful.

SCALP.

Scalp. The scalp or skin of the head is subject to a variety of diseases and pains, somewhat peculiar to it, which are thus arranged.

——— Pain and soreness in it, use Lach. Lauroc. Led. P. Muri. ac. Nux V. Petrol. Ranan. B. Spig. Sulp. Verat. Valera. or Caust.

——— do. in the bones, Auru. or Nitr. ac.

——— do. in the front part, Staphy. Sulp. Sulp. ac. or Verat.

——— Creeping or itching in it, Caust.

——— Hair falling off. (See this article in its place.)

——— Paralyzed numb feeling, Coni. Lach. Petrol.

——— Very sensitive, use Lach. Sabi. Sarss. Selen. Spig. Spong. Sulp. Sulp. ac. or Zinc.

——— Spasms in, Nitr. ac. Phos. ac. or Nux V. (See Neuralgia.)

——— Tingling sensation, Nitr. ac. Petrol. Phos. ac. Rus. Tox. or Sulp.

——— Tumors on, give Petrol. Silec. or Sulp.

——— Ulcers or abscesses on, Ars. Coni. Sep. Sulp. ac. or Zinc. will be among the most useful remedies.

SCROFULA.

Scrofula. This disease is an impaired state of the system, arising from a peculiar morbid condition; it is described as an affection of the glands in different parts of the body, particularly those of the neck, under the chin, behind the ears, and in other parts, such as the mesenteric glands; there is impaired digestion. They become hard, enlarged, and form indolent tumors, not very painful, but slow in their progress. If not arrested, they proceed on to suppuration, when an indolent ulcer is formed, which discharges a thin serous whitish whey-like matter. The general health is impaired, attended with a feeble, enervated state of body, the skin is pale and flabby. This disease sometimes locates on the joints, producing a tedious disease, rather difficult to cure, frequently destroying the joint.

The most advisable remedies for it, are Ars. Auru. Bell. Baryt. Calc. C. Caust. Coni. Ferr. Iodi. Kreoso. Merc. Muri. ac. Nitr. ac. Phosphate of Iron; this latter medicine in many cases is efficacious; or Silec. Spong. or Sulp.

When there is a scrofulous constitution, by a long continued use of some one or more of these medicines, in small or highly attenuated doses, a cure may generally be effected, or the case will be very much benefited.

If the joints or bones are diseased, Sulp. ac.

Calc. or Silec. or Iodide of Mercury, or Auru. or Phos. will be very useful. It will be of service to examine other diseases which may have aided in bringing on the complaint, or which are connected with it.

——— Bones diseased; when this is the case, give Asa. F. Auru. Carb. Veg. Ferr. Phos. Silec. Lyc. Merc. Mezere. or Silec. are the useful remedies.

——— Ulcers. When the diseased part proceeds to ulceration, it is generally advisable to dress the ulcer with exciting stimulating articles, and such as communicate oxygen to them, and to continue the internal use of the medicine; much depends on this. One of the best remedies to use to raise up a healthy action in these ulcers, is the Oxalis Acetosella (wood sorrel.) It should be gathered when green and fresh, pound it till a pulpy mass is formed, then mix with it an equal quantity or more of Indian or oat meal. It is best to moisten it with sour milk or whey; in this form of a poultice, apply it to the ulcer; it soon causes so much excitement and pain, that it will be necessary to add more meal to it. The ulcer soon changes the flabby livid appearance to a more florid healthy color.

It was the opinion of Dr. Bedoes, that by the use of this article, Oxygen was directly communicated to the ulcer.

This article has been used in some parts of the

country by the people for such indolent ulcers with much success.

The sorrel may be gathered when fresh, and formed into an electuary, so as to retain its properties for use at periods and places when the fresh herb cannot be had.

SCURVY.

SCURVY.—This disease is distinguished by debility, pale and bloated countenance, œdemateous state of the inferior extremities, livid spots on the skin, foul ulcers, bleeding from the part, offensive urine, fœtid stools, the gums are spongy, and bleed easily.

The most useful remedies for it are Ammo. Muri. Caust. Carbo. Veg. Nitr. ac. or Sulp. or Ars., together with a free use of vegetables and vegetable acids.

SEA SICKNESS.

SEA SICKNESS.—For this troublesome and distressing disease, the following remedies are recommended, Ars. Cocc. Kreoso. Nux V. Versico. Petrol. The latter medicine has obtained considerable reputation to check or cure this affection.

SKIN.

SKIN.—There are a large class of diseases which affect the skin; many of them are noticed under Herpes, and there are many others, such as the following:—

Skin, blotches on. Silec. Sulp. ac. Tabac. Tarax. or Tart. Anti.

——— do. Gangrenous. Use Carb. Veg. Lach. Sec. C.

——— Blue spots on or lead color. Lach. Nux M. Plumb. Acet. Sec. C. Sulp. ac. Thuy. or Verat.

——— Boils. To prevent or cure them, give Led. P. Lyc. Mag. C. Mur. ac. Nitr. ac. Nux V. Phos. Phos. ac. Phytol. Puls. Rata. Sec. C. Silec. Staph. Stramo. Sulp. Thuy. or Zinc. These remedies are the proper ones.

——— Burning excrescences on. Ars. Coni. Mosch. Morph. Mur. ac. Nitr. ac. Oleand. Petrol. Phos. Phytol. Puls. Rus. Rad. Sabad. Sarss. Sec. C. Sol. Nig. or Staph.

——— Cold or smarting sensation of. Use Auru. Baryt. Borax. Camp. Caust. Ipe. Iodi. Lauroc. Merc. Oleand. or Tart. Anti.

——— Icy sensation of. Tart. Anti. Verat. or Zinc.

——— Creeping sensation. Phos. ac. Sabad. Scill. Sec. C. Spong. Stramo. or Sulp. ac.

——— Dry, rough, or chapped situation.

Natr. C. Nitr. ac. Nux M. Petrol. Plumb. Acet. Sabad. Sang. Sec. C. Sulp. or Tart. Anti.

——— Ecchymosis. Sec. C. Sulp. ac. Thuy.

——— Eruptions, fine on. Caust. Merc. Natr. C. Nitr. ac. Oleand. Phos. Ran. Rulb. Rus. Rad. Rus. Tox. Sabad. Sang. Selen. Sep. Silec. Spong. Staph. Stramo. Sulp. Tarax. or Zinc.

——— Hot or Itching, or Red Rash. Kali. Iod. Kalmi. Lat. Lyc. Morph. Merc. Viv. Oleand. Ol. Anima. Phos. ac. Puls. Rus. Rad. Sarss. Sep. Sulp. ac. Tereb. or Verba.

——— Exanthemata or Vesicles on. Kreoso. Lach. Led. P. Merc. Mur. ac. Nux M. Oleand. Ox. ac. Phos. ac. Phytol. Plumb. Acet. Puls. Ran. Bulb. Sang. Sarss. Staph. Sulp. Tart. Anti. Tereb. Thuy. or Zinc. or Ars.

——— Itching or pain. Agar. Alum. Arg. Ars. Baryt. Caust. Coni. Iodi. Kalmi. Lat. Iodi. Led. P. Lyc. Mag. S. Morph. Nitr. ac. Nux V. Nux Jug. Phos. Plati. Ran. Bulb. Rus. Tox. Sang. Selen. Stann. Sulp. or Verat.

——— do. great. Silec. Spong. Staph. Sulp. ac. Tart. Anti. or Zinc., or the above medicine.

——— Itching and Inflamed. Use Acon. Ammo. C. Ammo. M. Anacard. Arg. N. Canth. Caust. Colocy. Kali. Bic. Kali. Iod. Kalmi. Lat. Merc. Nitr. ac. Nux V. Oleand. Phos. Plati. Rus. Rad. Rus. Tox. Sabad. or Scill.

——— do. In various parts. Scill. Spong. Stramo. Sulp. Tarax. Thuy. or Verat.

——— Numb sensation. Oleand. Opi. Petrol. Sabad.

——— Petechia. Sec. C. or Sulp.

——— Pustules and Vesicles, or spots on. Give Rus. Rad. Rus. Tox. Sep. Sol. Nig. Stramo. Sulp. Thuy. or Tereb. or Ars.

——— Pricking sensation in—use Rus. Tox. Sulp. ac.

——— Sensitive, Morph. Oleand. Phos. Podoph. P. Rus. Rad. Sec. C. Silec. Thuy. or Zinc. or Caust.

——— Shingles, (Zona,) ther emedies for this are, Acon. Bell. Graph. Merc. Puls. Rus. Rad. Rus. Tox. or Silec. (See Erysipelas.)

——— Soft, to make it so, Podoph. P.

——— Spots on, red, or nettle rash, Bell. Coni. Rus. Rad. Rus. Tox. Sabad. Sang. Sulp. Sulp. ac. Tereb. Verat. or Zinc. (See Herpes.)

——— do. Yellow, Sep. or Stramo.

——— Sweating to excess, Sol. Nig. Stramo. Sulp. ac. Tarax. Tart. Anti. or Tereb.

——— Tumors gangrenous, Carb. V. Sec. C. Scill. or Sulp. ac.

——— do. on vertex, painful, Morph. Phytol. Plati. Rus. Rad. or Zinc.

——— Urticaria, Led. Pelust.

——— Vesicles on, give Caust.

SLEEP.

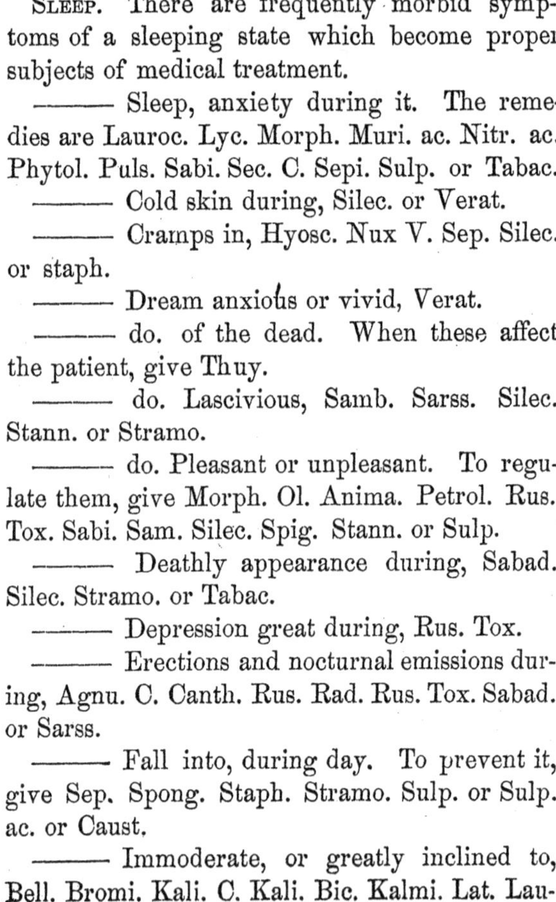

Sleep. There are frequently morbid symptoms of a sleeping state which become proper subjects of medical treatment.

——— Sleep, anxiety during it. The remedies are Lauroc. Lyc. Morph. Muri. ac. Nitr. ac. Phytol. Puls. Sabi. Sec. C. Sepi. Sulp. or Tabac.

——— Cold skin during, Silec. or Verat.

——— Cramps in, Hyosc. Nux V. Sep. Silec. or staph.

——— Dream anxious or vivid, Verat.

——— do. of the dead. When these affect the patient, give Thuy.

——— do. Lascivious, Samb. Sarss. Silec. Stann. or Stramo.

——— do. Pleasant or unpleasant. To regulate them, give Morph. Ol. Anima. Petrol. Rus. Tox. Sabi. Sam. Silec. Spig. Stann. or Sulp.

——— Deathly appearance during, Sabad. Silec. Stramo. or Tabac.

——— Depression great during, Rus. Tox.

——— Erections and nocturnal emissions during, Agnu. C. Canth. Rus. Rad. Rus. Tox. Sabad. or Sarss.

——— Fall into, during day. To prevent it, give Sep. Spong. Staph. Stramo. Sulp. or Sulp. ac. or Caust.

——— Immoderate, or greatly inclined to, Bell. Bromi. Kali. C. Kali. Bic. Kalmi. Lat. Lau-

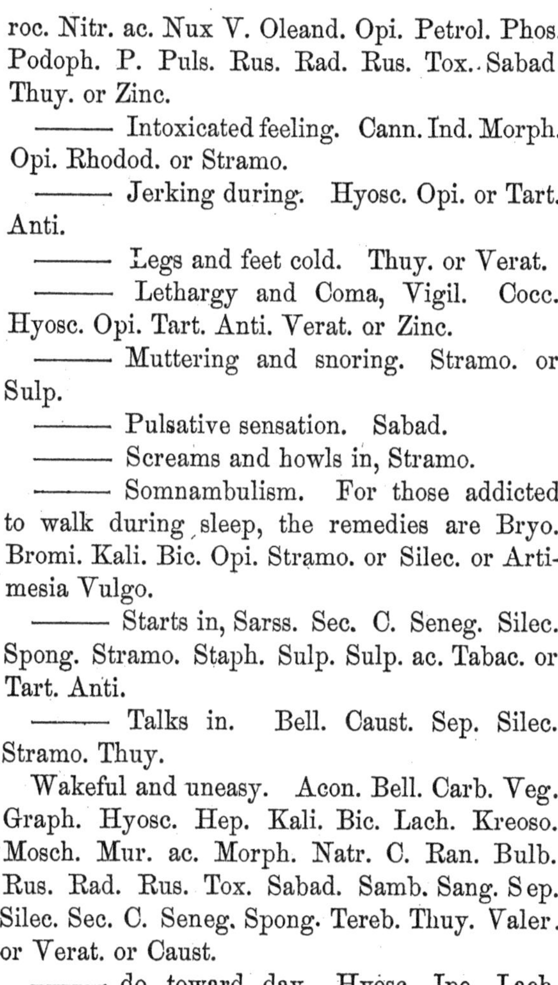

roc. Nitr. ac. Nux V. Oleand. Opi. Petrol. Phos. Podoph. P. Puls. Rus. Rad. Rus. Tox. Sabad. Thuy. or Zinc.

——— Intoxicated feeling. Cann. Ind. Morph. Opi. Rhodod. or Stramo.

——— Jerking during. Hyosc. Opi. or Tart. Anti.

——— Legs and feet cold. Thuy. or Verat.

——— Lethargy and Coma, Vigil. Cocc. Hyosc. Opi. Tart. Anti. Verat. or Zinc.

——— Muttering and snoring. Stramo. or Sulp.

——— Pulsative sensation. Sabad.

——— Screams and howls in, Stramo.

——— Somnambulism. For those addicted to walk during sleep, the remedies are Bryo. Bromi. Kali. Bic. Opi. Stramo. or Silec. or Artimesia Vulgo.

——— Starts in, Sarss. Sec. C. Seneg. Silec. Spong. Stramo. Staph. Sulp. Sulp. ac. Tabac. or Tart. Anti.

——— Talks in. Bell. Caust. Sep. Silec. Stramo. Thuy.

Wakeful and uneasy. Acon. Bell. Carb. Veg. Graph. Hyosc. Hep. Kali. Bic. Lach. Kreoso. Mosch. Mur. ac. Morph. Natr. C. Ran. Bulb. Rus. Rad. Rus. Tox. Sabad. Samb. Sang. Sep. Silec. Sec. C. Seneg. Spong. Tereb. Thuy. Valer. or Verat. or Caust.

——— do. toward day. Hyosc. Ipe. Lach.

Lyc. Merc. C. Mag. M. Mur. ac. Nux V. Opi. Mur. ac. Ox. ac. Rus. Tox. Sabad. Sep. Silec. Spig. Staph. Thuy.

——— Weeping in. Thuy.

——— Yawning in. Rus. R. Rus. T. Sabad. Sang. Sec. C. Seneg. Sepi. Silec. Spig. Spong. Stann. Staphy. Sulp. ac. Tabac. Tart. A. Valler. or Verat. or Caust.

SMALL POX. (Variolus.)

Small Pox. The serious character of this disease is pretty well known; it is considered the most contagious of any one in the catalogue of morbid affections. It commences with the general symptoms of inflammatory fever, attended with a chill, high fever, headache, pain in the back and limbs, skin hot, thirst great, pressure at the stomach, nausea, eyes sensitive to the light, mind impaired, prostration of strength; this stage continues about three days, when the eruption begins to appear; first, on the face, then on the body.

It cannot be fully determined whether the case is small pox or not until the eruption appears; when it shows itself, the fever and pain considerably abate; this has been considered a very tedious, loathsome, and dangerous disease, and there have been good grounds for such an opinion.

After the pustules appear, they pass on increasing in size, to about the ninth day, when they arrive to their maturity, containing purulent watery fluid or lymph; then they begin to turn brown; first on the face, and continue to do so over other parts of the body; they generally dry, and if the patient does well, the scabs begin to peel off, and a gradual recovery ensues.

When the case is very severe and the progress unfavorable, the fever is high, stupor and delirium take place, congestion of the brain forms, and a typhoid state comes on, the scabs or surface turn brown or black, and from the eleventh to the fifteenth day, the patient probably dies.

Treatment during the febrile or promonitory stage; the treatment should be active, and such as that for inflammatory fever; give Acon. Bell. Ipe. Anti. or Camp.

In addition to these medicines, a valuable antidotal preventive has been discovered and introduced as a remedy, which promises much to mitigate this disease, and remove from it a great portion of its danger and malignancy.

We take occasion to mention for this purpose, the VARIOLIN. The antidotal properties of this article were discovered by experience; it is based entirely upon the Homœopathic mode of ascertaining the properties of drugs, and the law of cure on which they are founded.

We proceed to give an account of the remedy and its effects, as we have had an opportunity of using it. It appears that this medicine given early in the case has the property of neutralizing or correcting the virus of the disease in the system, so as to check the progress of the disease.

Sometimes the case stops short, in a manner so that the pustules do not fill, or if they progress, they are in a manner moderately sore and painful, and small in size; therefore, as soon as the case is suspected or ascertained to be Varioloid or *Small Pox*, then begin to give this remedy; at the time omit the use of all other medicines. The dose proper to give is about one or two grains of the 2d trituration, or three or four drops of the second dilution; the dose at first should be repeated every three or four hours; some Homœopathic practitioners may prefer giving much higher attenuations, and at much longer intervals, but these are such as we have used and found to answer the purpose.

After about forty-eight hours, the time of giving the doses had better be lengthened to about six hours; the remedy should be continued until the eruption is checked, and it begins to flattten, and turn brown on the face; then, or soon after, it may as well be discontinued, for it may now be inferred that the antidotal effects have been introduced; the flattening of the pustules, or a check to their enlarging, often takes place by the fifth or sixth day, then, of course, they do not fill with lymph, but dry and shrink up, and prepare for peeling off; sometimes, however, the disease continues until the eighth or ninth day, when lymph forms, but the patient has very little pain, fever, or suffering during the time.

In the first stage of this disease, there should be caution used in giving hot or stimulating articles to bring or drive out the eruption, as it is termed, for it is an old maxim well established, that the eruption and severity of the disease will be very much in proportion to the mildness or inflammatory premonitory symptoms; thus attempting to drive out the eruption by such heating means is an error, and a remnant of former opinions long since exploded.

The patient should be kept moderately cool, and allowed to drink cold water, to gargle the throat, and to have it applied to the eyes.

If there should be severe symptoms during the use of the Variolin, some suitable medicine may be given for them; for instance, if there is much fever, use Acon. or Ipe. If there is headache or flushed face, Bell.; but these remedies are seldom needed.

If the Variolin cannot be obtained, the Vaccina may be used in lieu of it, with very good effect and great advantage.

In March, 1852, we read a paper before the Hahnemann Academy of Medicine on Small Pox, in which attention was directed to the Variolin,

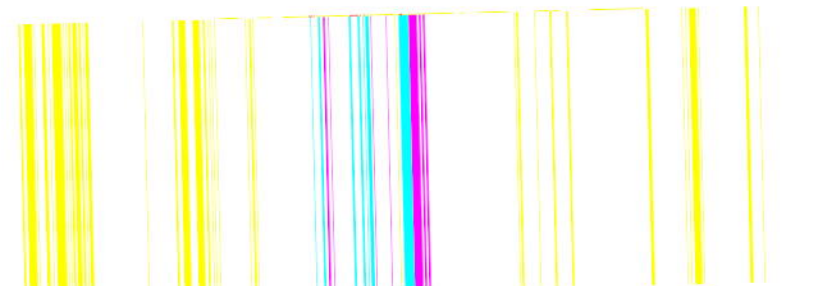

as an antidotal remedy for it. In that paper, several cases were related.

The Academy at the time passed this resolution:—

"That the thanks of the Academy be tendered to Dr. Sherrill, for the interesting and valuable paper read; and that a copy of it be requested, to file among the archives of the Academy."

An outline of one case, it is presumed, is worthy of a place here.

In January 6, 1852, Miss M., aged sixteen years, had not been vaccinated. After being very sick with fever, pain, &c. on the fourth day, she broke out with Small Pox; the eruption was very thick, and it soon became confluent on the face. On the third day of the eruption, the face and eyes were swelled so that she was blind; became delirious; was restless; hoarse, and had sore throat, and was seized with a severe stricture of the chest.

After considerable pains, we procured some Variolin; this was given her in this manner—a dose of about the first dilution every three hours. All other medicines were left off, except cold water, as a drink. In twelve hours, she was quite calm; the delirium had subsided, and in twenty-four hours the fever was gone; had very little thirst; pain allayed; pustules on the face drying. In about two days more, the pustules on the face began to flatten and turn brown; they continued to recede and dry up. About the twelfth day, they began to scale off, and she regularly improved to a recovery. It was a gratifying circumstance to observe that the face was very slightly pitted, although it was covered with a general scab. This has been the result in all the other cases.

In a former edition of this work, several cases of Small Pox are recorded, which was treated by the use of Vaccina; the success in them was complete. Since the time mentioned of treating the preceding case, about forty cases of Varioloid and Small Pox have come under our care; about an equal number of each. The treatment above detailed has regularly been pursued in all of them. Whenever the remedies have been used early, and fully continued, the patients have recovered.

In several cases of children who have had the disease, and who took the medicine early, were not much in bed, but continued up and about the room. The pustules sometimes recedes and dries away by five or six days.

The other Homœopathic remedies for this disease are Rus. T. Stramo. Sulp. or Merc. Nux V. Puls. Zinc. or Ars.

If there arise secondary symptoms of œdematous swellings, give Ars. Baryt., and such other medicines as are placed under Dropsy for Anasarca.

There is a prospect that the Variolin may be useful, that is, as a profylactic agent to protect the system against an attack of Small Pox when exposed to its virus, on a similar principle and plan, by which Belladonna prevents the Scarlet Fever. For this purpose, a grain of the second trituration, given once a day, appears to have the effect of guarding the person against an attack. In several families, where Small Pox prevailed, by taking those powders not one real case of Small Pox has come to appearance.

As far as we know, the case here related is the first that was treated in this city in the manner detailed above. There was an imperfect account published, that the Variolin had been used by some of the Homœopathic physicians of Germany, which furnished a hint that it might answer a useful purpose here.

To Dr. Sherrill:

Sir—I here give you the result of the action of the Variolin you kindly furnished me, and a short account of the case. Mrs. Mariott, aged thirty-four years, had severe symptoms peculiar to small pox; an eruption came out, which proved to be the worst kind of that disease, of a confluent form. I treated her six days in the usual way, when the face and eyes were swelled so much that she was blind. One scab covered the whole face; she was in a state of stupor; very uneasy and feverish. The case seemed most likely to prove fatal, when you called my attention to the Variolin. I gave one grain of the second trituration every three hours; the eruption matured well; she soon became calm; the fever left her; the swelling of the face subsided; the desquamation regularly took place; she had no secondary fever, and passed readily on to recovery. The face is but slightly pitted or disfigured.

Yours, respectfully,

HENRY S. FIRTH, M. D.

April 1, 1854.

SPASMS. SPASMI.

SPASMS.—There are a large number of diseases which pervade the body, and are attended with convulsive or spasmodic action. It would be a difficult task to explain their nature and point out the remote or proximate cause of them. Much has been written respecting them, explanatory of their nature, founded partly on facts and partly on hypothesis, without arriving at a very satisfactory explanation of their pathological nature.

The attempt made here will be merely to notice

the varieties of the symptoms, and point out the most useful remedies for them.

Spasm is defined "a sudden and more or less violent but brief contraction of one or more muscles or muscular fibres. Spasm is either chronic or tonic. In chronic spasms, the muscles contract and relax in quick succession, (as in convulsions.) In tonic spasms, the muscles contract in a steady and uniform manner, and remain contracted in a regular and comparatively long time."—*Webster.*

The general remedies for them are Acon. Anacard. Arg. N. Arnic. Ars. Bell. Cann. Ind. Calend. Camp. Chin. Cocc. Cicuta. Colocy. Coni. Hyosc. Ignat. Iodi. Kali. Iod. Kreoso. Lauroc. Merc. Mosch. Morph. Nux V. Opi. Phos. Prus. ac. Rus. T. Silec. Stramo. Strong. or Verat.

——— If they take place in consequence of mechanical injury, the preferable remedies are Arnic. Iòdi. Hyosc. Opi. or Mosch., with the treatment detailed under Injuries Mechanical, which see.

——— Agitation. If this condition occurs without general disease, give Acon. Arg. Nitr. Bell. Cann. Ind. Lach. Mosch. Nux V. Stramo. or Staph.

——— Chronic cases. When the patient has been a long time subject to spasmodic affection or fits, as it is termed, the remedies found the most useful are Ars. Ammo. C. Arg. Nitr. Cham. Canth. Cupr. or Stramo. or Colocynth.

——— Convulsions. This seems to be a general name used for spasmodic attacks, more so when they take place in infants and children. The remedies are the same as for spasms generally, such as Agar. Acon. Ammo. C. Cham. Cupr. Hell. Ignat. Kreoso. Merc. Nux V. Opi. Puls. Sabad. Sec. C. Silec. or Sol. Nig. These are to be used according to the symptoms presented. For information on this subject, reference is made to Emotions and to Neuralgia.

CATALEPSY.

Catalepsy.—This happens to be a rare disease, though when it does occur, it is a serious affection. When this work was about thus far printed, the work of Dr. Frilegh came into our hands. We take leave and pleasure to gather some aid from it in relation to this disease. In this it is described thus: "It is a sudden suspension of motion and sensation, the body remaining in the same position that it was in when seized." In the course of our experience, the following case came under our observation: An unmarried female, of about twenty-six years of age, was suddenly seized; she was motionless and insensible; the spells or fits lasted fifteen or twenty minutes, or even eight or ten hours, when she came to, and remained quiet awhile. Afterwards she had another attack; the breathing was slow and labored; the pulse was very little changed; the limbs could be placed in any manner, and there they would rigidly remain; the body could be easily raised to any position, and there it would firmly continue; it might be elevated to an angle of forty-five degrees; when there it stationary continued. These positions could be changed by an assistant.

The remedies recommended for this disease, are Acon. Arg. Nitr. Bell. Cham. Cann. Ind. Nux V. Stramo. or Ferr., or some others may be useful, which are named for spasms.

In the case above mentioned, after using a number of remedies without much effect, the patient was depleted, and put on the use of Argent. Nitr. In a short time she got well.

If there is hippocratic countenance, give Cham.

If there is a full flushed face, Bell. or Hyosc.

If the patient has a sunken, deathly appearance, Lauroc. Asa. F.

If the patient has fits of passions or anger, Hyosc. Hell. Stramo.

Should it be caused by disappointed love, Hyosc. Ignat. (See Emotions.)

If there is stupor or wildness, Stramo. Staphy.

If there is a continued rigidity, Argent. Nitr. Cann. Ind.

COREA SANITA VITA. ST. VITUS' DANCE.

COREA SANITA VITA.—This disease is described as an irregular action of the limbs; sometimes there are convulsive motions, though it is generally of an involuntary movement, without convulsive action; it affects one or both sides indiscriminately; sometimes it is attended with pain, though generally there is very little pain attending it; sometimes the patient is feeble and dejected; at other times they are not so, but tolerably cheerful.

The remedies are Asa. F. Ars. Caust. Chin. Cocc. Cupr. Hyosc. Ignat. Rus. T. Stramo. or Sulp. or Argent. Nit.

In treatment, we have observed the best results from Ars. and Cuprum.

If there is debility, Chin. or Ferr.

If it occurs at the age of puberty, Puls. Sabi. or Ars.

If there is distress of the head or determination of blood to it, Bell. Cocc. or Opi.

If there is eruptions on the skin, or these suppressed, Rus. T.

If there is an impaired mind, with wildness, Hyosc. Stramo. or Cuprum.

If the case partakes of Hysterics, Asa. F. (See Emotions, for other remedies.)

Coffee and Colchicum, in alternation, are stated to have been successful in curing some cases.

In the *North American Homœpathic Journal*, No. ix. p. 81, some cases are reported to have been cured by Artimesa Vulgaris.

ECLAMPSIA RAPHANA. MORBUS CERALIS OR TYPHOIDES.

ECLAMPSIA RAPHANA.—This disease is noticed under fevers; it seems to partake of the character of Typhoid Fever and Spasmodic Affection. It is thus defined:—"A sensation of splendor—brightness, effulgence; a flashing or light scintillation; a sparkling which affects the eyes. Sometimes in Epilepsy or in obstinate cases of Typhoid disease." Hahnemann is of opinion that Sol. Nig. Hyosc. Stramo. or Cupr. Acetis, are the most useful remedies for it, or Plati. or Sec. C. may be used to advantage.

EPILEPSY, EPILEPSIA.

EPILEPSY, EPILEPSIA. This malady consists in spasms of the chronic kind; it comes on in fits; the patient is seized with violent convulsions; a loss of consciousuess and voluntary motion; they generally froth or foam at the mouth; from their falling down quickly, it has obtained the name of FALLING SICKNESS.

A girl of 15, in the hospital, had them in rapid succession; the attendants stated that she had 600 in less than two weeks; she finally recovered. In other instances, there is a fit once a week, or month, or at longer periods.

The medicine mostly indicated, and found useful, are Acon. Agar. Asa. F. Artimes. Astor. Rub. Bell. Cann. Ind. Cupr. Silec. or Phos. ac. Sulp. or Argent. Nitr.

The remedies should be selected and used according to the symptoms presented.

In full plethoric habits, especially if there is a determination to the head, give Acon. Bell. Nux V. Opi. Puls. Sulp. or Verat.

If it is connected with a loss of blood and exhaustion, Chin. Phos. ac. or Calc. C. Millefo. Silec. or Sulp.

Should it arise from worms, Cina. Ferr. Hyosc. Merc. Spig. Stann. or Sulp.

If it is connected with hysterics, Asa. F. Cocc. Ignat. Mosch. Nux V. or Stramo.

If it is caused by intoxicating drinks, give Nux V. Ignat. Cupr. or Cham. See articles Drunkenness and Delirium Tremens.

In other cases, care should be taken to consult the diseases with which they may be connected under the proper heads, such as Emotions, Dyspepsia, Neuralgia, Suppressed Eruptions, &c.

In chronic and protracted cases, Argent. Nit. Cupr. and Ars. are some of the best remedies.

In the *N. A. Journal of Homœopathy*, No. IX.

several cases are related as having been cured by Artimesia Vergaris.

HYSTERIA.

HYSTERIA. This disease is peculiar to females. The symptoms are anxiety, shedding of tears, dyspnoea, nausea, palpitation of the heart, fullness of the chest, rising to the throat as though a ball was raising up, (globus hystericus,) spasms, jaws set, moving and agitation of the body, crying or involuntary laughter, screaming, foaming at the mouth, &c.

The best medicines are Agar. Ambr. Asa. F. Bell. Cocc. Coni. Hyosc. Mosch. Nux V. Phos. Puls. Sepi. Stramo. Verat. Viola. Odorata.

If the attack arises from suppression of the catamenia, Puls. Sepi. Asa. F. Hyosc. or Coni. Sabi. &c.

If from Menorrhagia, Millefo. Hamameli. and other remedies for this affection.

If there is a contraction of the muscles of the jaws and cold skin, Verat. In various conditions, the other remedies will be useful, which may be determined by examining the other nervous affections, and sometimes the pathogenesis of the medicine.

SPEECH AND THE JAWS AFFECTED BY SPASMS.

SPEECH AND JAWS AFFECTED BY SPASMS. Jaws arising and falling involuntarily, Lach. Morph. Opi.

——— Impaired or impeded. Bell. Caust. Euphob. Graph. Merc. Nux V. Stramo. or Verat.

STOMACH.

STOMACH. This part is subject to cramps and spasms; which may be very distressing and become serious. In most cases, one of the best remedies is Nux V.

If it is produced by dyspepsia or from intemperance, use Ignat. Nux. or Ars.

If it is from constipation or a contraction across the stomach, or attended with nausea, Ipe. Anti. or Nux V. or Sulp.

The other remedies useful in such cases, are Hyosc. Iod. Kali. C. Lach. Lauroc. Verat. or Colocy.

TETANUS OR SUBSULTUS.

TETANUS OR SUBSULTUS. This disease is characterized by a rigid contraction of the muscles; there are four varieties of it, named as follows: when the jaws are firmly set, it is termed LOCK-JAW. When the body is bent backward, it is termed Opisthotonos. When the body is bent forward, the name is Emprosthotonos. If the body is bent to one side, Pheurosthotonos.

The remedies found most useful for this affection, are Acon. Anacard. Bell. Camp. Cham. Caust. Hyosc. Ignat. Lauroc. Merc. Mosch. Nux V. Rus. T. Sol. Nig. Stramo. or Verat.

First, endeavour to ascertain and remove the direct cause.

If there is fever, with a flushed full face, give Acon. or Bell.

If it is the effect of mechanical injury, Arnica, and other remedies for such symptoms as may succeed, as Opi. or Hyosc.

If there is a wound, apply Arnica to that.

If there is a great bending of the body, Ignat. Rus. T.

If the stomach is affected, and other severe spasms, Nux V.

If there is agitation or trembling, Lauroc. or Sol. Nig.

If there is wildness or passionate disposition, Hyosc.

The other remedies named, will be useful in some conditions, and worthy of a trial.

STAMMERING.

Stammering.—The medicine best adapted for the cure of this affection are Cann. Ind. Caust.

Lach. Merc. M. Plati. Plumb. Sec. C. Stramo. or Verat.

While using a medicine, care should be taken to reform the practice and endeavor to change the habit of the patient.

STINGS OF BEES OR INSECTS.

Stings.—It is stated that Ledum P. or Guaco. is a specific to cure in such cases. The poison from the stings of insects or scorpions is cured by the same means.—*North American Journal of Homœopathy.*

STOMACH.

Stomach.—This organ is very sensitive to morbid derangement, and subject to a variety of affections. Some of them are treated of under other heads; some others will be noticed here, with the remedies for the symptoms.

——— Burning sensation in. Ambr. Auru. Calc. C. Camp. Caust. Colocy. Hep. Hyosc. Lauroc. Lobel. Mosch. Nux V. Puls. Rus. R. Sabad. or Sulp.

——— do. Horrid sensation. Sabad. Sabi. Silec. Stramo. or Caust. Colocy. or Verat.

——— Cancer of. Ars. Coni. Kreoso. Nux V. Silec. (See Cancer.)

——— Distension of. Give Coni. Caust. Nux V. Petrol. Plati. Sulp. Sulp. ac. or Thuy.

——— Empty sensation. Oleand. Sabad. Sepi. Stramo. Sulp. ac. Verba. or Zinc.

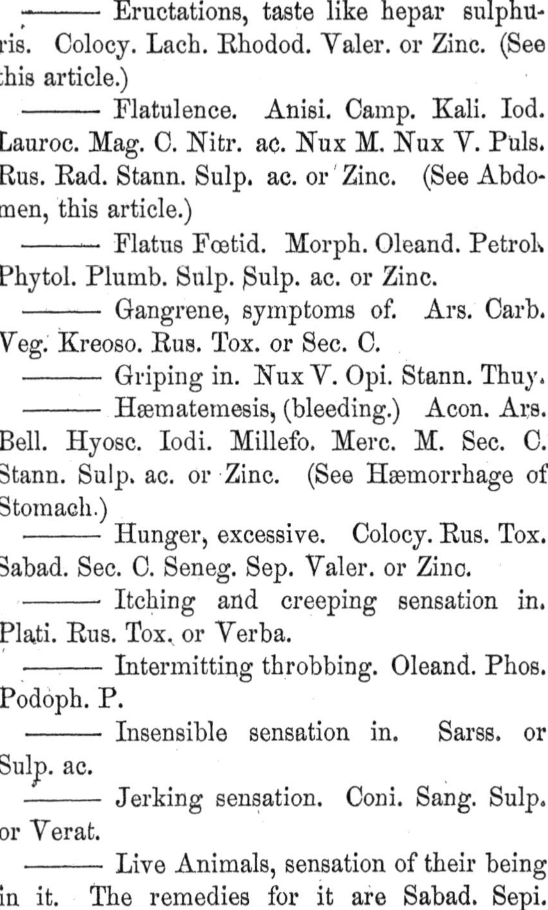

——— Eructations, taste like hepar sulphuris. Colocy. Lach. Rhodod. Valer. or Zinc. (See this article.)

——— Flatulence. Anisi. Camp. Kali. Iod. Lauroc. Mag. C. Nitr. ac. Nux M. Nux V. Puls. Rus. Rad. Stann. Sulp. ac. or Zinc. (See Abdomen, this article.)

——— Flatus Fœtid. Morph. Oleand. Petrol. Phytol. Plumb. Sulp. Sulp. ac. or Zinc.

——— Gangrene, symptoms of. Ars. Carb. Veg. Kreoso. Rus. Tox. or Sec. C.

——— Griping in. Nux V. Opi. Stann. Thuy.

——— Hæmatemesis, (bleeding.) Acon. Ars. Bell. Hyosc. Iodi. Millefo. Merc. M. Sec. C. Stann. Sulp. ac. or Zinc. (See Hæmorrhage of Stomach.)

——— Hunger, excessive. Colocy. Rus. Tox. Sabad. Sec. C. Seneg. Sep. Valer. or Zinc.

——— Itching and creeping sensation in. Plati. Rus. Tox. or Verba.

——— Intermitting throbbing. Oleand. Phos. Podoph. P.

——— Insensible sensation in. Sarss. or Sulp. ac.

——— Jerking sensation. Coni. Sang. Sulp. or Verat.

——— Live Animals, sensation of their being in it. The remedies for it are Sabad. Sepi. Stramo. Sulp. or Thuy.

NAUSEA AND VOMITING. This proceeds from various causes, and appears under different conditions. There are a large number of medicines indicated for it. The most useful ones will be enumerated. Acon. Ammo. C. Chin. Caust. Calc. Camp. Cann. S. Hep. Hyosc. Ipe. Kali. Iod. Lobel. Mag. C. Merc. Nitr. ac. Nux V. Oleand. Phos. Rus. T. Sabad. Silec. Sulp. Sulp. ac. Valer. Verat. or Zinc. (See Nausea and Vomiting.)

——— Nausea and vomiting of black matter, (black vomit.) Ars. Cupr. Carb. V. Guaco. Sec. C. or Verat.

——— Pain and inflammation of the villous coat. Acon. Camp. Coni. Colocy. Plumb. Acet. Puls. Stramo. Stron. Sulp. Tart. Anti. Thuy. or Verat. (See Cholera and Gastralgia.)

——— Paralysed state. Nux V. Puls. Rus. T.

——— Pressure on. Chin. Coni. Mosch. Muri. ac. Phos. ac. Puls. Rus. T. Sabad. Silec. Spong. Sulp. Tereb. Thuy. Verat. or Zinc.

——— Regurgitation. Lach. Nitr. ac. Nux V. Oleand. Rus. T. Tart. or Anti.

——— Rumbling in. Stann. Sulp.

——— Scirrhous or cancerous affection. Ars. Kreoso. Morph. Natr. C. Nitr. ac. Nux Jug. Nux V. or Phos.

——— Sensation like a ball in it. Valer.

——— Sour belching from. Ferr. Mangan.

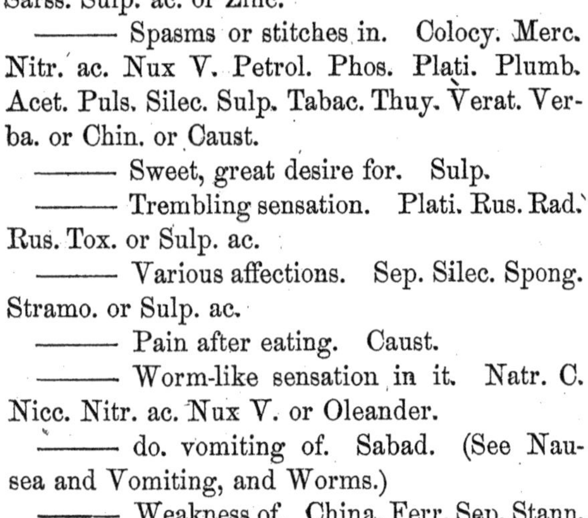

Mosch. Natr. C. Nitr. ac. Oleand. Phodod. Sabad. Sarss. Sulp. ac. or Zinc.

——— Spasms or stitches in. Colocy. Merc. Nitr. ac. Nux V. Petrol. Phos. Plati. Plumb. Acet. Puls. Silec. Sulp. Tabac. Thuy. Verat. Verba. or Chin. or Caust.

——— Sweet, great desire for. Sulp.

——— Trembling sensation. Plati. Rus. Rad. Rus. Tox. or Sulp. ac.

——— Various affections. Sep. Silec. Spong. Stramo. or Sulp. ac.

——— Pain after eating. Caust.

——— Worm-like sensation in it. Natr. C. Nicc. Nitr. ac. Nux V. or Oleander.

——— do. vomiting of. Sabad. (See Nausea and Vomiting, and Worms.)

——— Weakness of. China. Ferr. Sep. Stann. Sulp. ac.

STUPOR.

Stupor. This is a state of insensibility and loss of consciousness. It takes place in a large number of diseases, to wit, in Apoplexy, Drunkenness, Mechanical injury of the Brain, Low and Typhoid states of Fever, &c. It is very similar to Coma, which see. The remedies for it are pointed out under the various affections with which it is connected.

SWEATING.

SWEATING.—There is a constant exhalation from the surface of the body of a fluid in the state of vapor or perspiration, which is essential to health. When this is increased to a considerable extent, it becomes sweating.

In febrile diseases, in the first or active stage, it is of very great importance to produce a free perspiration or sweating, when it can be done by mild unexciting remedies. The treatment generally used has a tendency to increase the perspiration or produce sweating; this commonly takes place at the termination or crisis of a paroxysm of fever.

This discharge from the skin, however, sometimes is so large and excessive as to become a disease, and subject to medical treatment.

When it is the effect of debility from exhausting disease, means to restore the general health and strength will be required, such as Angust. China. Ferr. Quini. Sulp. ac., and good nourishment, &c.

If it is connected with hectic fever, then the remedies for that disease would be proper.

If it is the effect of some general morbid condition of the body, that state will require treatment. The remedies recommended for it are Acon. Bryo. Ipe. Sambu. Sep. Sulp. ac. or Chin.

Ferr. &c. Those remedies which are termed sudorifics, are some of the most useful for it.

In the great Epidemic, sweating sickness, which in Europe prevailed about the year 1484, small and repeated bleedings, and the use of those medicines termed sudorific, proved the most successful treatment.—*Donaldson's History of Epidemics.*

Some of the French writers have compared this Epidemic to that of Epidemic Cholera; in that the serous portion of the blood passed off by the skin, while in Cholera it is discharged by the alimentary canal. Blood drawn in small and repeated quantities, in either case, seemed to correct the morbid state of the blood-vessels and restore the system to a more healthy grade of action, so as to check the evacuations.

——— of the Feet. When this takes place to excess, or in a troublesome manner, the feet should be frequently bathed in warm water; this, if continued, will sometimes effect a cure. It will, also, be very serviceable to use a lotion of a weak solution of Arnica. Iodine. or Rus. Tox. Internally give Silec. Rus. Tox., a few pellets, or a high attenuation of one or the other, every day, or at longer periods. This is considered the best course; but other useful medicines are Baryt. C. Graph. Calca. Merc. or Lyc. Plumb. ac. Carbo. Veg. or Nitr. ac.

It is attended with danger, in such cases to

use much cold bathing or violent astringents to the feet.

SYPHILIS. Lues Venereæ.

Syphilis.—The character of this disease, as it appears, and the mode of treatment merely, will occupy a place here. It is now understood that there are two kinds of venereal affection which considerably differ in their nature: one is known by the term at the head of this article; the other by that of Gonorrhœa. Both of these diseases are communicated by intercourse of a healthy person with one who is affected with either of them; though it does not entirely depend on this manner of infection, as accidental or casual application of the virus to the genitals, or to a sore or raw surface of the skin may produce it.

This variety is described "a morbid poison, which, when applied to the body, has the power of propagating itself and acting both locally and constitutionally." The virus generally first attacks the glans penis of the male, and the labia of the genitals, or parts just within them, of the female. First, a small pimple or rawness occurs, then it spreads and becomes larger. This is termed *Chancre*. From this the virus is carried along the absorbents, or small vessels, to the groin, where it causes irritation and swelling of the glands, and produces a *Bubo*. From here the virus enters the system. This is the most common way; but to this course there are exceptions, though if the disease is not arrested, the system becomes generally affected.

When the chancre is discovered, it is best to apply to it a powder of about one-fourth part of Muriate of Mercury to three-fourths of prepared Chalk, or some other mild substance dusted on, or a little Calomel used in the same way. Some recommend the chancre to be gently touched with Lunar Caustic. By these means the virus may be destroyed, and the sore changed to a healthy condition, so as to heal up.

Internally, give Mercurius Solubus, the first or second trituration, half a grain or a grain, two or three times a day.

Some practitioners use less or higher potencies, but this seems to answer well. By this course the chancre generally soon heals. After using the powder externally two or three days, it may be discontinued, and the sore dressed with a simple ointment. The mercury should be continued until the ulcer is healed, or if it does not heal readily, it may be better to omit the mercury, and give Nitr. ac. Hep. or Sulp., or alternate one of these with the mercury.

BUBO.

Bubo.—If the above treatment does not check or eradicate the virus, the glands in the groin become diseased with inflammation and swelling—forming this disease—then it is an object of much importance to check and disperse the swelling. The mercury should be continued internally, and to allay and arrest the inflammation and swelling, cloths wet in cold water, or a cold solution of Acetate of Lead or Arnica should be applied to the swelled part, or a poultice made with the solution of the above named medicine, may be applied cold.

If there is a good deal of pain in the part, the surface of the poultice should be moistened with Tincture of Belladona or Laudanum.

If, however, the swelling does not subside, and is likely to suppurate, warm poultices should be applied to promote that process, and the mercurial remedies should be continued.

If there appears a flushed redness about the swelling or on the skin, a few doses of Belladona had better be given alternately with the mercury.

If the suppuration is tardy in coming to maturity, the exhibition of Hep. Silec. or Sulp. will hasten the process; also, those medicines will have a favorable effect towards healing the ulcer.

If the gums become sore and spongy, not from

the effect of the mercury, for the quantity given would not be likely to produce such an effect, but from the action of the disease, use Carbo. Veg. or Carbo. Ani.

In protracted cases, much benefit will be derived by giving Nitr. ac. Auru. Staphy. or Sulp. or Cinibar. This latter medicine is highly recommended in the *North American Journal of Homœopathy*. By continuing this course, it is represented by writers that the disease may be generally soon cured.

If it is not cured, and the general system becomes affected, producing a protracted or secondary stage, then constitutional symptoms take place.

There are many cases in which the treatment in the early stage has not fully cured the case and eradicated the virus from the system, when a train of general symptoms are exhibited, such as obstinate spreading ulcers in the groins, from a bubo not being cured, or ulceration of the throat; ulcers and blotches on various parts of the body; also nodes and other diseases of the bones; and frequently an affection of the lungs, inclining to or running into a consumptive disease.

It is admitted by many Allopathic authors, and it is a general opinion of Homœpathic writers that a great deal of the disease and suffering succeeding venereal affection is owing to the large quantity of mercury injudiciously given in the early stage, producing a mercurial poisonous condition of the system. (See Dr. Chapman's opinion, page 261.)

LUES VENEREA.

Lues Venerea.—The following abbreviated outline of a plan of treatment for this state of the disease is collected from medical authors and arranged for this purpose. The remedies recommended are Mercurius Vivus, Mercurius Cor. Sub. Nitric acid, Hepar Sulphuris, Phosphorus, Sulphur, Silecia or Arsen. Carbo. Veg. Lach. or Thuy. They are to be used thus:—

When the sore has a hard base or margin, Mercury is the best remedy; give Merc. Viv., one-fourth of a grain to two grains of the second or third trituration once or twice a day; some practitioners would give much less. Continue this treatment a few days till good pus is formed, when the taking of medicine should be stopped a few days, and then it may be given again.

If granulations do not appear, give three or four doses of Sulphur, the second or third trituration.

If the granulations are flabby and pale, give Nitr. ac.

Should the ulcer remain hard on the edges, irritable, and bleed easily, give Ars.

If there is a good deal of pain and inflammation, after the foregoing remedies have been used, give Acon. and Sulp. in alternation, every ten or twelve hours.

When the ulcer has a raised and rough edge, give Nitr. ac. Hep. S. Sulp. Ars. Silic. or Mercurius in alternation, with one of those preceding.

For a more full and detailed mode of treatment in protracted cases, the reader is recommended to more elaborate Homœopathic treatises on this disease.

Secondary states of the disease: "This form of the disease, so called, generally is the effect of the patients having taken large quantities of mercury, and frequently is more a mercurial disease than one produced by the natural operation of syphilitic virus."

The remedies found best for the various features of this condition of the system are the antidotes for mercurial disease, such as Hep. S. Nitr. ac. Bell. Lach. Sulp. Silec. Thuy. or Ars. Alumina or Lycop. They should be used as directed and indicated under the various heads laid down in this Repertory, under which the diseased state and the symptoms are treated.

SYCOSIS.

SYCOSIS.—The syphilitic disease at times produces this affection; the remedies advised for it are Staphy. Silec. or Thuy.

Warts and excrescences are among the secondary symptoms which form on the skin. The remedy for these is Thuy.

TABES MESENTERICA.

TABES MESENTERICA. The remedies for it, are Ars. Baryt. Caust. Calc. Iodi. Merc. Muria. ac. or Sulph.

This disease is similar to Marasmus, which see.

TEETH.

TEETH. There are a great number of diseases which affect the teeth and gums. A number of them are enumerated here.

——— Black appearance of them. Scill. or Verat.

——— Caries and painful. Use Baryt. Euphorb. Ignat. Lach. Merc. Petrol. Silec. Sulp. or Zinc.

——— Gums, subject to bleeding. Ammo. C. Bell. Carb. V. Colocy. Iodi. Merc. Muri. ac. Nitr. ac. Rus. T. Silec. or Tart. Anti. (See Mouth.)

——— Grating of them. Ferr. Ignat. Plumb. Nux V. Spig. Sabi. or Zinc.

——— Loose or lengthened sensation. Prun. Sp. Natr. C. Nux V. Opi. Phos. Plumb. Sang. or Spong. or Iris. Versico.

——— Odontalgia, (Toothache.) The most useful remedies for it are Acon. Ars. Bell. Coccinell. Hep. Hyosc. Kali. Iod. Lyc. Merc. Iodi. Nux V. Puls. Rus. T. Tart. Anti. Verat, &c.

If there is fever and swelling of the gums, Acon. Bell. Anti.

If there is pain without fever, Ars. Coccin. Hyosc.

If there is throbbing or jerking pain, Kali. Iod. Nux V. or Stramo. or Hyosc. Great relief may be obtained by wetting a little cotton with Tinct. of Bell. Hyosc. or Nux V., and applying it to the pained part. When the saliva should be swallowed, the remedy ought to be diluted with water, so as to consist of one-fourth of tincture.

If there is jerking pain, Sabad.

If there is jerking or beating sensation, Spong. Stann. or Zinc.

THROAT AND FAUCES.

Throat and Fauces. The throat and fauces are subject to a great variety of diseased affections; some of the symptoms are connected with other diseases; others are peculiar to these parts.

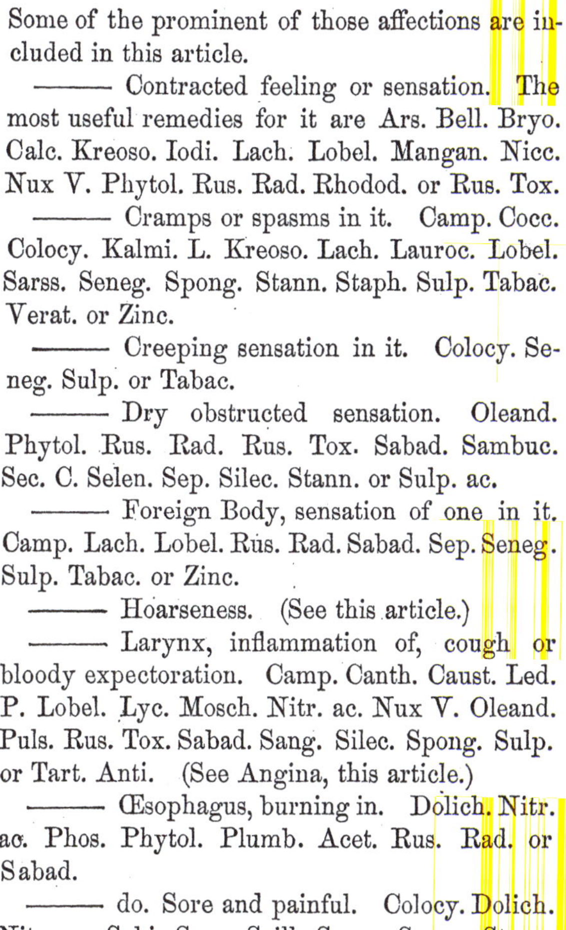

Some of the prominent of those affections are included in this article.

——— Contracted feeling or sensation. The most useful remedies for it are Ars. Bell. Bryo. Calc. Kreoso. Iodi. Lach. Lobel. Mangan. Nicc. Nux V. Phytol. Rus. Rad. Rhodod. or Rus. Tox.

——— Cramps or spasms in it. Camp. Cocc. Colocy. Kalmi. L. Kreoso. Lach. Lauroc. Lobel. Sarss. Seneg. Spong. Stann. Staph. Sulp. Tabac. Verat. or Zinc.

——— Creeping sensation in it. Colocy. Seneg. Sulp. or Tabac.

——— Dry obstructed sensation. Oleand. Phytol. Rus. Rad. Rus. Tox. Sabad. Sambuc. Sec. C. Selen. Sep. Silec. Stann. or Sulp. ac.

——— Foreign Body, sensation of one in it. Camp. Lach. Lobel. Rus. Rad. Sabad. Sep. Seneg. Sulp. Tabac. or Zinc.

——— Hoarseness. (See this article.)

——— Larynx, inflammation of, cough or bloody expectoration. Camp. Canth. Caust. Led. P. Lobel. Lyc. Mosch. Nitr. ac. Nux V. Oleand. Puls. Rus. Tox. Sabad. Sang. Silec. Spong. Sulp. or Tart. Anti. (See Angina, this article.)

——— Œsophagus, burning in. Dolich. Nitr. ac. Phos. Phytol. Plumb. Acet. Rus. Rad. or Sabad.

——— do. Sore and painful. Colocy. Dolich. Nitr. ac. Sabi. Sang. Scill. Seneg. Spong. Stann. Tart. Anti. or Thuy.

——— Pharynx dry with hoarseness. Bromide of Potash, Caust. Lach. Seneg. Sepi. Silec. Spig. Spong. Sulp. ac. Tart. Anti. or Zinc.

——— do. Itching and sore. Colocy. Kali. Iod. Kali. C. Kreoso. Merc. Merc. Iod. Muri. ac. Morph. Nux V. Petrol. Phos. Puls. Rus. Rad. or Tart. Anti.

——— do. and Trachea seems burnt. Colocy. Seneg. Sep.

——— Rattling in. Plumb. Acet. Puls. Ran. Bulb. Rapha. Rus. Rad. Sabi. Sep. or Tart. Anti.

——— Stricture on. Arg. N. Arnic. Caust. Cann. S. Canth. Gum. Gtt. Hyosc. Ipe. Kreoso. Lach. Led. P. Lobel. Nux V. or Sabad.

——— Suffocating Sensation. Mosch. Opi. Silec. Spong. Sulp. or Verat.

——— Swallowing impeded, Pharynx paralysed. Give Arg. Arnic. Bromide of Potash, Caust. Canth. Caps. Dolich. Hyosc. Ignat. Kalmi. Lat. Merc. Nux V. Puls. Rus. T. Tart. Ant. Verat. or Zinc.

——— Thirst excessive. Camp. Sec. C. Spig. Verat. or Zinc.

——— Titillation in. Bell. Scill. Seneg. or Sulp. or Caust.

——— Tonsils burning in. Lach. Tart. Anti. Thuy. or Zinc.

——— do. Swelled, enlarged, or ulcerated. Iodi. Lyc. Merc. Viv. Phos. Silec. or Verat. (See Tonsils, in Angina.)

Those persons who are very liable to have inflammation of the throat and quinsey, may prevent the attacks by taking every day or two a small dose of Ferri. or Baryt. C., or what is more sure Sepi. See those articles in *Jhar's Symptomen Codex.*

——— Trachea, burning sensation in. Bell. Ignat. Ol. Anima. Rus. Rad. Sabad. Selen. Tabac. Tart. Anti. Verat. or Zinc.

——— Inflamed and sore. Acon. Bell. Caust. Dolichos. Hep. Ipe. Kali. Bic. Kreoso. Merc. Iodi. Nux V. Puls. Rus. Tox. Sabad. Scill. Seneg. Sep. or Tart. Anti.

——— and Larynx, tingling sore sensation in. Baryt. Dolichos. Kali. C. Merc. Viv. Merc. Oleand. Phos. ac. Phytol. Plumb. Acet. Rhodod. Rus. Tox. Seneg. Spong. Stann. or Zinc.

——— or Trachea paralyzed. Coni. Lach. Nux V.

——— Ulcers or mucus in. Camp. Lach. Merc. Nitr. ac. Samb. Thuy. Verat. or Zinc.

——— Uvula swelled or elongated. Bell. Seneg. Tart. Anti. Thuy. or Chin.

——— Sore. (See Angina, Quinsey, &c.)

TREMOR OR TREMBLING.

Tremor or Trembling. This state is produced from nervous weakness or sensibility, and in a feeble state of health. The remedies are, Coni. Selen. Seneg. Sepi. Stramo. or Verat. or Ferr.

TUMORS.

TUMORS. These are a preternatural enlargement or swelling of a part. They are of various inds, and may be formed of different matter and texture. The following are those most commonly met with, and the Homœopathic remedies detailed, which are found to be the most useful as a curative.

——— of the bones, composed of bony matter, such as exostoses. They may be connected with a rickety constitution, or they may proceed from the effect of venereal virus; they are termed nodes, or tophs, or exostoses.

If they are produced by rickets, the remedies for that disease will be proper.

When they are the consequence of venereal contamination, the appropriate remedies are those for Lues Venerea. (See Bones and Syphilis.)

——— Encysted. Under this head, are placed those termed Wen. The remedies for them, are Baryt. Caust. Calc. Kali. C. Kali. Iod. Silec. or Ammo. Causticum.

When they become large and troublesome, it is advisable to remove them by an operation.

——— of or about the knee. These at times occur, formed of a gelatenous or indurated material; the remedies are Silec. or Iodine. Externally, a lead or soap plaister and compression.

——— Fungus Hæmatoides, or bloody mass or excrescence, composed of a fungus or flabby excrescence, and partly of blood, which they frequently emit. The remedies most useful for this disease are Calca. C. Kalmi. L. Millefo. Phos. Silec. Rus. T. or Thuy.

——— Inflammatory. All inflammatory and painful swellings and tumefactions will come under this head. The remedies are those used for inflammations generally, such as Acon. Bell. Bryo. Canth. Ipe. or Tart. Anti., together with such local remedies and applications as may seem to be required by the nature of the affection.

——— do. of the Joints, or White Swelling. In the first or early stage, use Acon. Bell. Bryo., and in the advanced stage, Coni. Iodi. Silec. Staph. Rus. T. (See Extremities, Joints, Acute Rheumatism, &c.)

——— Lymphatic. These are frequently connected with a scrofulous predisposition or constitution. The leading remedies for them are Ars. Baryt. Calc. Hep. Iodi. Phos. Sep. Silec. Spong. or Merc. or Kali. Iod. Phosphate of Iron is a very useful and efficient remedy. (Consult Scrofula.)

——— Scirrhous. Ars. Calendu. Coni. (See Cancer.) It is stated in *Jhar's Symptomen Codex* that scirrhous and cancer may be produced or aggravated by the use of Scilla. It may be inferred from this fact that squills would be a useful remedy for this disease.

TOE NAILS, Incurvated or Turned in.

Toe Nails, incurvated or turned in. Many persons are troubled with this painful affection, who have consulted surgeons and taken counsel, and used a variety of remedies without obtaining very material permanent relief. We have the confidence to believe that here we can furnish such sufferers with a permanent remedy. The difficulty in this disease consists in the nail being too broad, and from the edges turning down, so that they grow into the skin and flesh. Two indications are required for a cure: first, to produce a narrower nail; second, to have it grow flat.

Scraping or paring the nail down in the centre will sometimes induce it to grow so flat as not to curve down into the skin on the sides. But a more sure and certain plan is to cut a piece out of the centre, in the shape of a V; thus, let it run half or two-thirds of the length of the nail, and occasionally pare off a little of the inner edges of the V; this produces a contraction of the nail in width; the edges are drawn out of the flesh or skin, and the nail becomes more flat, and the trouble is obviated.

We have had the pleasure of relieving many cases of this painful affection by this simple operation.

ULCERS.

ULCERS. There are a variety of those affections and of different natures; the prominent ones among them with the appropriate remedies will be pointed out under this head.

The general medicines which are the most important to dispose them to heal, are Ars. Bell. Calc. Carb. Veg. Coni. Cinebar, Cupr. Graph. Lyc. Merc. Puls. Silec. Selen. Sepi. Sulp. or Zinc. These may, with benefit, be used in the following manner:—

If the ulcer has a livid appearance, bleeds easily, or has an ichorous bloody discharge, hard edges and burning pain in it, give Ars. or Carbo. Veg.

If it emits a fœtid effluvia, is spreading, or is of a dark hue, use Carbo. Veg. or Lach.

When the ulcer is deep, and forms a thin offensive matter, use Mercurius, Silec. Sulp. or Ars.

When there is itching, or burning, or smarting, Sulphur will be very useful.

In chronic ulcers, with hard edges, and having

a thin serous discharge, use Silec. Nitr. ac. Sepi. Lyc.

——— If proud flesh or fungus form on them, give Silec. or Ars. Sepi. or Sulp.

——— If there is ulceration of the alimentary canal, the proper remedies are Ars. Coni. Kreoso. or Nux V.

——— If bleeding from them takes place, Ars. Lach. Millefo. Sulp.

——— Callous. They frequently form hard, indurated, or callous edges or surfaces; in such cases give Calendula, Coni. Canth. Iodi. Phos. Sepi. Silec. or Aster. Rub.

——— Cancerous. The leading remedies for these have been laid down under Cancer, (which see.)

——— Carious. For this affection of the bones, use Asa. F. Merc. Nitr. ac. Rus. T. Silec. Staphy. Silec. or Sulp.

——— of the face. Ulceration and blotches on the face may generally be cured by Ars. Bell. Graph. Hep. Nitr. ac. or Petrol.

——— Fistulous. These may be very much benefitted or cured by using Arnic. Calc. C. Caust. Phos. Silec. Sulp. or Tart. Anti. By continuing one or other of these medicines a length of time, those ulcers may generally be cured.

——— Fungus. For these use Calca. Graph. Iodi. Petrol. Sepi. or Sulp.

——— Gangrenous. When they take on this

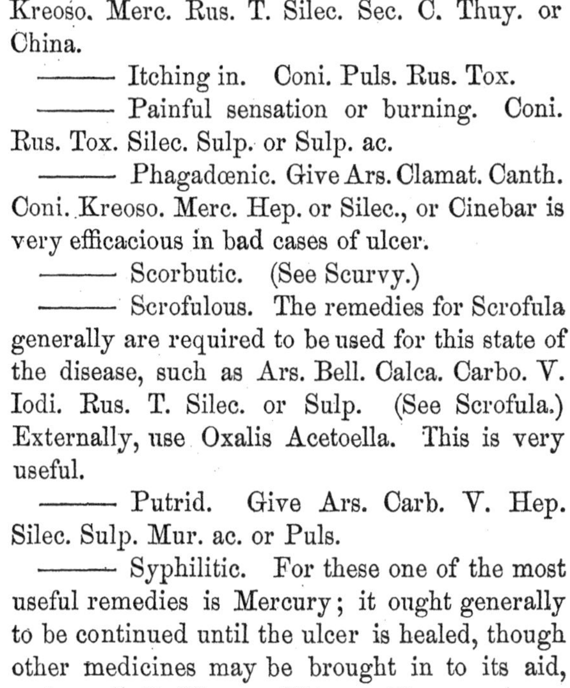

appearance, give Ars. Bell. Carbo. V. Hep. Kreoso. Merc. Rus. T. Silec. Sec. C. Thuy. or China.

——— Itching in. Coni. Puls. Rus. Tox.

——— Painful sensation or burning. Coni. Rus. Tox. Silec. Sulp. or Sulp. ac.

——— Phagadœnic. Give Ars. Clamat. Canth. Coni. Kreoso. Merc. Hep. or Silec., or Cinebar is very efficacious in bad cases of ulcer.

——— Scorbutic. (See Scurvy.)

——— Scrofulous. The remedies for Scrofula generally are required to be used for this state of the disease, such as Ars. Bell. Calca. Carbo. V. Iodi. Rus. T. Silec. or Sulp. (See Scrofula.) Externally, use Oxalis Acetoella. This is very useful.

——— Putrid. Give Ars. Carb. V. Hep. Silec. Sulp. Mur. ac. or Puls.

——— Syphilitic. For these one of the most useful remedies is Mercury; it ought generally to be continued until the ulcer is healed, though other medicines may be brought in to its aid, such as Iodi. Mezere. Nitr. ac. Thuy. or Auru. (See Syphilis.)

——— of the Throat. These may take place from various causes, and as being produced by different diseases or connected with them; which ought to be examined and referred to in regard to the treatment. The remedies most generally useful are Bell. Iodi. Hep. Merc. or Lyc. Silec. Sulp. or Thuy.

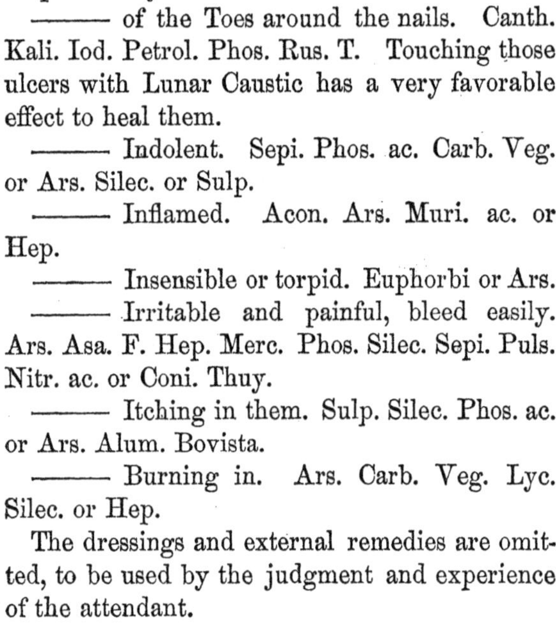

——— of the Toes around the nails. Canth. Kali. Iod. Petrol. Phos. Rus. T. Touching those ulcers with Lunar Caustic has a very favorable effect to heal them.

——— Indolent. Sepi. Phos. ac. Carb. Veg. or Ars. Silec. or Sulp.

——— Inflamed. Acon. Ars. Muri. ac. or Hep.

——— Insensible or torpid. Euphorbi or Ars.

——— Irritable and painful, bleed easily. Ars. Asa. F. Hep. Merc. Phos. Silec. Sepi. Puls. Nitr. ac. or Coni. Thuy.

——— Itching in them. Sulp. Silec. Phos. ac. or Ars. Alum. Bovista.

——— Burning in. Ars. Carb. Veg. Lyc. Silec. or Hep.

The dressings and external remedies are omitted, to be used by the judgment and experience of the attendant.

VACCINATION.

Vaccination. Since the discovery of the law of cure by Hahnemann, an opinion has been held that Vaccination was based on the Homœopathic principle, as an instance that like remedies cure like diseases.

An opinion also prevails, that the vaccine and variolus virus are of a similar nature, but different in degree, so much so, that the action of one on the body prevents the operation of the other. Some recent experiments seem to show that the internal use of the virus counteracts or neutralizes the morbid influence of the variolus-matter on the system.

Vaccination may be performed at all periods of life—the child had better be a month or more old before it is done; if there is danger of infection, it had better be done sooner. Pure lymph should be obtained and used for the purpose: the mode of doing it is well known. In about four days after vaccination, a redness appears at the place; a pustule rises up, and by the ninth day, it comes to maturity, though this varies to a day sooner or later. Now there is a fluid watery lymph in the pustule; this is the time to take infection; it should be taken soon after it is formed; after it gets of a purulent appearance, it is more uncertain to communicate the disease. After this period, a circular inflammation and swelling forms round the pustule, and sometimes it is quite sore. After a few days, the swelling abates, the disease recedes, and passes off.

To prevent the eruptions and affections of the skin which sometimes succeeds Vaccination, give

Sulphur of high attenuation, one dose a day for three or four days; this also renders the virus more pure and free from a Psoric contamination. After the close of the case, give a small dose of Sulphur a day, for three or four days;—it prevents eruptions and sores.

VARICELLA. Chicken Pox.

Varicella. This disease considerably resembles Small Pox, though it is a much more mild affection, not very contagious, neither does it appear in very numerous cases. It requires very little medical treatment; an attention to the diet and regimen generally is all that is required; although in some cases there is high fever and headache. The eruption fills with a watery fluid, and does not have the purulent nature of Small Pox.

If there is much fever, use Acon. or Ipe.

If the face is flushed, attended with headache, Bell. or Sol. Nig.

If there is irritation or a general uneasiness, Nux V.

VARIOLOID.

Varioloid. This is a modified state of Small Pox. It takes place after the patient has had kine pock or Small Pox. It is a secondary action of the Variolus virus, after the system has been once subjected to the operation of one of those viruses, from the body not being fully acted upon by the vaccine infection, or from its *running out* as it is expressed. There are a few instances, where the subject takes this disease; if the cases are compared with the great number vaccinated, those cases are very few. Formerly, this disease, when it appeared in nurses and those engaged about Small Pox patients, it was termed *Nurse Pox.* At length, the disease became more prevalent, and better understood, and this distinction was made, and name given to it.

It appears very much like Small Pox, only generally in a milder form, and the pustules are different, in this they raise up with a pointed top, which is hard on the point; they fill up with a watery lymph, and come to a height in five to seven days; then they recede, dry up, and frequentty pass off in a branny scurf.

Though in some instances the case progresses to about the appearance of Small Pox, and to the same length of time, when the pustules fill very much in the same manner; so that it will be very difficult in some cases to fix on a line between the two diseases.

It is considered that a second or third vaccination protects against this disease. Dr. Bell, in an Essay on it, states that the vaccine infection may operate four times, when the system is fully protected from the variolus.

In 1823—24, the varioloid prevailed to a considerable extent along the Hudson River. We collected some sketches and facts respecting it, which were published; and what was then written, has been supported by subsequent observation. By those statements it appears, "that the pustules are small, not attended with the circular inflammation of Small Pox. They have a peculiar horny prominent top; before the ninth day, they generally recede, and return to the skin, or go off in branny scales. The following conclusions seem to be warranted:

1st. That Varioloid will produce Varioloid.

2d. That in a subject that has not had kine pock or Small Pox, Varioloid will produce Small Pox.

3.d That Vaccination, in most all cases, is a preventative of Small Pox and of this disease.

4th. That the Varioloid will attack after Small Pox or kine pox."

The treatment for this disease should be similar to that pointed out for Small Pox.

VERTIGO.

Vertigo is a dizziness and giddiness of the head; it is a variety of headache. In selecting the medicines for it, much benefit will be gained by examining the article Headache. It may be occasioned by a great variety of causes, which it will be advisable to ascertain, if it can be done. The remedies generally used, and found the best, are the following: Acon. Ammo. C. Arg. Nit. Asteria. Rub. Bell. Bromi. Camp. Hyosc. Ignat. Merc. Kali. Bic. Kalmi. L. Lauroc. Merc. Mosch. Mur. ac. Nux V. Oleand. Opi. Petrol. Phos. Puls. Rus. Tox. Sep. Sol. Nig. Stann. Sulp. Sulp. ac. Thuy. Verat. Verba. (See the head, this article.)

——— If it proceed from a disordered state of the stomach, the medicines are Arnic. Nux V. Cham. Puls. Chin. Cocc. or Rus. T.

——— If from diseased irritation of the brain, Nux V. Arnic. Bell. Cham. Hep. or Puls.

——— Should it be in consequence of suppressed eruptions, give Hep. Calc. Puls. or Sulp.

——— When it is brought on by riding or irregular motion, Cocculus, Hep. Petrol. or Sulp.

——— If it is caused by rush of blood to the head or congestion of the brain, Acon. Alœ. Bryo. Arnic. Bell. Coni. Lach. Merc. Nux V. Opi. or Sulp.

——— If it is increased by raising the head or stooping, Acon.; or if it is attended with nausea or vomiting, Iris. Versico.

——— If there is nausea or impaired appetite, Antimo. Ipe. or Iris. Versico.

VIPER BITES.

Viper Bites.—Viper bites and stings, or scorpions, musquitoes, &c., Cedron or Guaco cures with great certainty.—*N. A. Hom. Journal*, No. 11, p. 272, 274.

WARTS.

Warts.—The remedies for this disease are Arnic. Caust. Calc. Dulcam. Natr. C. Natr. M. Rus. T. Sang. Sepi. Sulp. Thuy.

——— Fig. Thuy.

WHITE SWELLING.

Wh te Swelling.—This term is used for the tumefactions and diseased states that take place in the joints, when there is little or no discoleration of the skin. At first this disease may be of a dropsical rheumatic, scrofulous, or inflammatory nature. Under one of those heads the treatment is pointed out.

WORMS.

Worms.—*Ascarides*, (Pin or Flat Worms.) They are situated in the lower part of the rectum. The remedies for them are Acon. Agnu. C. Aloœ. Merc. Nux V. Petrol. Puls. Sabad. Stann. Tereb. Viola. Odorat.

—— *Lumbrici*, (common round worm.) The most useful remedies for these are Acon. Bell. Calc. China. Cina. Cicut. P. Ferr. Filax. Mas. Ignat. Merc. Nux V. Sabad. Silec. Spig. Sulp. It is advisable to use them as follows:

When there is fever, irritation, or itching at the rectum, give Acon. Ignat. or Merc.

If the bowels are irregular, the appetite poor, and the health feeble, give China. or Ferr. The latter is one of the most useful remedies for worms.

If there is frequent inclination to stool or tenesmus, use Merc. Nux V., or one of those in alternation with Ferr.

If there exists a relaxed state of the body, or a snuffling of the nose, or catarrhal affection, or rumbling of the bowels, the remedies are Dulcam. Sulp. Calc. or Sabad.

When the digestion is impaired, or there is nervous crampy symptoms, use Ignat. Nux V. or Ferr.

If those remedies do not cure, some of the others named had better be used, selecting them according to the circumstances of the case and the pathogenesis of the drug.

WORM TÆNIA. (Tape Worm.)

Worm Tænia.—The medicines which have been found to be most useful to expel this worm, are Filax. Mas.; this has gained considerable reputation; also, Sabad. Graph. Fragaria Vesica has been used with success in some cases. The Guaco, a remedy latterly come into notice, is represented to be very efficacious; other remedies recommended are Carbo. Anima. Carb. Veg. Kali. C. Phos. Petrol. Plati. Stann. Terebinth. or Sulphur.

In selecting a medicine, a regard should be had to the peculiar group of symptoms, so as to use a remedy, as much as possible, adapted to the case.

WOUNDS.

Wounds.—The general treatment for these will be found under Injuries, Mechanical; the detail for a particular treatment properly belongs to Surgery.

WRY NECK.

See Neck, Stiff.

FEMALE DISEASES.

Diseases peculiar to females will be considered in this division of the work.

The conformation and habits of females, and the important operations which they are designed for by Nature to pass through in the process of generation and the procreation of the human species, is such that there are some habits peculiar to the sex; which for their welfare and safety it is necessary to attend to, so that a regularity in some of the habits may be preserved. Among the most important of the peculiar habits and functions, next to the procreative operations, is the process of *Menstruation*. This evacuation is liable to be interrupted or suspended from various causes, when it becomes the subject of medical treatment to restore it, or to bring about a natural and periodical evacuation. This condition is termed

MENSTRUATION.

Menstruation.—This affection is generally divided into two varieties: First, that which relates to a beginning of menstruation of young females at about the ages of thirteen or fourteen, termed "the age of puberty;" Secondly, that which attends females during a subsequent period of life. In perhaps the majority of instances in young females, this process commences without much difficulty, but in many cases it is retarded beyond the proper period. When the health becomes impaired, sometimes seriously so, this state is called

CLOROSIS OR EMANSIO, MENSIUM.

Clorosis or Emansio.—The symptoms attending it are paleness of the face, flushes of heat, depraved appetite, longing for chalk, charcoal, and other uncommon articles; there is a languor, lassitude, weakness, emaciation, and œdematous swelling of the feet and legs, tumid abdomen; disordered stomach, headache, cough, irritation of the lungs, expectoration; and, if not relieved, these symptoms increase, and there is often an approximation to disease of the lung, which may end in consumption.

The medicines most useful for this condition are Acon. Ammo. C. Ars. Bryo. Cali. C. Ferr. Lyc. Puls. Sulp. or Graph.

If there is indigestion or semi-lateral headache, use Puls.

If there is congestion of the head, red flushed

pale face, oppression of the chest, use Graph. Sepi. or Sulp.

If there is hysterical symptoms, pale countenance, or dark spots on the skin, use Sepi. Puls. or Carb. C.

When there are symptoms of fulness of the head, bleeding of the nose or lungs, Bryo. Millefo. Sabi.

When there is pain in the back of the head, or eruptions of the skin, Sulp. or Lyc. or Rus. T.

If there is œdema, with debility, Calc. C. Ferr. Sulp.

In some conditions, other remedies for amenorhœa will be useful, to be selected by the experience and judgment of the prescriber.

The patient should rise early and take free exercise in the open air.

AMENORRHŒA. Suppression of the Menses.

Amenorrhœa.—After the habit is once formed, and menstruation has taken place, if it becomes interrupted or suppressed, it is known by this term. These evacuations, to be regular and healthy, should appear about every thirty days, although a few days, sooner or later, has no material effect to cause disease. The period of its continuance varies in different females, from three to six days. All authors recommend to the sex to observe special care to preserve this habit and periodical affection as regular as possible, for on this the health greatly depends.

The general remedies for it are Acon. Agnu. C. Ammo. C. Ars. Auru. Baryt. Berba. Vulg. Bryo. Calc. Caust. Coni. Cupr. Dulcam. Ferr. Hyosc. Kalmi. L. Iodi. Kreoso. Lauroc. Lyc. Nux V. Plati. Petrol. Podoph. Puls. Rus. T. Sabi. Sec. C. Stramo. Sulp. or Verat.

When the suppression is in consequence of a chill or exposure to cold, use Acon. Bryo. Puls. or Nat. C. Dulcam. Sepi. or Sulph.

If it is brought on by a fright, Acon. should be used first; after this, Lach. or Verat.

In chronic cases of weak debilitated subjects, give Sulp. or Sepi. or Coni. Ars. China. or Ferr.

When there is an irregularity or subsiding of the menses, or as it is called a *turn of the life*, the proper medicines are Cocc. Coni. Caust. Bromi. Colocy. Iodi. Graph. Nitr. ac. Nux V. Phos. Puls. Plati. Sang. Sec. C. Sepi. Sulp. Verat. or Zinc.

If there is not a full suppression, only an irregularity, use Sulp. Verat. or Ferr.

When there is indigestion, headache, palpitation of the heart, Puls. is indicated, or Bryo. Lyc. or Sulp.

If there is congestion of the head or chest, cold hands and feet, or flushed face, Graph. Bell.

When there is fulness of the head, bleeding of

the nose, dry cough, or spells of shivering, Acon. Bryo. Millefo. are the remedies.

In cases of pressing pain at the back of the neck, humming in the head, eruptions on the face, fulness of the stomach, irritable and angry disposition, give Hep. Sepi. Sulp. or Hyosc.

If there is dyspnœa or swelling of the feet and legs, use Calc. or Ferr. or Lyc. or Sepi.

If there is stricture of the throat or chest, Valer.

If the abdomen is enlarged or tumid, Lach. or Ars.

UTERUS.

Uterus.—The diseases peculiar to this organ or connected with it, will here be considered.

Barrenness.—In many instances, in a matrimonial state, there is a failure to be favored with an offspring—sometimes on account of interests or family connections or influences—it may be very desirable to have an heir.

When conception does not take place, the use of remedies by the female may predispose the uterine organ to conceive. The remedies most useful and recommended are Agnu. C. Caust. Auru. Borax. Plati. or Sulp. One or two attenuated doses of some one of these medicines continued a length of time will likely bring about such a result.

CONCEPTIONS, TO PREVENT.—This probably may be a more desirable result to produce than the preceding one. The remedies most useful are Ol. Sabi. Canth. Sec. C. or Plumb. These should be taken in the same manner as is pointed out for the preceding affection.

DISTENSION OF THE ABDOMEN.—When in an unmarried state, from several causes, this takes place, it is commonly attended with a suppression of the menses.

The remedies generally for it are Ars. Lyc. Sabi. or Merc. Nux V., &c.

If it is connected with a suppression of menses, pursue the treatment to be found under Amenorrhœa.

DYSMENORRHŒA. MENSTRUAL COLIC.

DYSMENORRHŒA.—There are many young females who suffer very much from this disease during the menstrual period; frequently they have severe pain and pressing down of the uterine parts, with cramps and spasms, vomiting, headache, and various other symptoms of suffering. One of the most useful remedies for it is Nux V.; a proper dose would be grr. of the second trituration, repeated every one or two hours till the pain is mitigated; or in moderate cases, if it is repeated every two or three hours, it may do. This form of giving Nux appears to be more efficient than to use the dilution; but the dilution of Nux may be used with good effect; two or three drops, or the second or third attenuation, given in the manner mentioned for giving the trituration, would be proper. The other remedies which are indicated and used, are Puls. or Coff. Hyosc. Sepi. or Cocc; and also the others recommended are Caust. Opi. Petrol. Kalmi. L. Rus. T. or Iodine.

It will be very desirable to use means to prevent such attacks, and guard the system against such an affection. Some medicine used during the interval may do much to afford such relief; the most advisable for this purpose are Caust. Sepi. Kalmi. L. or Nux V.; a dose or two of one of these articles, given every day or two during the interval, or beginning ten or twelve days before the time of the sickness, are likely to afford relief and facilitate the menstrual process. By this course, the habit after awhile may be changed, so that such treatment would be unnecessary. If the body can be protected against such severe attacks, it will prove a great comfort and blessing to delicate and suffering young females.

——— Groins, pain in them during the catamenia, give Nux V. Sepi. or Tart. Anti.

Hysteria. Uterine Spasms.—This disease is placed under Spasms.

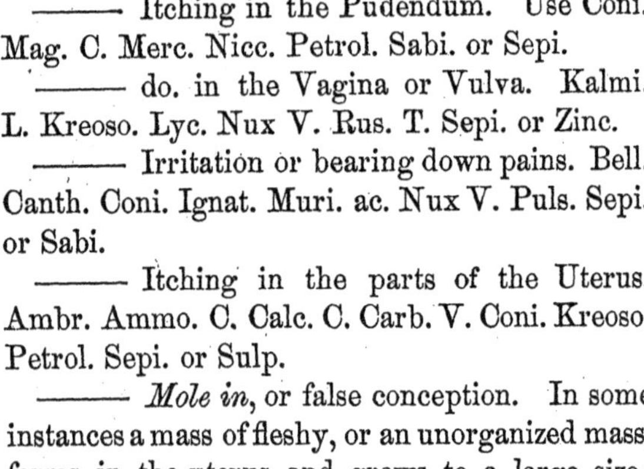

——— Itching in the Pudendum. Use Coni. Mag. C. Merc. Nicc. Petrol. Sabi. or Sepi.

——— do. in the Vagina or Vulva. Kalmi. L. Kreoso. Lyc. Nux V. Rus. T. Sepi. or Zinc.

——— Irritation or bearing down pains. Bell. Canth. Coni. Ignat. Muri. ac. Nux V. Puls. Sepi. or Sabi.

——— Itching in the parts of the Uterus. Ambr. Ammo. C. Calc. C. Carb. V. Coni. Kreoso. Petrol. Sepi. or Sulp.

——— *Mole in*, or false conception. In some instances a mass of fleshy, or an unorganized mass, forms in the uterus and grows to a large size; the female may suppose she is pregnant. At the proper period, life of the fœtus is not felt; still the case progresses to the period when labor is expected. But here again is a disappointment; labor or delivery does not take place, and at times the female is doomed to carry the uncomfortable and unwelcome burthen. The remedies recommended for this affection are Plati. Sec. C. Sabi.

——— Mons Veneris, pain in it. Tereb. Thuy. or Verat.

HÆMORRHAGE METRORRHAGIA.

Hæmorrhage.—When the discharge of blood from the uterus becomes more free and copious than that attending common menstruation, it is a diseased state, and receives this name, and becomes a subject of medical treatment.

It is generally attended with pain in the back, in the uterus, and some pressing down, though not always, for sometimes flooding occurs with little or no pain, or pressing down.

The remedies are Acon. Arnic. Bell. Calc. C. Ferr. Hyosc. Ipe. Millefo. Nux V. Rus. T. Sepi. or Verat. or Hamameli. Millefo. and Hamameli seems to be the most useful; there are many other medicines recommended, which are useful in some conditions.

——— When the discharge is excessive, with pain resembling labor pain, give Ipe. Millefo. Sabi. Nux V. Cham. Plati. or Sulp.

——— If the discharge is dark colored, give Mill or Hamameli.

——— If it is bright red, and in a full habit, prone to miscarry, and labor-like pains, Sabi. Sec. C. or Millefo.

When there is great debility, give Chin. or Ferr.

When the flowing frequently comes on or continues a long time, or is attended with cramps, Nux V. or Calc. or Plati. or Hamameli.

If it recurs in hysterical subjects, Ambr. Ignat.

If it is attended with bearing down pains, Platina.

If the menses come on too early, attended with diarrhœa, Verat. Muri. ac. Sabi. or Sepi.

When there is excessive discharge, with clots or offensive fetor, Millefo. or Kreoso. are proper medicines.

The other medicines will be useful in many cases.

LEUCORRHŒA. Fluor Albus. (*Whites.*)

Leucorrhœa.—This is a very common and unpleasant affection, with which many females are troubled; it is a discharge from the vagina, or os uteri, of a white yellowish matter, though frequently the matter is of a mucus character; it does at times affect infants and young females, but it is generally confined to grown women.

Treatment.—In full habits, give Acon. Agnu. C. or Ambr.

If the discharge is reddish, Cocc. or Ammo. C.

Should the parts become excoriated, or there is a greenish discharge, use Merc. Sepi. or Puls.

If there is a whitish corrosive discharge, Calc. C. Sulp. or Ammo. M.

If the discharge is of a cream color, Puls. or Calc. C.

If it is a whitish matter, particularly in children, give Calc. C. Sulp.

If it is attended with hæmorrhoids, Nux. V. or Merc. or Sulp. Other remedies, which are useful, are Ars. Auru. Cann. S. Caust. Coni. Copaib. Bals. Ferr. Nitr. ac. Petrol. or Plati.

In weak, debilitated patients, the general health should be improved by the use of Chin. Ferr. or Ars., and a generous diet, with exercise in the open air.

If the internal use of some of the remedies named do not succeed in curing, it would be advisable to inject cold water into the vagina, or a solution of Sulphate of Zinc or Acetate of Lead or Nitrate of Silver.

NYMPHOMANIA.

NYMPHOMANIA.—The remedies for this affection, and to allay and quiet the veneral orgasm, are Bell. Canth. Cann. S. Hyosc. Sulp. ac. or Zinc.

OVARIA INFLAMED.

OVARIA INFLAMED.—When it is ascertained that this is the case, use Acon. at first; after the fever is reduced, Bryo. Canth. or Rus. T.

——— do. Enlarged or indurated, give Ars. Baryt. Iodi. Merc. Sepi. or Sulp.

——— Os Tinsa, or os uteri, indurated. Ars. Coni. Natr. C. or Sep.

PROLAPSUS, OR PROCIDENTIA. FALLING OF THE MOTHER, (SO CALLED.)

PROLAPSUS.—From long diseased action or weakness of the parts, the uterus settles down into the vagina; in some cases it passes so low that the os uteri is out even with or beyond the labia. Among females, there is a good deal of anxiety about this affection; but from what they are told, sometimes by one of the medical profession, who may be willing to work upon their excited feelings, they are of opinion that they have prolapsus, when it is not so.

When, however, there is a prolapsus, the remedies for it are Ars. Auru. Bell. Nux V. Plati. Sec. C. Sepi. or Stann.

By a steady continuance in the use of some one of these medicines, the patient may be greatly relieved or cured. We have known both results to take place.

A great variety of pessaries, abdominal supporters and instruments have been introduced and recommended for this disease; a great portion of them do not answer much purpose, further than to afford some temporary relief. Patients are often deceived by flattering representations in their favor, and by such means females are imposed upon. The only reliable and permanent remedies are those for internal use.

PUDENDUM OR LABIA.

Pudendum or Labia.—Burning pain in it, use Sepi. Silec. Staphy. Sulp. Tereb. Thuy. or Verat.

——— do. Inflamed and swelled. Acon. Bell. Kreoso. Muri. ac. Nitr. ac. Nux V. Sepi. Thuy. or Verat. It will be serviceable to apply to the part cold liquid applications of Arnica or Acetate of Lead.

——— Sexual embrace, great inclination for. This is similar to Npmphonamia. Canth. Sabi. Sarss. or Sulp.

——— do. Deficient inclination. Agnu. C. Canth. Iodi.

Scirrhous, or Cancer of the Womb.—This organ, as well as other parts of the body, is liable to be effected with this disease. It comes on by slow degrees, attended with pain through the uterus; pressing down; a prominent state of the abdomen; the menses are irregular; there may often be a slight flowing from the vagina; the pains become shooting and burning; the health is greatly impaired.

The most advisable remedies for this disease are very similar to those for scirrhous and cancer, pointed out under Cancer, such as Ars. Auru. Baryt. M. Coni. Kreoso. Phos. ac, in the advanced stage of this disease. Phosphate of iron is a valuable remedy; it quiets pain very much, and affords relief otherwise; or use Sepi. Silec. or Thuy.

To show the salutary influence of the use of those remedies, some notes of a case contained in the previous edition of this work, are transferred.

In August, 1842, Mrs. C., after suffering three years with uterine disease, had an enlargement of those parts. The abdomen extensively distended; frequent hæmorrhages; prolapsus uteri; violent pain; about every six weeks an abscess formed in the uterus; it burst out, and there was a copious flow of pus, blood and water; the uterus was indurated and very large. She was confined to bed; had been under Allopathic treatment over two years, and she was now pronounced incurable. In this condition she came under my care. She took Ars. Nux V. Cann. S. Silec. Agar. Bell. Kreoso., generally in the second attenuations, varied, and adapted to the symptoms as near as judgment directed.

She soon began to improve, and continued on. In six months she was up, walking about; in nine months was fully cured, and has enjoyed good health till this time, 1854.

——— Throbbing or jerking in, sensation of. Prunus Sp. Sepi. or Zinc.

PREGNANCY

Diseases of Pregnancy.—In the early period of this condition, as well as sometimes in advanced states, females are troubled with a loss of blood from the uterus, and other diseases.

If this state is attended with occasional discharge of blood, or somewhat like menstruation, use Cocc. Millefo. Phos. or Plati.

If these medicines do not answer to check or regulate the evacuation, some of the other medicines set down for Uterine Hæmorrhage, should be used.

When they are troubled with morning sickness, or nausea, or vomiting, give Ipe. or Nux V. Kreoso. or Ars. Coni. Nitr. ac. or Mag. C. or Phos. Bryo. Lyc. or Acon. Bell. Hyosc. Sep. Sulp. or Tart. Anti.

It will sometimes be required to vary and try several of those medicines to meet the peculiarity of the symptoms. Kreosote and Petrol. has obtained a good deal of reputation for sickness at this period.. For fainting and hysterical affections. (See these articles under their proper heads.)

Toothache and affection of the jaws, (see these articles in their place.)

Swellings of the legs and veins of the legs. When there is inflammation and pain in them, give Puls. Sulp. or Acon.

If this affection is connected with hæmorrhoids or costiveness, give Ignat. Nux V. or Sulp. after the others, or in alternation with them.

If there is blueness of the veins of the legs, use Ars. or Carb. V.

If an erysipelas or blotchy eruption comes out on the legs, give Bell. Rus. T. or Thuy., or Agar. Graph. Carb. V. Sepi. are useful in these affections.

Pregnancy Uterus.—Abortion threatened. To restrain this disposition, give Bell. Canth. Cham. Chin. Kali. C. Nux V. Opi. Sabi. Sec. C. Sepi. or Sulp. Great benefit is gained by introducing a small piece of opium into the vagina, and giving Ferr. or China.

——— Abortion or catemenia, to produce during the time. The most certain medicines are Artimes. Kreoso. Nux M. Plati. Plumb. Sabi. Silec. or Sec. C.

——— Appetite deficient during. Chin. Cham. Mag. M. Natr. C. Petrol. or Tart. Anti.

——— Convulsions or spasms in. Bell. Cocc.

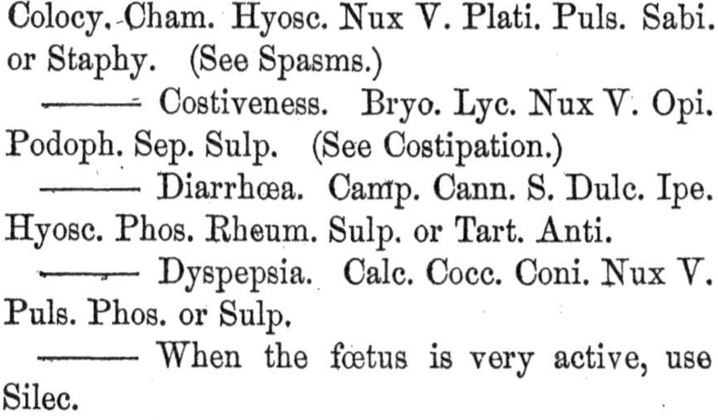

Colocy. Cham. Hyosc. Nux V. Plati. Puls. Sabi. or Staphy. (See Spasms.)

——— Costiveness. Bryo. Lyc. Nux V. Opi. Podoph. Sep. Sulp. (See Costipation.)

——— Diarrhœa. Camp. Cann. S. Dulc. Ipe. Hyosc. Phos. Rheum. Sulp. or Tart. Anti.

——— Dyspepsia. Calc. Cocc. Coni. Nux V. Puls. Phos. or Sulp.

——— When the fœtus is very active, use Silec.

——— Moral affections impaired. Acon. Bell. Cupri. Plati. Puls. or Stramo.

——— Pain and bearing down. Natr. C. Nux V. Puls. Sabi. Sec. C. or Sepi.

When there is severe cutting pain about the uterus, Colocy. has afforded great relief.

——— Pain in abdomen. Bell. Bryo. Cham. Nux V. Sepi.

——— Spasms epileptic. Mosch. (See this article in Spasms.)

ACCOUCHEMENT AND THE DISEASES SUBSEQUENT TO IT.

Accouchement.—In the majority of cases of labor, it begins with moderate pains in the uterine region or in the back. These increase more or less; sometimes they are very slow and lingering; at others, the pains are in quick succession and pressing down. There is generally some anxiety with the patient or nervous excitement, for which it will be of service to give a few doses of Coff. or Nux V.

If the pains are lingering or irregular, or if there is a full habit of body, or a feverish state, give Acon. or Bell.

When the labor lingers with feeble pains, use Iodi. Puls. Sepi. or Secale C.

If there is an irritable state of mind or habit, Cham. Nux V. or Staphy.

In latter years, the Sec. C. has probably been used to promote parturient pains more than any other article. As this may be attended with some danger, and produce injury to the infant, it is proper to remark and give a caution respecting it. In large doses it produces a stupifying effect and torpor of the child. In *Dr. S. Bard's Midwifery*, some precautionary remarks are made, in substance thus: "That before giving Ergot, the uterus should be well dilated; there should be caution in not giving very large doses, that a large dose, and continued action of it, might stupify and destroy the child."

In *Jhar's Symptomen Codex*, by the late Dr. G. W. Cook, it is stated that before giving Sec. C., the accoucher should be well satisfied that the uterus is amply dilated and the presentation natural. The mode of giving it here mentioned is to make a decoction of one drachm in a gill of water, and give a table spoonful every five minutes till three spoonfuls are taken. This is enough to answer the purpose, and is capable of producing very salutary effects.

If the labor is protracted, and attended with severe and distressing pain, Bell. Coff. Nux V. or Opi.

If there are cramps, and if so, they are likely to partake of hysteria, give Asa. F. Ambr. Hyosc. or Nux V.

Sometimes the labor is protracted; the pains severe; the patient has severe headache, and she finally gets congestion of the brain, with stupor. In such cases, give Bell. Cocc. or Opi. Writers on midwifery recommend bleeding freely in such cases. It is a question whether the attendant would do justice to the patient to omit this remedy. The child should be delivered as soon as possible. If this cannot be effected by ordinary means, by manual assistance, (recollect the pains are suspended,) then recourse should be had to the use of the forceps. Success in such cases depends on prompt and correct action.

If the course here suggested, by using the forceps, is pursued, the child may be delivered alive, and probably the mother saved. Such has been the result of our experience.

Now, a word on the use of the forceps. They may, and often have been used, without materially injuring the child, and it may by them be brought forth alive; but in many cases where it may be advisable to use them, the infant is dead beforehand, then the sooner it is delivered the better. In such cases of difficulty, there generally are causes which deprives the child of life, without referring it to the use of instruments.

It is gratifying to be able to state that very few cases occur where such means are required.

The first thing after delivery is to bring away the *placenta*, or after-birth, by making a gentle extension on the cord. This may generally be done in 10 or 15 minutes, and seldom any inconvenience ensues by this course. If there is a delay, it will be proper to wait for some expulsive pains, and give the patient some of the remedies named bove, to promote the pains of labor.

TREATMENT AFTER DELIVERY.

Treatment after Delivery.—The patient should be quietly placed in bed, and have a bandage applied around the waist; give her some doses of Arnica in an attenuated form; this relieves the soreness and quiets the after pains; or give Bell.

FLOODING OR METRORRHAGIA.

Flooding or Metrorrhagia.—It is customary and necessary for there to be some discharge from the womb after delivery, but this sometimes becomes free and excessive, so as occasionally to produce serious and alarming effects; then the case requires medical treatment. The most useful medicines for this purpose are Millefo. Hamameli, Ipe. or Sepi. Tincture of Cinnamon is highly recommended, four or five drops given as a dose, and to be repeated several times. It seems this would be best adapted to passive or advanced stages of the case; we have observed good results from it.

LOCHIA.

Lochia.—This discharge from the uterus, after delivery, varies very much in quantity in different females; the quantity may be very small, though it is important that there should be some evacuation. If it is checked or suppressed within six or seven day or more, pain and uneasiness ensue, fever sets in, and sometimes a train of serious symptoms take place. The remedies to restore this evacation are Puls. Sabi. Nux V. Sec. C. or Hyosc.; fomenting across the abdomen, with alkaline solutions, are very useful.

MILK.

Milk.—This nutrifying matter for the infant sometimes is furnished in excessive quantity, when care should be taken to have the breasts drawn, or there will be danger of inflammation and gathering of them. The patient should be kept on low diet, and given two or three doses of Calc. in a day.

The milk is often deficient in quantity to supply the demand of the infant; this may be increased by giving Agnu. C. Carbo. Animalis or Caust. two or three times a day. Carbo. Ani. has a great influence to increase the quantity of milk. Another article comes highly recommended for increasing the milk—it is Ricinus Communis or Bofœra. The leaves or juice of this plant applied to the breast produces a great increase of milk in the female.—*N. A. Journal of Homœopathy*, No. 1, p. 386.

It has been suggested that the oil from the plant rubbed on the breast might answer the purpose.

INFLAMED BREASTS.

Inflamed Breasts.—One of the great difficulties from which females suffer after parturition, is inflammation and suppuration of one or both breasts. There are a variety of exciting causes which tends to bring on this disease; these we do not undertake to examine, but proceed at once to give the proper treatment.

It may be remarked that this disease is very often aggravated and rendered tedious by the injudicious use of hot stimulating articles. Nurses and good old women have some specifics of this kind, and cures for ague of the breast, and some doctors are too much inclined to such a practice.

It should be borne in mind that this is an inflammatory disease, attended with fever, and ought to be treated as such. The proper remedies are Acon. or Bell.; use one of these until the fever and heat of the breast is moderated; then Bryo. will be proper.

If there are shooting or twinging pains, Ignat. or Nux V.

Apply cloths wet in cold water to it, or to the water add Arnica, Acetate of Lead, or Muriate of Ammonia, or ice. By these means, early used, the disease may be checked and the case cured; but if it progresses, and there is a prospect of suppuration taking place, it will be proper to apply warm poultices to it; also give Hep. Merc. or Sulp.

If suppuration takes place when it is matured, if the pus does not form an opening for itself, it will be advisable to open it: the incision had better be large, for after that the ulcer more readily heals.

INDURATED BREASTS.

Indurated Breasts.—When a breast becomes inflamed, if the disease is not fully relieved by resolution or suppuration, a hard indurated state frequently takes place in some part of it or in the whole substance of it. If this progresses, a scirrhous tumor may be formed. The remedies for it are Baryt. C. Calc. C. Coni. Phos. Silec. or Sulp.

NIPPLES, SORE.

NIPPLES, SORE.—This is a very annoying and painful disease for nursing females to endure. The internal remedies for it are Arnic. Calc. C. Hep. Iod. Merc. Nux V. Silec. or Sulp. In addition to those, external applications to the nipple may be used to advantage. For this purpose a great number are introduced, and among the best are the following: Moisten the nipple often with a diluted tincture of Arnica, or Iodine, or a weak solution of borax in brandy; or this preparation is very soothing: Make a solution of Borax of moderate strength, add to it Oil of Almonds and a little Carbonate of Soda; form a linament, which apply to the part.

PHLEGMASIA DOLENS, OR MILK LEG.

PHLEGMASIA DOLENS.—This is a general swelling of one or both legs, which sometimes takes place during child-bed state; the skin is white, not discolored; it is of the nature of Anasarca, of a peculiar nature; sometimes it is painful; at others it is not very much so. The remedies found most useful for it are Acon. Arnic. Ars. Hell. Iodi. Nux V. Rus. T. or Silec.

If there is considerable fever, Acon.

After this the most prominent remedy is Arnic.

If there is general weakness and a spongy swelling or burning pain in the leg, Ars.

If there is a deficiency of the lochial discharge, Puls. or Rus. T.

If there is nervous irritation or crampy feelings of the leg, Nux V.

For the weakness which ensues, give Chin. Iodi. Silec., &c.

PAINS AFTER.

Pains after.—After confinement, the patient is subject to a continuance of pain similar to those of labor; some have them very mildly, others very severely.

Directly after delivery, and the good lady is made comfortable in bed, give Arnic. or Bell.; a few doses, one every two or three hours, more or less, as the pain and soreness may be; this relieves the soreness, and, in some measure, prevents or lessens the after pain.

If they continue severe, give Coff. Nux V.; these generally are sufficient. When they continue severe, a free evacuation from the bowels will be of great service.

PUERPERAL FEVER, OR INFLAMMATION OF THE WOMB.

Puerperal Fever.—In many instances this disease succeeds the time of parturition. Like other diseases, this sometimes is only an occasional and mild affection. At other periods it is very prevalent, seizing on a great number, and exhibits an epidemic character. It frequently is attended with great severity, and under some modes of treatment is very fatal.

A number of Allopathic writers, such as Denman, Gordon, Hey, Armstrong, and Drs. Bard and Hosack, consider this an inflammatory disease. The many cases we have seen well confirms those opinions. It commences with chills or rigors; tenderness and pain of the abdomen; a distension of the abdomen, which is tender to the touch; the lochia suppressed. In addition to these symptoms, we have observed others with violent pain in the head, back and sacrum, and terrible screaming; sometimes there is congestion of the uterus. In some instances, and in particular localities, it is represented that this disease partakes of a typhoid nature. This may be in some measure induced by a mode of treatment.

Treatment.—The Homœopathic remedies for this disease are:—

If there are chills or fever, give Acon. After using this awhile, or until the symptoms are somewhat moderated, it will be proper to give Arnic. Bell. or Bryo.

If there is nervous irritation or spasms, Nux V., either alone or in alternation, with one of the preceding medicines.

If the first period has passed, and there is soreness through the part, and uneasiness of the urinary organs, Canth. Colocy.

When the active symptoms are moderated, some of the other remedies will be required, to wit:—

If there is irregular chills or perspiration, Merc. or Puls.

If there is anxiety of mind and uneasiness, give Cham. Ignat. Coff. or Bryo.

In feeble constitutions, where there has been loss of blood, give China. or Quini.

Should there be great sensibility of the uterus, give Nux V. Sepi. Bell. Cham. or Coni. Cocc. Kreoso. Mur. ac.

Should cramps or spasms supervene, use Cocc. Ignat. Hyosc. (See Spasms.)

If ulceration at the os tinica takes place, Carbo. V. Graph. Sulp. or Silec. or Ars.

——— Pot-bellied or protuberant abdomen, Lach. Sec. C. Silec. or Sep.

INFANTS.

There are a series of diseases which affect infants. A consideration of them will form the matter of this division, without entering into an examination of the causes or their pathological nature. The plan will be followed in this work of noticing the diseases, symptoms, and detail the treatment.

ACIDITY OF THE STOMACH.

Acidity of the Stomach.—Infants are very liable to have sour belchings from the stomach or throwing up flatulent acid matter, or the milk turned sour. The remedies for it are Bell. Borax, Calc. Rheum. or Sulp. Select one that appears to be most indicated; if this does not cure, choose another.

APTHEA OR THRUSH.

Aphthea or Thrush.—A great portion of infants are attacked with this disease. It begins with slight soreness of the mouth; a white scurf or scum appears in it; this frequently is only in small patches. In other cases it is very generally spread over the mouth on the tongue, in the fauces, and even, it is said, to extend to the stomach and through the bowels. In this way it is a serious disease.

The most useful medicines for it are Borax, Merc. Sol. It is better to give them in powder put on the tongue. One may be given by itself or in alternation. The case generally improves during their use. In addition, it may be advisable to give Sulp.

If the apthous scurf assumes a dark or gangrenous appearance, use Ars. Nitr. ac. or Sec. C.

ASPHYXIA.

ASPHYXIA.—Infants are liable to a sudden suspension of the circulation of the blood and apparent cessation of breathing. Sometimes this takes place at birth or directly after; when they only at intervals draw a sighing breath; then place the child in warm water, and soon as possible endeavor to aid the breathing by pressing on the chest, and dilate it again, or blowing in the mouth; this may bring the lungs into action. During the process, apply warm vinegar to the nose, or some volatile article. If the child is plump and full, and there is a purple appearance, or symptoms of congestion, Dr. S. Bard used to recommend dividing the umbilical cord, and discharge three or four teaspoonfuls of blood. This may aid much in bringing about breathing; it may relieve the lungs and enable the heart to act. By perseverance in this course, the infant may frequently be brought to.

——— In cases afterwards. The further remedies are Acon. Cham. Chin. Mosch. Opi. Sambu. or Tart. Anti.

In the first stage, put a drop or two of the first dilution of Mosch. or Anti. on the tongue. This should be repeated every ten to twenty minutes.

If there is not an improvement in half an hour, Opi. should be used in the same way.

If the affection continues, and the face is pale, China. or Quini. in dilution; one or two drops should be put in the mouth, and this may be repeated in ten or fifteen minutes.

If the child revives and becomes feverish or has a red flushed face, Acon. or Bell. will be useful.

The child should be placed in warm water, or it may be wrapped in a warm flannel.

ASTHMA.

Asthma.—This disease affects infants somewhat differently from that of adults. At the attack a suffocation is experienced; they give a shrill cry; often have a livid color of the face; the breathing is hurried and laborious; they struggle and gasp for breath.

——— Ambra is one of the best remedies for this affection. If this does not cure or arrest it, the other remedies proper are Ipe. Sambu. Cham. or Ars. In protracted cases, Colchi.

———of Millar, is described a sudden spasmodic contraction of the top of the windpipe, like spasmodic croup, producing a crowing, strangling noise, causing great distress. The remedies which seem best adapted to its cure, are Acon. Ipe. Ars. Mosch. Asa. F. or Puls. Hep. Spong. or Sambu. Generally, the first should be Acon.

If there is a rattling in the throat, give Ipe. alone or in alternation with Acon. At first, if the symptoms are severe, the doses ought to be given every half hour, perhaps oftener during this stage. The addition of Mosch. or Asa. F. would be serviceable.

If there come on, prostration, or cold sweating and loss of strength, give Ars.

If the respiration becomes whizzing, the face blue or inclined to lethargy, give Sambu. At the latter stage, to remove the hoarseness and soreness about the larynx, Hep. or Spong. will be useful.

CHAFING AND EXCORIATIONS.

Chafing and Excoriations.—Little children are very liable to have chafed, raw, and sore places on the skin, particularly so in the groins and on the neck. In such cases, care should be taken to keep the part clean and dry. There are remedies for internal use, which aids materially in curing this affection; they are Borax. Ignat. Merc. or Hep. S.

If some of these do not effect a cure, those named under Herpes may be very useful. Externally apply scorched flour, hair powder, or some other absorbing, drying article. It may be advisable to moisten the sore part with diluted Arnica or Iodine.

CHOLERA INFANTUM.

Cholera Infantum.—Infants as well as adults are subject to have diarrhœa, particularly so during the hot season, when it is called Summer Complaint or Infantile Diarrhœa.

The symptoms are: the child's bowels become irregular; the stools very often, with grumbling of the bowels and painful uneasiness; the stools are slimy, watery, or greenish, or frothy, with an offensive fetor. The child looses strength, and becomes pale and feeble.

The remedies are Acon. Bell. Cham. or Rheum.

Ipe. or Camph. Calca. C. Cinnamo. Merc. Sol. or Verat. or Zinc.

In the first stage, or if there is fever and soreness of the bowels, give Acon. Ipe. or Camph.

When the above-mentioned symptoms are moderated, use Cham. Calc. or Merc. Solub.

If the diarrhœa continues, still it will be advisable to give Rheum. Cinnamo., or continue Merc. Sol.

If the stools are green, or there is an exhaustion, Ars.

If there are cramps or a cold skin, Verat. or Nux V.

If the diarrhœa continues after the more acute symptoms are removed, use Zinc. or Plumbi.

It will be advisable to endeavor to improve the strength by mild nourishing diet, and by applying a bark bandage around the body.

COLIC.

Colic.—This disease is indicated by pain of the bowels and griping, worrying and crying. It is a common affection of infants.

The remedies most useful are Acon. Bell. Ipe. or Cham.

If there is fever or soreness of the bowels, give Acon. Ipe. or Cham.

If there is flatulence or rolling of the bowels, Borax, Colocy. Senn.

If there are cramps, Nux V. Staphy. or Opi.

CORYZA.

CORYZA.—A catarrhal affection, when the nose and head are stopped and stuffed up, (as it is termed.) Dulcam. is the best remedy. After it use Ars. Nux V. Puls. Sulp. (See Angina Catarrhalis.)

CONVULSIONS.

CONVULSIONS.—Infants and small children frequently are subject to have convulsions or fits, as they are termed, which create a good deal of anxiety in the family. When the fit comes on, give the child free air; keep it as still as possible, and in a horizontal position; soon as possible put their feet and legs in warm water, and rub them; but do not put mustard or any volatile stimulant in the water, nor have them about the child: they deprive the lungs of vital air, which is very much needed. (See our observations on Epidemic Cholera.) Such remedies are more objectionable when the treatment detailed in this work is adopted.

Let the warm bath be continued twenty or thirty minutes. After this it may be useful to give injections of warm water, or water with milk and molasses. The medicines most proper are Bell. or Nux V. or Ignat. In most cases this course will check the spasms or effect a cure in a short time. If these should fail after a fair trial, recourse should be had to Acon. Cham. Opi. or Stramo., or some of the other medicines placed under *Spasms* will be beneficial. The teeth should be examined to see if a swelling of the gums may not be an irritating cause.

If the stomach seems to have some indigestible matter in it, or there is vomiting, it will be well to attend to that; something given, such as warm water or other article, to evacuate and relieve the stomach, will frequently be very useful. (See Nausea and Vomiting.)

Children subject to fits, may be benefitted to keep the fits off, by taking a dose of Ferr. or Nux V. every day, or in two or three days.

COSTIVENESS.

Costiveness.—All that is necessary to recommend in this article may be found under *Constipation.*

CROUP.

Croup.—For the treatment of this disease, see Angina Membrana.

CRYING EXCESSIVELY.

Crying Excessively.—This, in a moderate degree, is considered a healthy exercise for the lungs; but sometimes it is excessive, and then medical treatment becomes proper and necessary. Care should be taken to see whether a pin or some other cause does not irritate the child. The medicines most useful are Bell. Cham. Jalapi. Ipe. or Senn.

If some of these remedies do not relieve the case, recourse may be had to others mentioned under Abdomen, where one may be found to apply to the symptoms.

FEVER REMITTENT.

Fever Remittent.—Infantile Remittent Fever. At the attack, use Acon.; or if there is nausea or vomiting up of the food, Ipe. at first may do best.

If there is much pain and uneasiness of the bowels, give Cham. or Puls.

Should there be considerable heat and redness of the face or skin, or distress of the head, give Bell.

If there is an irritable crampy condition, Nux V. or Mosch.

In the progress, if there is pressing down or tenesmus, Sulp. or Nux V.

When there is bilious affection, use Merc. Sol.

alone or in alternation, with Cham. or Bryo., or such other medicine as may be indicated.

If there is a disposition to costiveness, give Merc. Sulp. or Podoph.

Should inflammation, or irritation, or painfulness continue or affect the bowels, Lach. or Opi. will be advisable.

If the patient is of a delicate and feeble constitution, or the disease is attended with prostration, use Ars. Cocc. Chin. Silec. or Sulp.

If there is great prostration, give Ars. Carb. V. or Quini.

If the face is pale with languor, or if there are symptoms of worms existing, use Silec. Cina. or Sabad.

If there is a dullness of the head or inclination to stupor, give Bell. Cocc. Lach. or Opi.

In the advanced stage care should be taken to support the strength; for this purpose nutritious injections will be very useful; also apply a bark bandage around the body, and wet it with brandy every day. This we have observed to produce very salutary effects.

ITCHING.

ITCHING.—Infants are frequently troubled with an irritable or itching state of the skin, which produces uneasiness and fretfulness. There are some remedies which may be given to allay this affection; those are Sulp. Rus. T. Sulp. or Verat., or some of those to be found under Herpes.

LUNGS, INFLAMMATION OF.

LUNGS, INFLAMMATION OF.—In this disease, they have fever, pain in the chest, difficulty of breathing, and a dry cough.

Remedies.—In the early stage, Acon. or Bell. After these have been given, and the fever moderated, Bryo. Ipe.

In the somewhat advanced stage, if there is rattling, Puls. or Sang. may be advisable. Examine Inflammation of the Lungs.

MILIARY ERUPTIONS.

MILIARY ERUPTIONS.—A fine running red rash sometimes affects the skin. Nurses call it Red Gum. The remedies are Sulp. or Bell. or Rus. T.

NEVI MATERNI, OR MOTHER'S MARK.

NEVI MATERNI.—Infants often have some marks, spots, or excrescences on the skin when born. They bear this name. Sometimes they are not attended with inconvenience further than in sight; they cause deformity. In other instances, they grow and form a kind of excrescence or spongy tumor. The remedies recommended for them are Calca. C. Carb. V. Silec. or Sulp.

OPHTHALMIA.

Ophthalmia.—The remedies for the diseases of the eyes of infants may be found under Eyes.

RATTLING OR CRAMPY HOARSENESS.

Rattling or Crampy Hoarseness.—Infants frequently have a cough of a tight, dry, and rattling kind, similar to moderate croup. The remedies are Hep. Spong., or if there is fever, Acon. or Ipe.

RED GUM.

Red Gum.—A fine spreading rash, or inflammation of the gums. Use Ars. Auru. Dulcam. Merc. or Sulp.

RICKETS.

Rickets.—See this article in the general list.

SLEEPLESSNESS, OR A CONTINUED WAKEFUL STATE.

Sleeplessness.—The remedies to relieve it are Bell. Cham. Cocc. or Opi.

TEETH AND GUMS.

Teeth and Gums.—The remedies for these affections may be found under those heads in their alphabetical place.

13

TABES MESENTERICA.

Tabes Mesenterica.—In this disease, the child looses flesh and strength; is feeble and languid; the bowels are irregular; more generally costive; there is a frequent craving after food, but it does not afford nourishment and support; the patient decays and wastes away. There is an enlargement of the glands of the neck, groins, and sometimes of other parts.

The remedies found most useful are Sulp. Calc. or Iodi.

If they are much emaciated, and the mesenteric glands appear to be enlarged, with mucus thin stools, give Calc. Ars. or Baryt. C.

If the skin is dry, shiny and hard, with hollow eyes, use Ars.

If there are worms, or involuntary passing of urine, Cina. Spig. or Borax.

If there is a whitish diarrhœa and moist skin, China. or Ferr.

Should there be bloody discharge from the bowels, Millefo. Hamameli. or Rus. T.

URINE EXCESSIVE, OR INCONTINENCE.

Urine Excessive.—Asa. F. Borax. Canth. or Caust.

URINE SUPPRESSED OR DIMINISHED IN QUANTITY.

Urine Suppressed.—Acon. Camph. Cann. S. Uva. Urs. (See Bladder.)

WETTING THE BED.

(See Enuresis, Bladder.)

WORMS.

(See the remedies, which are placed under Worms.)

COLDS, STOPPAGE OF THE HEAD, SNUFFLING.

Colds.—This is frequently a very troublesome affection to little children. One of the best remedies for it is Dulcam.; but other remedies, recommended for colds and catarrh, under Angina Catarrhalis, wil be very serviceable.

If the nose is dry, and there is only a slight discharge from it, and worse at night, give Nux V. or Hyosc.

If there is thick mucus stopping up the nose, with cough or wheezing, give Sambu.

If there be a watery discharge and sore eyes, Cham.

When there is fever, watery discharges, sore nostrils, and red cheeks, Carb. V. Calc. C. Puls. or Sulp.

REGURGITATION OF MILK.

Regurgitation of Milk.—Nursing children are often troubled with throwing the milk off the stomach. For it, use Ipe. Puls. Anti. or Nux V. Flatulence is likely to attend it, for which use Cham. Carb. V. or Sulp.

MILK CRUST, SCABS AND BLOTCHES ON THE HEAD.

Milk Crust.—The proper remedies for this affection will be found under Herpes, Dow Worm, and Scald Head.

JAUNDICE.

Jaundice.—Infants are frequently affected with a yellowness of the skin; the eyes are of a yellow tinge; they become dull and languid; the bowels irregular. The remedies are Cham. Merc., or if they are costive, or have pain or cramps, Ignat. or Nux V.

ERYSIPELAS.

Erysipelas.—This is a spreading red eruption on the skin, attended with fever; sometimes it is slight, at other periods it is severe, and may become a dangerous disease. The remedies are Acon. Bell. Camp. or Rus. T. or Ars. or Sulp.

If there is much fever, use Acon.

If there is a fine red rash, Bell.

If there are large eruptions or vesicles, give Rus. T. or Silec.

In the advanced stage, if there is hard lumpy places on the skin, or a puffy swelling, give Ars.

If there is a torpid state or irregularity of the bowels, use Sulp. or Clematis. Graph. or Silec. (See Erysipelas.)

LOCKJAW.

Lockjaw.—During convulsions, infants and children are liable to have the jaws firmly locked together. The remedies for it may be found under Convulsions, Tetanus, and Spasms.

HOT RED SPOTS, OR SPREADING RASH.

Hot Red Spots, or Spreading Rash.—By nurses this is called *Hives*. The rash is fine and red; there is a little reddish watery fluid in them; sometimes they form incrustations, attended with mild fever. The remedies are Acon. Rus. T. or Sulp.

TEETH.

Teeth.—This period is frequently a trying one for little children. There is some pain of the jaw; they become irritable and uneasy; there is a pressure of blood to the head, producing an irritable state of the brain and nerves; the teeth coming forward, presses on the gums; this causes some soreness and swelling. In this state the child is liable to have spasms.

If there is fever attending this state, give Acon. Bryo. or Ipe.

If there are cramps or spasms, Ignat. Nux V. or Cupr.

If there is much swelling or pain of the gums, Bell. or Coff.

Should the symptoms be severe, examine the gums, and if a tooth is near coming out of the skin, cut the gum down to it.

During teething, giving one or two doses a day of Ignat. or Nux V.; these will allay much of the distress and aid the process.

HYDROCEPHALUS. Dropsy of the Bra n.

Hydrocephalus.—The character of this disease is an affection of the head. The symptoms of it, as stated in *Hull's Laurie*, are headache, particularly of the front part; nausea, vomiting, dilated pupil, slow pulse, stupor, and convulsions. Scrofulous children, and those having large heads, are most liable to have it. This description applies mostly to the idiopathic or chronic form of the disease.

The acute states of disease, which terminates in what is called Dropsy of the Brain, is ushered in with inflammatory fever and inflammation or congestion of the head. In this state the skin is dry, pulse quickened; the child is worse at night; it is peevish; grinds the teeth, and screams; becomes indifferent or stupid; pupils dilated, eyes red, and sometimes there are cramps. This disease is very likely to take place where the fever, which the child has had at first, is treated by calomel and opium.

The remedies for the first kind of dropsy of the brain are Acon. Hell. Iodi. or Ars., and such as are indicated for the constitutional disease which the child may be laboring under.

For the latter type, the proper remedies are those which are prescribed for fever generally, and for inflammatory affection or congestion of the brain, such as Acon. Bell. Bryo. Cham. Let the bowels be freely evacuated; this has a great influence to relieve affections of the brain.

When the fever has moderated, and the urgent symptoms lessened, use Hell. Ars. Nux V. or Phos.

It will be of great service to place the feet in

warm water often, or to put hot cabbage leaves on them wet.

Cloth wet in cold water should be applied to the head, and cold water given as a drink.

Consult the articles Fever, Head, and Brain, in other parts of the work, where the remedies for the various symptoms are pointed out.

APPENDIX.

[A.]

It may be inferred that the remarks made in this work on blood-letting are not warranted by experience or results. To guard against such an opinion, we have quoted from medical history to substantiate our observations.

It is inferred that the object of the use of remedies and the practice of medicine is to cure the sick, and a plan of treatment which does that in the most effectual manner, and in the greatest proportion of cases in a given number, is the most advisable. This is to be ascertained only by statistical results.

It may be objected by Homœopathists that these statistics are taken from Allopathic writers, but as far as health and life are concerned, they are not the less important for that, and they may be useful to Homœopathic practitioners, as they show the benefit of occasionally using a remedy which has heretofore had great influence in curing diseases. Without presuming to include much of our own opinions or recommendations, the selections are principally those from other writers. These are calculated to show the superior success in treating severe and epidemic diseases where *blood-letting* has formed a prominent remedy compared with other modes under Allopathic management. It is doubtful whether it is advisable or justifiable entirely to reject a remedy, as some have done, which has for ages proved eminently useful in curing diseases. We have witnessed cases, and have noticed accounts of others, which have proved very unfavorable under Homœopathic treatment, which appeared might have been cured by the same treatment, provided there had early been a judicious abstraction of blood.

In a period of time, called the dark ages, previous to the 16th century, an opinion very generally prevailed that in violent diseases, particularly in those of an epidemic or malignant nature, there took place in the human system, at the attack, or soon after, a condition of direct debility and loss of muscular and vital powers, and a tendency to a typhoid, gangrenous state, "that in those cases," says Dr. Rush, "malagnancy and putrefaction were associated together." This led to a method of treatment which was, by the use of such remedies as were supposed to have the greatest influence to guard against debility and a disposition to gangrene. The remedies selected for this purpose appears to have been of an exciting, heating, sweating, spicy, and stimulating nature. By this course, it seems, there was no allowance made for an inflammatory, depressed, or obstructed state of the system, which it might be necessary to remove before using such exciting remedies.

Under the use of such a course of treatment by the great Plague of London, in 1665, there were 60,000 died and 28,000 carried off by other distempers.

A physician, who has had some renown, known as SYDENHAM, objected to the then prevailing opinions and mode of practice, and recommended *blood-letting* and a refrigerant course to be pursued. As far as his recommendations were followed, it appeared that the treatment was much more successful. "Inflammatory diseases," says Sydenham, "were more frequent than ever before known."

About this time, some discerning person came to the

conclusion that those violent diseases, in their first stage, were of a "spirituous, inflammatory, or congestive nature, and those most violent ran their course soonest to a gangrenous putrefactive state, or a sudden congestion and fatal termination." In such a condition of the system, it is contended by able writers that spicy and stimulant opiate and alcoholic remedies, if given to a considerable extent in the early stage, the disease is hurried more rapidly, and the case is likely sooner to terminate fatally. The stimulant sweating plan was called the *Alexipharmic* method of treatment. Under this course the epidemics of that period were extremely fatal.

By the influence of this physician, a very material change was brought about in the management of acute and violent disease.

Some idea of this practice and the change which was produced, may be understood by referring to some remarks in Dr. Miller's Retrospect of the 18th Century He says—"To oppose the cardiac Alexipharmic doctrines of the Sylvian school, the illustrious Sydenham arose, (about 1660.) He was eminently suited for the purpose. The sagacity of this physician led him by almost seeming intuition to discover and obey the dictates of nature, and to afford every proper assistance, without urging her to useless and hazardous efforts. The effects of this revolution were immediately seen in the improved treatment of acute diseases of every description, when, instead of the fashionable Alexipharmic (stimulant) plan, intended to promote imaginary depurations by additional heat and stimulus, a safer antiphlogistic *bleeding* and cooling method was adopted to unload the oppressed, (congestive habit,) to reduce excessive action, and to preserve the strength of the system for future conflict." Like Hahnemann and others who have introduced improvements and innovations calculated to benefit mankind, Sydenham met with great opposition and reproach from the faculty and from various sources. In some instances, corporate bodies, it was said, and even governments, interfered to prevent the spread of his doctrine and practice.

A remarkable instance of this kind is related in Dr. Townsend's Journey through Spain. It states "that a violent malignant disease prevailed there. On the subject of treatment, the medical men widely differed. Some of them were in favor of the Sydenhamic method, whilst others were opposed to it. At length the government interfered, and they made out a prescription, composed of many articles, of a spicy, sweating, heating and stimulating nature. An edict was passed that the doctors should use for the epidemic this prescribed plan of treatment. Under this course, there was a total failure—nearly all the cases subjected to it were fatal. The government discovered that they had made an unfortunate prescription, and revoked the ordinance."

It may be a subject of regret that the Sydenhamic doctrines and practice has not been more followed out in modern times.

To elucidate this subject, it will be proper to furnish some facts and statistical statements in reference to some of the violent and epidemic diseases, by presenting the Alexipharmic stimulant plan on one side and the refrigerating and cooling method on the other.

In Dr. Rush's Treatise on the Epidemic of 1793, in Philadelphia, he advocates the Sydenhamic doctrine and practice by *bleeding* and other evacuations and sudorific means. In summing up the results of this plan, compared with the Alexipharmic stimulant method, he states "that under this mode of treatment the fatal cases were not over 1 in 50." "I lost not over 1 in 20 of those I saw on the first day." Again, in another instance, "I cured 99 in 100 of all who applied on the first day of the disease." "Out of 200 patients I lost but four." Dr. Griffith says: "By the same treatment (pursued by Dr. Rush) 49 in 50 were cured." Dr. Pennington said, "that by the same course, in 43 cases, none died." "About 6,000 of the inhabitants of Philadelphia probably owe their lives to bleeding and purging."

In this work, the results on the other side are also given. "Those treated by bark and wine, whole families were swept off." Dr. Compte states "that when those remedies (stimulants) were used, *death* was hastened in every case, and that under the use of bark, wine, opium, and stimulants, one-half died." "At the Hospital at Bush Hill, in Philadelphia," says Dr. Rush, "where bark, wine, calomel, opium, and alcoholic stimulants were the principle remedies, out of 807 cases, 448 died."

In Dr. Donaldson's account of the yellow fever which prevailed in New York in 1822, it is stated "that I treated 22 cases by free *bleeding* and refrigerating means, not one of them died." "Under the treatment, by mercurials opiates and stimulants, which were used by most of the practitioners, about one-half died."

In 1811, and some of the subsequent years, an epidemic disease prevailed in this country to a very great extent. It was not confined to cities or villages, but spread in streaks in many parts of the country, particularly in the Eastern States, extended westward to the Lakes, and proceeded southward. It was equally severe as the Cholera; about as fatal under some plans of treatment, and more difficult to cure.

Symptoms.

Among others, it was attended with the following symptoms:—"Sometimes it commenced with severe ague, violent pain in the chest, difficulty of breathing, intense pain in the head, also in some or all the limbs; nausea and vomiting, or severe diarrhœa; at times the pain of the chest was acute, at other periods, there was a stricture, heaviness, and inability to dilate the chest; the tongue in the progress generally was scurfed, and had lively red edges; there was great apparent debility to synchope or even full fainting; the most common pulse was small, flaccid, and at times nearly imperceptible; there was a disposition to assume a typhoid (gangrenous) type, particularly when evacuations were not early made; the face often had a lurid, dingy hue; in some cases the powers of life were suspended. Similar to Asphyxia, dissections showed the lungs, heart and brain distended and gorged with black blood. The pulse rose, and became more full and firm; after bleeding and other evacuations, the blood was generally, at first, dark and carbonated; after the evacuations, the blood became more florid and lively; the symptoms which followed depended very much on the mode of treatment.

An opinion became very prevalent that this disease was so much of a typhoid nature, that blood-letting was improper, and that the Alexipharmic course of treatment, with free use of calomel, opium, and alcoholic preparations, were only to be relied on. In many instances whiskey was given by the bottle, and at the funerals, to prevent *catching the disease*. The liquor freely went around, and drunkenness mingled in the scene.

"Under this mode of treatment, in some districts, one-half died. The Rev. L. Burch, of Stanford, who devoted his whole time among the sick, the dying and the dead, showed the writer a list he had taken of the number of that town. Of about 130 cases, of these, 62 were dead! The treatment he stated was highly Alexipharmic and alcoholic stimulants. Several physicians, of the middle and eastern part of the county, gave the writer very similar statements about the treatment, with corresponding results.

"An impression prevailed that the disease was directly of a typhoid nature, and this was so much in accordance with popular opinion that it required great firmness to resist the current that set from every direction against every species of depletion. Nurses, old women and others appeared with hemlock, and other essences, hot excitants and stimulants to lop off the head of the hydra epidemic—whereas, by a moderate use of blood-letting and other evacuating refrigerant means, the fatal cases did not exceed 1 in 20."—*Our History of the Epidemic in Duchess County.*

By the statistics furnished in this work it is shown that under the stimulant, calomel, and opiate treatment, about one-half died; and that by bleeding, sweating, and a refrigerating course, 19 in 20 were cured.

There was no record nor publication which showed what was the treatment in the county town, but the physicians and the people there represented it to be Alexipharmic, mercurial, and stimulating in a high degree. The writer was informed by some of the physicians and the people, that most all the severe cases were fatal.

The diversity of opinion about the treatment of such a raging disease, placed a juvenile member of the profession in a trying and responsible position, as being at first, *alone*, in advocating and using blood-letting and other refrigerating remedies, and opposed to the use, at first, of Alexipharmic stimulating articles. However, facts and favorable results of cases in his district furnished such convincing proof, that shortly opinion was changed in favor of the refrigerating depleting treatment.

In Dr. Mann's treatise on this epidemic, as it spread along the northern frontier, from Lake Champlain to Erie, and in the army, in 1812-13, it is stated " that by practitioners among the inhabitants in the vicinity of the army, a large portion used the Alexipharmic, mercurial, and alcoholic treatment"—" that under this course, one-third to one-half died"—" that the mode of treatment, under his direction in the army, was bleeding moderately or freely, according to circumstances, with refrigerating and sudorific means, the fatal cases did not exceed 1 in 16."

In Professor Gallup's account of this epidemic in Vermont, it is stated "that the Alexipharmic plan, with calomel, opium, and alcoholic articles, was the most popular; that under this plan, in some instances, about half died"—"by the bleeding and other remedies, similar to those recommended by Dr. Mann, 15 in 16 were cured."

In Dr. Lovel's Hospital Report, from Burlington, Vermont, it is stated "that in one month, in 1812, there was at no time less than 20 on the sick list of the epidemic; that in the time there was only three deaths; the treatment was similar to that recommended by Surgeon General Mann"—"that among the inhabitants in the vicinity, the Alexipharmic, mercurial and stimulant course was generally used; that during this month there were among the citizens, 72 deaths."

In a treatise on this disease by Dr. North, of Connecticut, it appears that the treatment he used in the beginning was Alexipharmic, and that this was increased to a high degree of stimulation. The Doctor lamented that by the use of very large quantities of permanent and diffusible stimulants, reaction could not be brought out, and the patients sunk and died. He overlooked the importance of unloading the blood-vessels and relieving the system from depression and inflammation before beginning to fill up with such powerful excitants.

In the Medical and Philosophical Register, Dr D. Hosack recommended a treatment similar to that of Dr. Mann.

Drs. Ackerly and Scofield, hospital surgeons at Staten Island, in their report confirmed a similar mode of treatment, and say that very few of the soldiers died.

The works referred to were all published after the epidemic subsided, so they were not of use in the treatment—each one had to rely on their knowledge and observation to pioneer his course.

It would seem that an accurate knowledge of the history of this epidemic might furnish indications enough to enable one to adopt a tolerable successful mode of treating Epidemic Cholera. In many respects, the symptoms and constitutional conditions were very much alike.

Now attention may be directed to a more modern disease—the EPIDEMIC CHOLERA. This has elicited a great diversity of opinion and an equally diversified mode of treatment. It is intended here merely to trace some of the prominent modes of treatment in Allopathic practise, and to give the results.

In this connection a prominent claim will appear in favor of the benefits of Homœopathic practice, as it shows that it may be used beneficially in the treatment of violent and epidemic diseases, without running a chance of injuring the patient and aggravating the case, by the use of large quantities of drugs which may be improper in the condition; for such a thing may happen as to hasten its fatal termination by improper remedies, and the patient not being permitted to die, "by the natural run of the disease," who can say that large quantities of such articles as Cayenne pepper and alcohol may not have had a great deal to do with rendering the cholera fatal.

There was a nostrum sold and puffed here in 1849, said to be composed of tincture of Cayenne pepper, spirits of camphor, laudanum and alcohol, to *prevent and cure the Cholera.* No doubt this nostrum cost the city several dozen of lives.

By the use of minute doses of medicine, it appears that those diseases have been cured, and the patient's life not jeopardized by large quantities of inconsistent drugs.

In the history of Epidemic Cholera, some important facts are disclosed which show a wide difference between one mode of treatment and that of another, as the following, among some of the results which have appeared will show, that when a free use of opiates, calomel, irritating and stimulating articles have been used in the early stage, the disease has been attended with great fatality. On the other side it is shown that when those articles have been in a measure excluded, and a refrigerating, diluting, or evacuating method adopted, the result has been much more favorable.

It is stated here in regard to this, as well as on all other occasions, it is the first stage of the case we refer to, for the treatment and remedies used then often forms the turning point of the case, and give shape to all that follow. In the advanced stage, in most cases, cordial and stimulant remedies may be advisable and proper.

In 1831, the British Medical Board, at Bombay, made a report "that the practice of blood-letting is the sheet-anchor of hope."—*Lon. Med. Jour.*

Dr. Corbyn, British Surgeon in Asia, says: "Believing as I do that Cholera to be incipient inflammation, blood-letting is the first remedy—indeed, it is the most important."—*Ib.*

A colonel in a British regiment stationed in Africa, in 1832, took the treatment in hand himself. By bleeding and giving freely of mild drinks he saved all the soldiers who were attacked with cholera.—*Ib.*

Mr. Baker, the British Consul General to Egypt in 1832, directed slow bleeding and a free use of mild drinks, which were attended with uniform success.—*Morn. Star.*

In France, Brussais and others used bleeding and cold water with favorable success. "Now, thank God," said he, "we give patients as much cold water as they wish."—*Ib.*

Dr. Cruvillier, of France, who had the charge of a large hospital, treated the cholera as a congestive and inflammatory disease with much success.—*Ib.*

Drs. Bell and Conde, in their treatise on Cholera, say "that the physicians in Russia, Poland and Germany, bled their patients with success."

In England and Ireland several doctors bled to great advantage.—*Lon. Med. Jour.*

All agree that the use of opiates, mercury, and stimulants were very unsuccessful.—*Ib.*

In America, as far as accounts have been published, it appears that the plan of treatment mostly pursued has been by the use of opiates, calomel, spicy vegetables, essences, vegetable and mineral astringents, alcoholic or diffusible stimulants, it is more than probable that those drugs sometimes increased the pressure on the brain and vital organs, so as to defeat the object of cure intended.

In 1832, Professor Chapman, of Philadelphia, published a paper on this disease, in which he recommended bleeding, and used it with success.

In 1832, Drs. Bell and Conde, of Philadelphia, published a treatise on Cholera, in which they say "there is inflammation and congestion"—"the blood was dark, but grew more florid after bleeding"—"the brain, intestines and liver showed congestion"—"the lungs were gorged with black blood"—"the stomach showed traces of inflammation"—"the treatment by bleeding has been more successful than any other plan"—"in all cases where blood-letting has been used, and the chest relieved, a recovery has ensued"—"opium increased the congestion"—"many denounced calomel as injurious"—"by the use of brandy, 32 out of 34 died."

Dr. Sterling, of England, says, "calomel has been used in all places, yet the patients have died."—*Lond. Med. Jour.*

Dr. Leo, of Russia, states that "calomel irritates the alimentary canal, and aggravates the disease."—*Ib.*

Dr. Wilson, of Belfast, says, "I cannot see on what principle calomel is used, for if the patients recover, their constitutions are ruined."—*Ib.*

Dr. Clot Bey, physician to the Pacha of Egypt, in 1832, after trying various remedies, all of which failed, he adopted blood-letting, and gave copious mild drinks, with warm applications to the skin. Great numbers were cured by this method. The common people adopted this practice, and by it cured themselves.—*Ib.*

In a report from one of the Cholera Hospitals in New York, in 1832, by Dr. Ferris, it was stated that bleeding was used in many instances, and that there were 9 out of 10 cured.

In Poughkeepsie, before the appearance of the epidemic in 1832, there had not been much published which was reliable, and pointing out any particular method of cure. When it commenced, the people, as they generally are when a violent or uncommon disease appears, were strongly inclined to the use of exciting and stimulating articles to prevent and cure it, and the medical men generally favored this practice. When they can rely upon medical authority, the people adopt such a course with avidity.

It will appear by the preceding observations that those stimulant articles have proved very unsuccessful. In the first case of what seemed to be cholera, we saw there was a group of symptoms presented which had been common, and often witnessed in previous epidemics, and which were described by writers. This led to the conclusion that without much regard to the alimentary evacuations, if the constitutional symptoms could be cured by treatment similar to what had been successful in other similar conditions of disease—the cholera might be cured.

With these views the treatment was commenced. By examining the cases at page 84, the treatment and the result will appear. The anticipations were realized by the success of the course. My feelings may be imagined, and were in a measure expressed in a letter to a friend, (extracted from the history of that disease,) thus:—"The result of those cases produced a pleasing train of reflections and a hope that for this epidemic, which had traversed over a great portion of the world, and spread desolation and dismay in its progress, there might be adopted a successful method of cure."

It will be perceived that the treatment was bleeding in small quantities, and that repeated or more freely, as the case seemed to indicate; by producing nauseating or gentle vomiting, a free use of mild drinks, (cold water was preferred,) and by warm applications to the surface of the body. Since that time we discover that the editor of the London Medical Journal recommends this mode of using nauseating remedies. The remedy for this purpose was equal parts of ipecac. and blood-root in infusion, given warm. It had a cogent effect to restore a warmth on the skin, and produce sweating. Bleeding was used in about half of the cases. After the first and severe stage was over, if the disease continued, other remedies were used which were proper for the symptoms. Under this plan of treatment, the fatal cases, as is shown in a register contained in our history of this epidemic, as it prevailed in Poughkeepsie, was only five per cent.

All the other medical gentlemen used the Alexipharmic, calomel, opium, and astringent plan, frequently with a liberal use of alcoholic articles. According to the reports of the Board of Health of the cases, under the latter mode of treatment, one-half were fatal.

An observation made in the account of the epidemic of 1812, will apply well here: "It required great firmness to resist the current that set in from every direction, (and even from the Board of Health,) against the depleting and refrigerating practice."

My Homœopathic friends will perceive that here accidentally, was adopted a Homœopathic principle of small bleedings to relieve congestion and nauseating remedies to cure nausea and vomiting.

In the County Almshouse, about a mile from the city, the epidemic prevailed with severity, which was under the management and treatment of those who used the Alexipharmic stimulant, calomel, and opiate remedies. By the register of the institution it appears that there were 95 in 100 died.

In the village of Barnegat, (the Lime Kilns,) on the banks of the river, six miles south—after the disease abated in the city, it appeared here with severity, few or none escaped the premonitory symptoms. The first eight cases were subjected to the calomel opiate treatment, and they *all died.* After this, a meeting of the citizens was held, when it was resolved that the whole village should be placed under my care. There were, beside those in the premonitory stage, about 30 confirmed cases; without an exception, they all recovered.

As an expression of gratitude, the inhabitants presented me with this testimony:—

"We, the subscribers, inhabitants of Barnegat, certify that the Cholera made its appearance in this place; that there were about 40 cases, many of which were so violent that they required much laborious medical attendance; that this was done by Dr. Sherrill and his assistants. For the efficacy of his services, we form a a high opinion from the fact that his patients all recovered.

[Signed,] WM. B. LAWSON, and nine others."

There are some reports and collections of facts which may be referred to, which show in some measure the treatment and results of the cholera in this city in 1849. The corporation established five hospitals for Cholera patients, furnished them with all the necessaries for the purpose, and to the Board of Health were added a large number of medical gentlemen to attend the hospitals.

By the report of the Board of Health, it appears that the remedies used were opium, camphor in large doses, mercury, spices, Cayenne pepper, cordials, stimulating sudorifics, alcoholic articles, vegetable and mineral astringents; externally mustard, capsicum, lotions, bags of hot water, &c. To this there was one exception: In one of the hospitals "bleeding from the arm was used in some cases with marked benefit." Post mortem examinations showed congestions, gorged, and stuffed conditions, of parts, similar to those described by Drs. Bell, Conde, and many others.

It appears by this report that the results collected from all the hospitals, the fatal cases were over 54 per cent.

From having a good opportunity to judge, and from making observations, it appeared that a great deal of the treatment in private practice was similar to that reported by the Board of Health. In the upper part of the city, where the stimulating treatment appeared to be freely used, nearly "whole families were swept off." The disease and the fatality was charged to the exhalations from the bone-boiling establishments. It is doubtful whether these had any influence on the disease one way or the other; the greater portion of the cases were more than a mile from them. It may be asked, what had those places to do with the treatment of the disease? Where the mode of treatment pointed out in this work was used, which it was pretty extensively in the upper and west parts of the city, there was not a single fatal case. The register in the City Inspector's office shows that there were 5,071 deaths by Cholera in the city in 1849.

There was an understanding among the Homœpathic practitioners to report their cases to the secretary of the society, Dr. Bowers. Probably these reports were not very complete. By the publication of them it was shown that the fatal cases were six per cent.

After the epidemic subsided, the Hahnemann Academy of Medicine appointed a committee to collect the cases attended by its members. They reported that from the best information obtained, the fatal cases were five per cent.

In the essay on the disease, heretofore mentioned, by

statements made, that according to the plan detailed in this work, the fatal cases did not exceed two per cent.

In Dr. Pulte's work, it is stated that under his Homœopathic treatment in Cincinnati, the fatality was three and a half per cent.

In 1849, the Cholera prevailed in Poughkeepsie again. From S. B. Dutton, Esq., President of the Board of Health for the township, we were informed "that the treatment was generally by tincture of Cayenne pepper and other spices, opiates, mercury; heating, sweating remedies, and alcoholic articles, all largely given, externally, was freely used; also, mustard and other acrid articles and diffusible stimulants. In the township, without the corporation, there were about 80 cases—three-quarters of them were fatal."

The Secretary to the Board of Health for the city corporation, C. Carman, kindly showed the writer his book. By the statements in that, and what he represented, the remedies used here were similar to those above-mentioned. The same medical gentlemen used them. "There were within the city corporation 400 cases, and out of these 280 deaths."

It appeared further that in the Duchess County Almshouse, about a mile from the city, and mostly under the same general medical attendants, there were 100 cases, and of these, there were 70 deaths.

The secretary observed that the stimulating remedies were used and approved of in the Almshouse to a very great extent, and even then the patients died.

There were two Homœpathic physicians in the place. The writer was informed that the cases treated by them were generally successful.

APPENDIX.

[B.]

FROM the position held as President, in the Duchess Medical Society, in 1825, the by-laws required me to deliver to them an address. The subject chosen was a review of the prominent diseases of that locality for the preceding year. The Remittent Fever, which frequently became typhus in the progress, had prevailed to a great and unusual extent. In that discourse expressions like these occur:—"I have not for a long time, until lately, observed cases of fever, which, in the early stage, exhibited the small, soft and obscure pulse which often took place in the epidemic of 1812. In this the attack was sometimes mild, and the disease slow in forming; at others it came on quickly. In some cases the pain was severe; the head dull and heavy; a sleepy dullness of the eyes; skin dry and husky; tongue fiery red on the edges; bowels torpid; a tired languid feeling; countenance lurid; great prostration.

"I believe attempts have been made to cure this state of disease by Alexipharmic sweating means, and by mercury and opium. This plan often fails, and if it does succeed, it is after a long, tedious and protracted illness. The patient gets a black tongue; a black scurf on the teeth; dilirium and nervous irritation, and a train of those symptoms called *typhus*.

Whither those fevers in the beginning are typhus, is a question; I believe they are rarely so. I am aware that in the treatment causes may occur to give them a protracted form of typhus, which may be *prevented* by early removing the compound inflammatory symptmos. Under the mercurial opiate or Alexipharmic treatment, the case often runs on two, three, four or five weeks; a train of aggravated typhoid symptoms succeed, and frequently ends in death.

"Those cases may be successfully treated by bleeding at first, and this should be followed by evacuating and sudorific means. If there is prostration or seeming direct debility, the bleeding had better be small at first, and repeated if necessary, as it frequently is; the blood in this state is dark, thick and heavy; whereas, in the advanced state of typhus, it is said to be dark and thin. In the first stage the blood runs slow; after bleeding, it becomes more florid, and exhibits signs of inflammatory action; after this abstraction, the pulse rises, is more full and firm, and then evacuations form the bowels, and sudorifics may beneficially be used. By this course, the case is cured in from five to seven days, (and then there are no typhus symptoms.) In this plan of treatment there has been no fatal case. When remittent fevers have been treated upon those principles, I have not had occasion to prescribe for a typhoid or a long protracted case."

In the disease here referred to, there were a great number of protracted and typhoid cases, and a large proportion of them were fatal. A similar contrast in the treatment of such fevers, and in the results, was observed for many years.

Had the cases been preserved since the time referred to, which occurred in that county, there would have been shown many dozens, which were treated by those different plans, with a similar difference in the result to that above stated.

In concluding the labors of preparing this work for the press, an extract is made from the address just referred to, to show the closing scene of life of a distinguished member of the profession, who at the time was President of the College of Physicians and Surgeons in this city. The character presented may furnish an example worthy of imitation by others.

"It was a peripneumonic attack that terminated the life of the first President of this Society, Dr. Samuel Bard. In passing this event, a short digression, it i presumed, will be excused, to cherish the memory of patron and friend. As a physician, he had an active, discriminating mind and discerning judgment, well calculated to detect the intricate and obscure operations of morbid action, and to devise means to effect their removal. Those who had an opportunity of meeting him within these walls, will readily bring to mind our then flourishing situation, when we were stimulated by his example, and edified by his maxims and his addresses. Although for many years retired from the city and from active business, he was not withdrawn from professional usefulness or benevolent purposes. He constantly, when required, gave counsel to those around him; and among the poor, sought out cases of sickness and want, on which to bestow gratuitous services. His wife, who was first attacked with the same disease, was his last patient, and he her last physician! He being soon attacked, was obliged to end his medical labors, and withdraw from her the day before she died—and in his turn became a patient. During his short illness, he displayed his usual vigor of mind and promptness of decision. He conversed with me and with his friends, with calmness, on the nature of his disease and the approach of death. During the last trying night he cheerfully said—'Ah, Sherrill, you are generally pretty lucky, but you have got your match now; you won't save me, More than once he expressed in substance a couplet that he had used on another occasion:—

'O God! direct my erring mind to things above;
Teach me to place my bliss in faith, and hope, and love!'

He dwelt on the importance of early subduing arterial action, and of preventing effusion in the lungs, which he anticipated would with him be the case. All he dreaded, he said, was the suffocating distress that that would give him. In the former opinion his anticipations were realized—in the latter they were not. Although effusion took place, he became calm, and died in full assurance of receiving a Christian's reward for a life well spent."

CATALOGUE OF MEDICINES

Used in Homœopathic practice, which have been proved on the healthy subject, and referred to in this work.

	Technical Names.	*Abbreviations.*	*English Names.*
1	Aconitum Napellus,	Acon.	Monkshood or W'fsbane
2	Æthusa Cynapum,	Æth.	Garden Hemlock.
3	Actea Spicata,	Actea.	Baneberry.
4	Agaricus Muscarius,	Agar.	Bug Agari.
5	Agnus Castus,	Agnu.	Chaste Tree.
6	Alœ Gummi,	Alo.	Aloes.
7	Alumina,	Alum.	Pure Clay.
8	Ambra Grisea,	Ambr.	Ambergris.
9	Ammonium Carb.	Ammo. C.	Carbonate of Ammonia.
10	Ammonium Murias,	Ammo. M.	Muriate of Ammonia.
11	Ammonium,	Ammoni.	Gum Ammoniac.
12	Amygdalæ Amara,	Amag. Amar.	Bitter Almond.
13	Anacardium,	Anac.	Malacca Bean.
14	Angustura Vera,	Angu.	Bark of Angustura.
15	Anisum Stellatum.	Anisi.	Anise Seed.
16	Antimonium Crude,	Anti. C.	Crude Antimony.
17	Anthrakokali,	Anth. K.	Anthracrite Coal.
18	Aphis,	Aphi.	Honey Bee.
19	Argentum,	Arg.	Silver.
20	Argentum Nitricum	Arg. N.	Nitrate of Silver.
21	Arnica Montana,	Arnic.	Leopard's Bane.
22	Arsenicum Album,	Ars.	Arsenic Ac.
23	Arsenicum Hydrogenisatum,	Ans. H.	Arsenated Hyrogen.
24	Artemisia Vulgaris,	Art.	Mug Wort.
25	Aurum Maculatum,	Arum.	Common Aurum.
26	Asa Fœtida,	Asa.	Gum Resin, Ferula.
27	Asarum Europæum,	Asar.	Asaret of Europe,
28	Asparagus,	Aspar.	Asparagus Common.
29	Athamenta,	Atham.	Mountain Parsley.

Technical Names.	Abbreviations.	English Name.
30 Aurum Foliatum,	Auru.	Metalic Gold.
31 Aurum Fulminans.	Aru. F.	Fulminating Gold.
32 Aurum Muriaticum,	Auru M.	Muriate of Gold.
33 Baryta Carbonica,	Bar. C.	Carbonate of Barytes.
34 Barryta Muriatica,	Bar. M.	Muriate of Barytes.
35 Belladonna,	Bell.	Deadly Night Shade.
36 Benzoic Acid,	Ben. Ac.	Flowers of Benzoin.
37 Berberis Vulgaris,	Ber. V.	Barberry.
38 Bismuthum,	Bism.	Nitrate of Bismuth.
39 Borax Veneta.	Bor.	Borax.
40 Rovisti,	Bor.	Puff Ball.
41 Branca Ursina,	Branc.	Bears Breach.
42 Bromine,	Bromi.	Nitrate of Bromine.
43 Brucea Antidysenterica,	Bruc.	
44 Bryona Alba,	Bryo.	White Bryona.
45 Caladium Seguinum	Cal.	Aurum.
46 Calcarea Caustica,	Cal. Cau.	Quick Lime.
47 Calcarea Carbonica,	Cal. Ca.	Carbonate of Lime.
48 Calcarea Phosphorica,	Cal. P.	Phosphate of Lime.
49 Calendula,	Calend.	Marigold.
50 Camphora,	Camp.	Camphor.
51 Cannabis, Indicus Resina,*	Cann. Ind.	Indian Hemp of Bengal
52 Cannabis Sativa,	Cann. S.	Hemp Common.
53 Cantharis,	Canth.	Spanish Fly.
54 Capsicum,	Caps.	Cayenne Pepper.
55 Carbo Animalis,	Carb. A.	Animal Charcoal.
56 Carbo Vegetabilis,	Carb. V.	Charcoal.
57 Cascarilla	Casca.	Croton Cascarilla.
58 Castoreum,	Cast.	Castor.
59 Causticum,	Caust.	Caustic.
60 Cedron Seeds,	Ced.	Cotton Seed.
61 Chamomilla,	Cham.	German Chamomile.

* In the New York Medical Journal for 1844, vol. iii page 390, there is an article on Cannibus Indicus, or Indian Hemp of Bengal. When this is given in a state of health, it produces a pleasant delirium and intoxication; it causes epilepsy, catalepsy, chorea, &c. On this account it is named as a remedy for these diseases. We have used it in a number of instances in diseases, with great benefit. It is hoped some one will furnish a good pathogonesis of it.

Technical Names.	Abbreviations.	English Names.
62 Chelidonium,	Chel.	Great Celendile.
63 Chenopodii Glauci,	Chen G.	Oakleaved Goose Foot.
64 China Officinalis,	Chin.	Peruvian Bark.
65 Chininum Sulphuricum,	Chin. S.	Sulphate of Quinine.
66 Chininum Hydrocyanicum,	Chin Hyd.	Hydrocyanate of Quini.
67 Cicuta Virosa,	Cie.	Water Hemlock.
68 Cina,	Cin.	Mugwort of Judea.
69 Cinnabaris,	Cinn.	Red Sulp. of Mercury.
70 Cinnamomum,	Cinn.	Cinnamon.
71 Cistus Canadensis,	Cist.	Rock Rose.
72 Citricum Acidum,	Citr.	Citric Acid.
73 Coccinella,	Cocci.	Cochineal.
74 Cocculus,	Cocc.	Indian Cockel.
75 Cochleara Armoracia,	Coch.	Horse Radish.
76 Coffea Cruda,	Coff.	Raw Coffee.
77 Colchicum,	Colch.	Meadow Saffron.
78 Colocynthis or Colycenthis,	Colyco orColyc	Bitter Cucumber.
79 Conium Maculatum,	Coni.	Hemlock.
80 Convolvulus,	Conv.	Bind Weed.
81 Copaivæ Balsamum,	Copab.	Balsam Compavia.
82 Corallium Rubrum,	Corol.	Red Coral.
83 Cortex Male,	Cort. M.	Pomegranate.
84 Cotyledon Umbilicus,	Cotyl.	
85 Crocus Sativus,	Croc.	Saffron.
86 Crotalus,	Crotal.	Rattlesnake Poison.
87 Cubelæ,	Cub.	Cubebs.
88 Cuprum,	Cupr.	Copper.
89 Cuprum Aceticum,	Cupr. Ac.	Acetate of Copper.
90 Cuprum Carbonicum,	Cup. C.	Carbonate of Copper.
91 Cuprum Oxydatum Arsenicum,	Cup. Ox. Ars.	Arsenate of Copper.
92 Cuprum Sulphuricum,	Cup. S.	Sulphate of Copper.
93 Croton Tiglium,	Crot.	Croton Oil.
94 Cyclamen,	Cycl.	Sow Bread.
95 Daphne Indica,	Daph. I.	Indian Daphne.
96 Digitalis Puerpera,	Digit.	Fox Glove.
7 Dictamus Albus,	Diet.	Bastard Ditany.
98 Drosea Rotundifolia	Dros.	Sun Dew.
9		

Technical Names.	Abbreviations.	English Names.
99 Dulcamara,	Dulc.	Bitter Sweet.
100 Elaterium,	Elat.	Wild Cucumber.
101 Eugenia Iambos,	Eug.	Malabar Plum Tree.
102 Eupatorium Perfoliatum.	Eup.	Thoroughwort.
103 Euphorbium Officinalis.	Euph.	Spurge.
104 Euphrasia,	Euph.	Eye Bright.
105 EvonymusEuropus	Evony.	Spindle Tree.
106 Ferrum,	Ferr.	Metalic Iron.
107 Ferrum Aceticum,	Ferr. Ac.	Acetate of Iron.
108 FerrumCarbonicum	Ferr Carb.	Carbonate of Iron.
109 Ferrum Iodatum,	Ferr. Iod.	Iodide of Iron.
110 Ferrum Magneticum,	Ferr. Mag.	Loadstone.
111 FerrumMuriaticum	Ferr Mur.	Muriate of Iron.
112 Ferrum Sulphuricum,	Ferr. S.	Sulphate of Iron.
113 Filix Mas,	Fila.	Male Fern.
114 Fluoric Acid,	Fluo. ac.	Fluoric Acid.
115 Galvanism,	Galv.	Galvanism.
116 Gentiana Cruciata,	Gent. C.	Cros-foot Gentian.
117 Gentiana Lutetia,	Gent. L.	Gentian Lutea.
118 Ginseng,	Gins.	Ginseng.
119 Granatum,	Grana.	Bark of Pomegranate.
120 Graphites,	Grap.	Black Leda.
121 Gratiola Officinalis	Grat.	Hedge Hysop.
122 Guiacum Officinalis	Guiac.	Resin of Guiacum.
123 Guaco,	Guaco.	New Drug, from Central America.
124 Gum Gutta,	Gtt. G.	Gumboige.
125 Hamamelis,	Witch.	Witch Hazel.
126 Hæmatoxylum,	Hæmat.	Logwood.
127 Helleboros Niger,	Hell.	Christmas Rose.
128 Helianthus,	Heli.	Sunflower Seed.
129 Hepar Sulphuris,	Hep.	Sulphuret of Lime.
130 Hydrocyanic Acid,	Hyd. Ac.	Prussic Acid.
131 Hydrophobin,	Hydro.	The Virus of Canine Madness.
132 Hyosciamus Nigrum,	Hyosc.	Black Hellebore.
133 Hypericum Perfoliatum,	Hyp. Per.	St. Johnsworth.
134 Jalapi,	Jala.	Jalap.
135 Jatropha,	Jatr.	Barbadoes Nut.

	Technical Names.	*Abbreviations.*	*English Names.*
136	Ignatia Amara,	Igna	St. Ignatius Bean.
137	Imponderabilla Electricity.	Elect.	Electricity.
138	Intropha,	Intr.	Infernal Fig.
139	Indigo,	Ind.	Indigo Plant.
140	Iodium,	Ioid.	Iodine.
141	Ipecacuanha,	Ipec.	Ipecacuanha.
142	Iris Versicolor,	Iris. V.	Blue Flag.
143	Juncus Effusus,	Junc.	Flowering Rush.
144	Kali Bichromicum,	Kali Bic.	Bichomate of Potash.
145	Kali Bromatum,	Kali. Bro.	Hydro-Bromate of do.
146	Kali Carbonicum,	Kali. C.	Sub-carbonate of do.
147	Kali Chloricum,	Kali. Ch.	Chlorate of Potash.
148	Kali Iodium,	Kali. Iod.	Iodide of Potash.
149	Kali Nitricum,	Kali Nit.	Nitrate of Potash.
150	Kalmia Latifolia,	Kalm. Lat.	Mountain Laurel.
151	Kreasctum,	Kreoso.	Kreasote.
152	Kausso,	Kuss.	Brayera Anthelmintia*
153	Lachesis,	Lach.	Lechesis, poison of serp't
154	Lactuca Virosa,	Lact. V.	Strong Scented Lettuce
155	Lamium Album,	Lami. A.	Dead Nettle.
156	Laurocerasus,	Lauro.	Cherry Laurel.
157	Ledum Palustre,	Led.	March Tea.
158	Lobelia Cardinalis,	Lob. C.	Scarlet Lobelia.
159	Lobelia Inflata,	Lob. I.	Indian Tobacco.
160	Lupulus,	Lup.	Common Hop.
161	Lycopodium,	Lyc.	Wolfsfoot.
162	Magnesia Carbonica,	Mag. C.	Carbonate of Magnesia
163	MagnesiaMuriatica	Mag. M.	Muriate of Magnesia.
164	Magnesia Sulphurica,	Mag. S.	Sulphate of Magnesia.
165	Manganum Oxydum,	Mangan.	Manganese.
166	Menyanthes,	Meny.	Buck Bean.
167	Mephitis,	Meph.	The Skunk Fetor.
168	Mecurialis Perennis,	Merc.	Dog Mercury.
169	Mercurius Murias,	Merc. M.	Corrosive Sublimate.
170	Mercurius Solubus	Merc. S.	Merc.Solu. Hahnemann
171	Mercurius Iodatus,	Merc. Iod.	Protoide of Mercury.
172	Mercurius Vivus,	Merc. Viv.	Quicksilver.
173	MercuriusAceticus	Merc. Acet.	Acetate of Mercury.

* See North American Homœopathic Journal, vol. i. p. 116.

Technical Names.	*Abbreviations.*	*English Names.*
174 Mercurius Precipitatus,	Merc. Precep.	Red Precipitate of Mercury.
175 Mercurius Dulcis,	Merc. Dul.	Calomel.
176 Mezereon Daphne,	Mezer.	Mezereon.
177 Millefolium,	Mill.	Millefoil Yarrow.
178 Moschus,	Mosch.	Musk.
179 Muriatic Acidum,	Muri.ac.	Muriatic Acid.
180 Murex Purpura,	Mur. Pur.	Purple Shell Fish.
181 Narcissus,	Narsc.	Narcissus.
182 Natrum Carbonic.	Natr. C.	Sub Carbonate of Soda.
184 Natrum Muriaticum,	Natr. M.	Muriate of Soda.
185 Natrum Nitricum,	Nat. N.	Nitrate of Soda.
186 Natrum Sulphuricum,	Natr. S.	Sulphate of Soda.
187 Niccolum,	Nicc.	Nickle,
188 Nitric Acid,	Natr. ac.	Nitric Acid.
189 Nitricum,	Nitr.	Nitrate of Potash.
190 Nitri Spiritis Dulic	Nitr. Sp.	Nitrous Æther.
191 Nux Juglans,	Nux Jug.	European Walnut.
192 Nux Moschata.	Nux M.	Nutmeg.
193 Nux Vomica,	Nux V.	Nux Vom. Poison Nut.
194 Oleander,	Oleand.	Laurel Rose.
195 Oleum Animale,	Ol. An.	Oil Animale of Dippelii
196 Oniscus Asellus,	Onis.	Woodlouse.
197 Opium,	Opi.	White Poppy Juice.
198 Opium Morphinum	Morph.	Morphine.
199 Origanum Vulgare,	Orig. V.	Origanum.
200 Ortheotoxicon,	Ortheotox.	Serpent Poison.
201 Oxalic Acidum,	Ox. Ac.	Oxalic Acid.
202 Pœonia,	Pæon.	Peony.
203 Paris Quadrifolia,	Par. Q.	True Love.
204 Petroleum,	Petrol.	Stone Oil Naptha.
205 Petroselinum,	Petros.	Parsley.
206 Phellandrium,	Phell.	Water Fennel.
207 Phosphorus,	Phos.	Phosphorus.
208 Phosphoric Acid,	Phos. ac.	Phosphoric Acid.
209 Phytollaca Decandria,	Phyt. D.	Poke Weed.
210 Pimpinella,	Pimp.	Pimpernel.
211 Pinus,	Pin.	Pine Tree.
212 Plumbum,	Plumb.	Lead.
213 Plumbum Aceticum,	Plumb. Ac.	Acetate of Lead.

Technical Names.	Abbreviations.	English Names.
214 Podopyhllum Peltatum,	Podoph.	Hog Apple or Mandrake.
215 Pothos Fœtidus,	Poth. Fœt.	Ictodes Fœtid.
216 Prunus Spinosa,	Prun. Sp.	Sloe Tree.
217 Pulsatilla,	Puls.	Pasque Flower.
218 Rananculus Bulbosus,	Ran. B.	Bulb. Root of Crowfoot
219 Ranunculus Scceleratus;	Ran. Sc.	Marsh Crowfoot.
220 Raphanus Sativus,	Raph.	Horse Radish.
221 Ratanhia,	Rat.	Ratany Root.
222 Ricinus Communis,	Rici. C.	Castor Oil Plant.
223 Rhabarbarum,	Rhab.	Rhubarb.
224 Rhododendron,	Rhod.	Yellow Rhododendron.
225 Rhus or Rus Radicans.	Rhus. R.	Ivy Vine.
226 Rhus or Rus Toxicodendren.	Rhus. T.	Poison Sumac.
227 Rhus, or Rus Vernix,	Rhus. V.	Varnish Tree.
228 Ruta Graveolens,	Ruta G.	Garden Rue.
229 Sabadilla,	Sabad.	Alder Buckthorn.
230 Sabina.	Sabi.	Savin Shrub.
231 Sambucus Nigra.	Samb. N.	Elder Shrub.
232 Sanguinaria Canadensis,	Sang. C.	Blood Root.
233 Sapo Domesticus.	Sapo.	Soap Common.
234 Sassaparilla,	Sass.	Sassaparilla.
235 Secale Cornutum,	Sec. C.	Ergot False Rye.
236 Selenium,	Selen.	Selenium.
237 Senega,	Seneg.	Rattlesnake Root.
236 Senna,	Senn.	Senna.
239 Sepia Succus,	Sep.	Scuttle Fish Juice.
240 Silicea,	Sil.	Silica.
241 Solanum Nigrum,	Sol. Nig.	Garden Night Shade.
242 Spigelia,	Spig.	Indian Pink.
243 Spongia,	Spong.	Sponge Burnt.
244 Scilla Maritima,	Scill.	Sea Onion.
245 Stannum,	Stann.	Tin.
246 Staphysagria,	Staph.	
247 Stramonium,	Stram.	Thorn Apple.
248 Strontiana,	Stron.	Strontiana.
250 Sulphur,	Sulp.	Brimstone.
251 Sulphuric Acid,	Sulp. A.	Sulphuric Acid.
252 Tabacum,	Tabac.	Tobacco.
253 Tancetum,	Tanac.	Tansy Common.

Technical Names.	*Abbreviations.*	*English Names.*
254 Taraxacum,	Tarax.	Dandelion.
255 Tartarus Emeticum,	Tart, E.	Tartrite of Antimony.
256 Taxus Bacata,	Tax.	Yew Tree.
257 Terebinthina,	Tereb.	Turpentine.
258 Teucrium,	Teucr.	Wall Germander.
259 Thea Sinensis,	Thea.	Imperial Tea.
260 Theridion	Ther.	Theridon of Curacoa.
261 Thuya or Thuja Occi	Thuy.	The Tree of Life.
262 Tongo,	Tong.	Tongo Bean.
663 Triosteum,	Troist.	Horse Ginseng.
264 Triongo,	Triong.	Tonquin Bean.
265 Urtica Urens.	Urt.	Stinging Nettle.
266 Uva Ursa,	Uva.	Bear Whortleberry.
267 Vaccina,	Vacc.	Kine Pock Infection.
268 Valeriana,	Vale.	Valerian.
269 Variolin,*	Vario.	Small Pox Infection.
270 Veratum Alba.	Verat.	White Hellibore.
271 Verbascum,	Verb.	Yellow Mullen.
272 Viperi Redi.	Vip. R.	Italian Viper.
273 Vinca Minor.	Vinc.	Perriwinkle.
274 Viper Torva,	Vip. F.	German Viper.
275 Viola Odorato,	Viol. O.	Sweet Violet.
276 Viola Tricolor	Viol. T.	Heart's Ease.
277 Zincum,	Zinc.	Zinc Metalic.
278 Zincum Sulphuricum,	Zin.	Sulphate of Zinc.
279 Zincum Oxidum,	Zin. O.	Oxide of Zinc
280 Zinziber	Zin.	Ginger.

* Variolin is the specific virus of small-pox. It is contained in the lymph of the pustules, and probably exhaled from the person while affected with it. To obtain it for use, take one drop of lymph from a pustule when at maturity; put this to 99 grs. of sugar of milk, triturate it an hour; this forms the first turitration. 1 gr. of this added to 99 grs. of sugar of milk, and triturated an hour, forms the second trituration, and in this manner any higher grade or attenuation may be obtained.

NOTE.—The names of several medicines are spelled differently in different works; and in some Homœopathic works they vary from what they are in some Allopathic books. In this work there are a few words spelled somewhat differently—both ways have good authority. On page 137, first line, for *fornication* read *formication;* and on page 352, line 25, for *grr.* read *gr.* 1.

NOTICES OF THE PRESS.

Notices of the Press and from individuals, of the Author's works on Epidemic Cholera, and on this Treatise.

Dr. J. W. Francis, of New-York, observes—"I have read with care Dr. Sherrill's Essay. The general principles which it sustains is in conformity with numerous facts, which observers must have noticed during the prevalence of cholera (of 1832.) His views are good, and the collateral illustrations are in point."

The former edition of this Repertory received from the President and Vice President of the New-York Homœopathic Society this recommendation:—"We having examined the manuscript, are of opinion that the Manual Repertory, by Dr. Sherrill, will be a useful and valuable work, and cheerfully recommend it to the patronage of the profession and the public."

The author's Essay on Cholera of 1849, was thus noticed by the Press:—

[From the Merchant's Day Book of October, 1849.]

"In his Essay, Dr. Sherrill attempts to prove that Cholera is—1st, An inflammatory and congestive affection; 2d, That stimulating and alcoholic preparations are improper and injurious remedies; 3d, That moderate bleeding is useful and efficacious: 4th, That by this mode of treatment the fatal cases have not exceeded two per cent. The points assumed are supported by a great number of authorities and statistical statements.

[From the Weekly Review, New-York, Jan. 9, 1849.]

"A very important agent, recommended in Dr. Sherrill's Essay, and brought into use—one directly supporting life, is oxygen air for patients to breathe while in a state of collapse, which 'is the best remedy that can be used.' It seems that attention was called to this remedy by the same writer during the cholera of 1832.

"By applying these doctrines and maxims to the treatment of this epidemic, it appears a method has been adopted, which has uniformly been successful—so much so that in a large number of cases in which no remedies were used, only such as are recommended in this Essay, less than three per cent. were fatal.

"On account of these statements and favorable results, this Essay is worthy of particular attention and careful perusal. Should this epidemic appear here again, as it undoubtedly will, this discovery may be a means of disarming it of its malignity and its terror.

"It is argued that the disease is inherently of an inflammatory or congestive nature, and that stimulating acrid drugs and a free use of opium, in the early stage, are injurious, and likely to render the case fatal." Opinions of numerous authors and statistics are furnished to sustain the opinions and statements given. It is urged that moderate bleeding in many cases is necessary, but by the use of the other remedies recommended, 'a great majority of the cases may *be cured* without it.' According to those statements and favorable results, this Essay will be of great importance to the community. The simple method of treatment and successful results shows it to be one of the best that has been laid before the public."

[From the New York Tribune, May 28, 1852.]

"CHOLERA AND ALCOHOL.—There is a very strong propensity among the people generally to resort to ardent spirits and other stimulating remedies for the cure of the cholera. Those who are attacked, drink bad brandy to cure the disease, and those *who are not, drink the same poison to* '*to keep it of.*' The prevalence of the Cholera at the South and Southwest, and the possibility of its approach to this city, have induced Dr. H. Sherrill to issue a second edition of a pamphlet essay, entitled 'A Temperance Method of Treating Epidemic Cholera.' The essay points out the injurious effects and fatal consequences of alcoholic mixtures in the treatment of Cholera, and suggests a comprehensive mode of treatment, in which all stimulating articles are proscribed. The opinions set forth in the essay are fortified by numerous citations from celebrated authors and by the exhibition of pertinent statistics. For instance, a large number of cases of Cholera which came under the care of Dr. S. during its prevalence in 1849, and in the treatment of which no alcohol or strong stimulant was used, not over two per cent. proved fatal."

[From the Organ, June 15, 1852.]

"The Essay points out the injurious effects and fatal consequences of alcoholic mixtures in the treatment of Cholera, and suggests a comprehensive mode of treatment, in which all stimulating articles are proscribed. The opinions set forth in the Essay are fortified by numerous citations from celebrated authors, and by the exhibition of pertinent statistics. For instance, it is said that of the many cases of Cholera which came under the care of Dr. Sherrill, during its prevalence in

1849, and in the treatment of which no alcohol or strong stimulant was used, less than three per cent. proved fatal."

The Philadelphia Medical Journal gives a flattering review of the treatise on the Cholera of 1832.

The London Medical Journal, in alluding to it and the principles and practice, states that "they are among the best that have been proposed."

The Boston Medical Journal, gave an approving and flattering notice of this treatise.

Dr. Barnes, President of the Yates County Medical Society, states—"The Essay of Dr. Sherrill, on Cholera is the first thing I have seen which is satisfactory in explaining the nature of the disease and mode of treatment."

Dr. Vail, of Kentucky, observes, "With Dr. Sherrill, I consider the cholera a congestive disease. I found the general method of treatment he recommends very successful on the Ohio river."

"We have examined the manuscript of the Repertory and Practice of Homœopathy, composed and prepared by Dr. Sherrill. The arrangement is very good, and is an improvement on others of the kind.

"It will make a convenient and useful book for ready reference for the profession and for domestic use. We should be gratified to have it in print.

Samuel B. Barlow, M. D.
M. Freligh, M. D,
Edward V. Brown, M. D.
Hannah Cook, M. D.
C. C. Kiersted, M. D.
Christopher Kiersted, M. D.
Henry S. Firth, M. D.

RULES FOR PRESCRIBING,

IN ADDITION TO THE DIRECTIONS ON PAGES 10 AND 19.

The quantity and manner of giving doses is so much alike in the various diseases, that generally the medicine proper in the case is named, and not the exact dose, for general rules are laid down for the quantity of the doses, and time of giving them, and then this is left very much to the opinions and experience of those who prescribe, aided by general directions.

If the triturated powders are used, half (½) to a grain may be given, and the dose repeated in an hour, or in 3, 6 or 8 hours, or at longer periods, according to the nature of the case. Severe cases require doses oftener than milder ones—or 2 or 3 grains of the powder may be put into a half gill of water, and a tea spoonful of this given, in the same way as above mentioned.

If the liquids (dilutions) are used, put 8 to 10 drops into a half gill of water, and give a tea spoonful of this, in an hour or two, or at longer or shorter periods, according to the nature of the case.

In cases of severe Croup, Epidemic Cholera, or Spasms, at first, the doses ought to be repeated every ten minutes, and then afterward at longer intervals.

If the pellets are chosen, 2 or 3 may be given at a time; or 8 or 10 may be put into a half gill of water, and a tea spoonful given at a time, repeating as pointed out in the previous directions.

The strength or attenuation of the medicine to be used, varies according to the opinion or fancy of the precriber, in this they use from the first attenuation to the thirtieth and higher, the higher the grade or number the less medicine is contained in it; all those who use different attenuations, claim to be successful. The nature of the case temperament, and peculiariti s of the patient ought to have an influence in selecting the grades and attenuations of the medicines.

INDEX.

ESSAY ON CHOLERA.

THE Homœopathic Society of Medicine which holds its sittings in the city of New York, established a rule some time since, requiring its members, at the regular meetings to furnish one or more cases of disease, with the method of treatment, whether successful or otherwise, or a short essay on a medical subject. The author furnished some remarks and a case which has since formed the basis of this essay, but which have been materially enlarged and improved as they appear here. At a period of the profession in which each Physician is expected to do his part, the writer is unwilling to apologise or to give any reason why this essay is published as an appendix, but will venture to say, that as the highest duty of the Physician should be to cure the sick—in the discharge of his duty, he has added the following humble effort, hoping that his professional brethren may be edified and that the lay reader will find that diseases which are sometimes supposed to be incurable, may be successfully treated.

I deem it proper to precede the cases which I am about to present with some preliminary observations—

It is now a long series of years that I have been engaged in investigating the nature of the diseases which affect the human body and in endeavoring to ascertain and devise means by which they best might be cured. During this period of time, at eight different seasons, I have met with violent, malignant, epidemic diseases, which spread extensively over the country, affecting great numbers of persons; which diseases I have been pretty extensively engaged in treating.

In making a detail of the names of some of them, the following diseases may be enumerated:—

In the years 1812 and 1813 and some of the succeeding seasons, an epidemic spread very extensively over the eastern states, and the state of New York. It extended to the west and south; it was termed Spotted Fever, Bilious Pleurisy, Winter Fever, Typhoid Pneumonia, Acute Inflammatory Disease, Congestive Fever, Congestion of the Lungs, &c. See page 397.

In 1825 the Puerperal or Child Bed Fever in an epidemic form spread extensively in many of the counties along the banks of the Hudson River. It was more general in attacking almost every female who passed through the process of child bearing, than it had been at any other period in the present century: the disease was frequently very violent, and in some districts extremely fatal; in others, the fatal cases were very rare; this result depended much on the method of treatment.

In 1826 the Dysentery appeared and spread in the same counties and in various districts along the Hudson River, more generally and severely than it had at any other season within the knowledge of the writer. In some sections a large number of cases were fatal, the cases frequently presenting highly inflammatory or congestive symptoms. Some account of those diseases and the plan of treatment which proved most successful, are detailed in my work on the epidemics of those seasons.

To that account of the Dysentery belong the following remarks: "In violent cases the symptoms assumed an aspect of severity. The pulse was sometimes firm and tense, but generally small, soft and compressible; this kind of pulse attends congestion of the abdomen, (and other parts). Blood-letting was attended by the most happy results. The quantity drawn was governed by the effects produced." During the prevalence of the disease, which was about three months, under the treatment detailed in those sketches there were three deaths, about equal to four per cent. of the number attended.

The epidemic Cholera appeared and spread over the country in 1832, 1834, 1849 and 1854. The history and pathology of the Cholera of 1832, which I composed and published has been alluded to in the remarks on that disease in the body of this work and some of the results mentioned.

In each of those epidemics I took notes and memoranda, which were published and extensively circulated. In each instance the results of my investigations and observations led me to pursue a method of treatment different from that generally adopted by my cotemporaries.

There was a great diversity of opinion as to the mode of treatment, and in many instances there seemed to be no particular plan or system of management pursued, but rather a haphazard experimental use of remedies, as the histories of them and some statistics in the sketches show.

In all the instances mentioned, by the use of the treatment recommended in those notes and memoranda, the cases almost uniformly yielded and the patients recovered.

In all these epidemical diseases, there was a similarity in some respects; in the early stage of the case an important feature of a pathological nature presented itself, each case exhibited symptoms more or less of a compound inflammatory, or a congestive condition of the system, and in many instances, of an aggravated state of inflammation. The cases were frequently attended with violent pain, great depression and obstruction to the circulation of the blood, difficulty of breathing, a dingy, lurid countenance, and small flaccid pulse, and it was discovered that those symptoms indicated an inherent inflammatory or congestive state of the system. Such a condition frequently induced practitioners in adopting a method of treatment of the epidemic of 1812 in the first stage of the case to resort to the use of exciting agents, or to opiates freely used, mercurials and heating sudorifics to quiet pain and to resist or counteract a tendency to debility or to a typhoid, gangrenous state, without reflecting or appearing to know, that in such a condition of disease those medical agents have a strong tendency particularly when used in the early stage of the case, to aggravate or produce that state of disease, and in such states, may, and often have, hastened the fatal termination of the case. In many respects, in some localities a similar course of treatment was pursued in the Child Bed Fever, and in Dysentery.

Unfortunately for the community, similar opinions have been embraced in relation to Epidemic Cholera, and a mode of treatment, corresponding with such opinions, has been pursued. In a great portion of the treatment, as it has been reported, there appears to have been a want of system, and no general governing indications of cure, and in many respects, a retrograde action in improvement has taken place. For in 1854, according to reports made, there were introduced into practice increased quantities of cayenne pepper, mercury in ponderous doses, spices, hot drops, powerful astringents and alcoholic libations, to which was added a new method of curing by *steam*—a new application of steam to remove disease and force on the powers of life.

Pause, gentle reader, and reflect on the dangerous effects of pouring such drugs in large quantities into a stomach, the inner surface of which is in a state of inflammation or a high degree of irritability.

According to statements and reports made, where this kind of treatment has been used, one half and more of the patients were dead! dead!

[See Appendix A.]

The histories of these diseases, and the result of treatment, show that the use of remedies best adapted to cure compound inflammation or congestion and to quiet irritation, in the early stage of the case, has in practice proved the most successful in the treatment of Epidemic Cholera.

In reference to this matter there is presented a forcible argument in favour of Homœopathic practice. For in this mode of treatment, if the remedies used do not happen to be most suitable to arrest the disease and effect a cure, they are not likely materially to aggravate the disease and hasten a fatal termination of the case, as large quantities of improper drugs erroneously given may do and have often done!

The peculiar symptoms presented to an intelligent Homœopathic practitioner will indicate the remedy and practice most proper and advisable to pursue. There is however a remedial agent which sometimes has been used with decided benefit in Allopathic treatment and which may be used with marked advantage in some conditions of disease combined with Homœopathic medicine, I allude to Blood-letting. In some states of disease this agent is claimed to be Homœopathic, the state of disease and the manner of using it is pointed out in another place in this book, in the article on congestion and in the chapter on Epidemic Cholera, and permit me here to state that I have not in any instance of a diseased condition of the human body observed that blood letting has had the effect to control disease and to check its progress so soon, so sure and so immediately as it does in Epidemic Cholera, as the cases here detailed, selected from a great number, show.

It is, however, to be understood, that there are but a small proportion of cases according to my experience of Cholera for which bleeding will be required, provided Aconite and Camphor be used with the other remedies as recommended in the article on Cholera in the work heretofore alluded to, at page 74, et sequor; also in the cases connected with this essay. In instances of great depression, when there is a lack of circulation of the blood in the early stage of the case, and the symptoms are of a doubtful nature, or there may be doubts about the abstraction of blood, a small quantity, say three or four ounces, may be taken at first, and the operation repeated in a few hours as I have often done, and which seems to be a safe and judicious course, the pulse rises, becomes fuller and firmer as I have frequently witnessed, "the blood changes its shade from a dark carbonated hue to a more florid vital colour" (Vide. my history of the Cholera of 1832.) Some cases which were successfully treated in this way may be seen at page 85.

There are many symptoms attending epidemic Cholera similar to those presented in other epidemics; for instance, in that of 1812, in the early stage of the case frequently there was a stricture of the chest without much pain, difficulty of respiration, lurid, dingy countenance, a dull, sunken eye, small compressible pulse, sometimes spasms and a torpid, doughy feeling of the skin. These symptoms are noticed by surgeon general Mann and by Professor Gallup in their treatises on that epidemic, also similar remarks are made in my account of that disease. It is also stated in those works that in such states of disease, by small abstractions of blood the pulse became more full and firm, and this practice contributed much to the cure in that epidemic.

In the epidemic Dysentery which has been mentioned, similar symptoms were exhibited, and they were controlled by the same course of treatment.

In the history of the epidemic of 1793, by Dr. Rush, similar symptoms are noticed for which small and repeated bleedings are recommended. With this information, and these facts presented to the mind, the practitioner or others may not be surprised that I used blood-letting in the first cases of epidemic Cholera, which came under my care in 1832, and with success.

During the four seasons in which the Cholera has prevailed in this country, I have been extensively engaged in the treatment of that disease, the successful results have added to the number of cases which have been placed under my care.

According to notes and memoranda made and preserved, it appears that, including cases of Cholerine and such as were fully formed, many of them of a very aggravated character, I have examined, advised for, and attended about two-thousand cases. Of those which were treated throughout by the method recommended, in my accounts alluded to, there were not over twenty cases which terminated fatally; in 1849 the fatal cases did not exceed two per cent. and in 1854, under the method of treatment pointed out in this work, there was not a fatal case.

I have detailed a few of the cases for illustration.

CASE I.

June 2, 1854, Mrs. J. of 20th street, was violently attacked with vomiting and diarrhoea, the discharges were watery and white, she had severe pain and burning at the stomach and a sinking sensation, with cramps and great prostration; the skin was cold, the eyes sunken. I took Aconite, 2d dilution, put 20 drops in a half tumbler of water, gave a teaspoonful every ten minutes. Also, mixed Spirits of Camphor in sugar and water, proportioned so as to give one tenth of a drop at a dose, a spoonful of this was given the intermediate five minutes between the doses of Aconite. Cold water was administered as a drink. After a short time the symptoms moderated, then the periods of giving the doses were lengthened to a half hour, and finally upwards. In the progress, to allay the cramps and pains, a few doses of Nux Vomica, 2d trituration, were given in alternation with the other medicine. In about four hours, the vomiting was checked, and the diarrhoea diminished, when the Acon. and Camph. were omitted, and Cuprum 2d trituration given, gr. 1 about every two hours.—June 3d. The disease was checked, the patient sat up, an occasional dose of Cuprum was given.—June 4th. Cured.

Note—In violent cases of Cholera, where there is severe inflammation or great irritability of the internal surface of the stomach, Camphor in doses of a drop or more, seems evidently too much, as is recommended and used by some persons—therefore I have found it advisable to reduce the dose to the fourth of a drop or less, generally to the tenth of a drop, and sometimes there has been given the first dilution of one hundredth of a drop, and this may be preferable in some cases.

As Camphor precipitates in water, it is better to add sugar to the water, so as to form a sort of syrup, to which the Camphor may be added in such quantity as may be desired to use.

CASE II.

June 26, C. J., Amos Street, of intemperate habits, was attacked severely with watery Diarrhœa and vomiting, followed with violent spasms of all the limbs, the skin was very cold, thirst very great, burning heat at the stomach, sinking depression, difficult, laborious respiration, sunken eyes, lurid countenance.

Acon. and Camph. were prepared and given as mentioned in the preceding case. Ice water was allowed as a drink. After continuing these remedies six or eight hours, Veratrum 2d trituration was given in alternation with Camphor, hot bricks wet with vinegar were applied to the feet.

27. The vomiting and Diarrhœa were very much checked, the pulse was small and flaccid, there was great oppression at the chest and difficulty of breathing, the eyes were sunken, the skin, particularly of the feet and legs, was very cold, there were violent spasms, so that it took two or three men to hold him, and added to which he had a dull, lurid countenance. He was bled 12 ounces—the blood ran very slowly, but by applying hot water to the arm, that quantity was obtained. The blood was black, it soon became coagulated, Verat. and Cupr. 2d of each, were given in alternation every hour, and vapour of hot vinegar to inhale. There was an urgent call for ice water, which was freely allowed. The vomiting and spasms soon after ceased, and the diarrhoea lessened, warmth of the skin came on, and sweating ensued.

28. The patient was very easy, and nearly free of the cholera symptoms. The Cuprum was continued.

29. Cured.

CASE III.

July 8th, E. Kenny, 39th St. At about 8 o'clock, P. M., was attacked with watery Diarrhœa, great burning and distress at the stomach, with severe vomiting, the stools were of a rice water appearance. She had severe spasms, the feet and legs were very cold; at 11 o'c., P. M. when I first saw her, two drops of Spts. of Camphor were put into a half gill of sweetened water, and two drops of Tinct. of Aconite were added to a like quantity of water, a teaspoonful of each was to be given in alternation every ten minutes, but it was immediately thrown up, the doses were diminished to one-fourth of a teaspoonful which was retained—icewater was freely given and eagerly taken—the doses were increased, so that in about an hour she could bear a teaspoonful of the mixtures—the vomiting was checked considerably, but the burning heat and pain continued in the stomach, and the thirst and spasms were severe, the oppression of the chest and difficulty of breathing increased, the pulse became small, tremulous and flaccid, the tongue was very red, the eyes sunken, the face livid and skin cold; the period had now arrived which required bleeding. At 2 o'clock A.M. on the 9th, I took 12 oz. of blood from the arm—the arm having been previously immersed in a vessel of hot water; the blood ran slowly at first, but perseverance obtained that quantity, the blood was blackish and soon coagulated firm as liver, the vomiting and spasms soon ceased and the Diarrhœa lessened; in three hours she lay quiet and easy: at 12 o'clock, noon, she was up and went down stairs—at 6 P. M. was about the house—cured.

I have added the testimonial of Dr. Sullivan, who kindly assisted in the case. It is gratifying to have so respectable a voucher and associate.

"The above mentioned patient being in the same house with me, I attended the case with Dr. Sherrill, and witnessed the above described successful treatment.

"Jno. L. Sullivan, M. D."

CASE IV.

July 14th. M. Borland, a rugged young woman in Wooster St., was severely attacked with cholera. The vomiting and diarrhoea were severe and copious, violent spasms came on, she had burning pain of the stomach, cold skin and urgent thirst. I gave her Acon. 3d, three drops every ten minutes, and spt. of camphor one-tenth of a drop every intermediate five minutes, this course was commenced at about 2 o'clock P. M.; also, she took cold water. At 9 o'clock, the symptoms had very much moderated, but she got no regular nursing nor medicine during the night, as the family were leaving the place, in the latter part of the night, the disease increased. At 9 o'clock, A. M., on the 15th, she was retching and had a copious watery Diarrhœa, great pressure at the chest, difficult breathing, severe spasms, cold skin, sunken eyes, lurid countenance, small compressible pulse. The patient was bled 14 oz., the blood was dark and deoxydated; it soon coagulated in the vessel to the firmness of liver, directly after this the spasms and vomiting left her and the diarrhœa lessened, the pulse became more full and firm: veratrum and cuprum, 2d triturations were given, also iced water to drink, which she took with great eagerness. As it became necessary to remove her from this place, she passed from under my care; but the disease was arrested so that she recovered.

The foregoing case occurred at a boarding house; there were in the house, six cases of cholera; some sickened there, others after they had left the house, the other patients were all treated by different allopathic Physicians, and all died! except the patient whose case I have detailed.

CASE V.

July 14th. J. Clough, a cabin boy on a Hudson River sloop, about noon was attacked with vomiting and Diarrhœa, which were succeeded by burning pain in the stomach and spasms. The vessel was run into the slip at the foot of Christopher St., to obtain medical aid. It was 10 o'clock, P. M., when I first saw the patient, he had a rapid rice watery Diarrhœa and vomiting, with pain and heat in the stomach, and severe spasms, the feet and legs were very cold and eyes sunken. I administered Acon. and Camph. in the same manner as is mentioned in the first case—with a free use of ice water as a drink, bottles of hot water were put to the feet.

15th. 6 o'clock, A. M., the vomiting and Diarrhœa were much lessened, the patient had severe spasms, the eyes were sunken, face purple, great difficulty of breathing, tongue cold, feet and hands cold, pulse very small and flaccid, skin torpid, great thirst and heat at the stomach. The arm was immersed in hot water, and 10 oz. of blood were taken, the blood was very dark and thick, apparently deprived of vitality.* It soon coagulated very firm, the use of Acon. and Camph. was continued every fifteen minutes in alternation, with a dose of veratrum 2nd, every three hours, and a copious use of ice-water as a drink, and vapour from hot vinegar to breathe. At 10 o'clock, A. M., the breathing was more free, the eyes becoming natural, the pulse was fuller and more firm, the spasms, vomiting and Diarrhœa had nearly disappeared, the skin was getting warmer, and perspiration followed. At 3 o'clock P. M., the patient was very thirsty, ate ice greedily, had some stools of a bilious appearance, the reaction of the system was exhibited beautifully.

I gave Acon. 2nd, every half hour and Cuprum 2d, every three hours. 8 o'clock, P. M. the patient sweat freely, the thirst was lessened, he was doing well.

17th. 7 o'clock, A. M., the patient had slept a good deal, there were diffused warmth and moisture over the body, the cramps and pain had ceased—continued the aconite and cuprum in alternation every three hours. 7 P. M. the patient was so far convalescent, that as the Captain was anxious to leave, and I considered the disease arrested, it was concluded that the master of the sloop might set sail and continue the voyage—Cured.

---

* Note—In 1832, as is mentioned in my history of that Epidemic, there were several cases in which the blood was so deprived of vitality, while remaining in the blood vessel that it did not absorb oxygen from the air when drawn and while standing in the cup, as blood generally does, nor change its color, nor coagulate. When some of it being drawn off by small and repeated bleedings, the lungs were relieved and enabled to act more freely, the circulation was increased, so that the vital air, which God himself had furnished in the circumambient atmosphere, rushed into the lungs, and uniting with the blood, it increased the florid color and the vitality, generated heat which was distributed throughout the system. In such conditions the blood becomes more florid after a small portion of it is abstracted. (See pages 77 and 85.)

This illustrates an important physiological principle which is stated in the history of the primeval state of human existence, that the vital air or oxygen by the pressure of the atmosphere was forced into the lungs, there united with the blood, and brought life into existence, which is beautifully expressed thus: "that when God created man, he breathed into the lungs the breath of life."

CASE VI.

July 18. R. Smith, 134 Amos St. was attacked with severe vomiting and diarrhœa, burning pain in the stomach, the pulse small and flaccid—I gave her acon. and camph. in alternation, in about the same manner as is mentioned in the preceding cases, with cold water to drink.

19th, 8 o'clock, A. M.—the vomiting had ceased, the diarrhoea lessened, but the patient had heavy obstructed breathing, severe burning pain in the stomach, violent spasms, with the skin cold and torpid, the face was blue and dingy, the eyes sunken, tongue cold, pulse small and compressible, general collapse had commenced—I gave Veratrum 2d trituration every 15 minutes, continued the cold drink and applied hot bricks, &c. to the feet and legs, and the fumes of vinegar to inhale.

12 o'clock, noon. The patient was not materially relieved, had great difficulty of breathiug. I now immersed the arm in very warm water, rubbed it awhile, then was able to raise a vein so as to take 12 oz. of blood; it ran very slow, and was extremely dark. Veratrum and cuprum, 2d trituration, were given in alternation with hot applications to the feet and legs, and cold water as a drink.

7 o'clock, P. M. All the symptoms were relieved, the pain and heat of the stomach were removed, the patient had neither vomiting, diarrhœa nor spasms, the pulse was fuller and firmer, a general warmth pervaded the skin, and she perspired freely—continued veratrum and cuprum each second, alternately, with light nourishment.

20th. The patient was free of disease, except a slight diarrhœa and debility.

21st. Dismissed—cured.

"The case of Rose Smith, occurred in my family, having much interest in it, I watched the treatment closely, and from my knowledge and belief, this is a true and correct statement.

"P. A. Bailey, 134 Amos St."

CASE VII.

Aug. 26th, M. S. Tucker, at 49th street, a male, after having Diarrhœa about 48 hours it became copious and watery, he had burning pain in the stomach and severe cramps came on with extreme thirst, he soon sunk into a prostrated collapsed state, the feet and legs were very cold; 3 P. M. I first saw him, and began by giving Aconite 2 drops of 2nd dilution every 15 minutes, and spirits of camph. one fourth of a drop half way between the other doses, and made a free use of ice water as a drink.

9 o'clock, P. M. the vomiting had ceased, the diarrhoea was nearly checked, the pain of the stomach was lessened, the pulse was better, he sweat freely, generally warm.

27th. The pain had about left the stomach and he was easy, skin natural, a slight diarrhoea only—gave Acon. and Cuprum in alternation every hour.

28. Dismissed, cured.

The discoverer of the law of cure and founder of the Homeopathic practice, Hahnemann, before he saw a case, as is stated, from a knowledge he had obtained from trials of medicine on the healthy subject, decided that in most cases of epidemic Cholera in the first stage, camphor was the remedy which ought to be given in very minute doses.

In the treatment of Cholera, in 1832, I early came to the conclusion that a primeval pathological condition of the patient, was an inflammation of the villous coat of the stomach, and alimentary canal, and that the system was inclined to congestion. Several writers have sustained similar opinions; among them may be named, Dr. Brussais, of Paris, Dr. Corbin, British Surgeon in Asia, the British Medical Board of Bombay, Dr. Bey, Physician to the Court of Egypt, Dr. Donaldson, treatise on Epidemics, Drs. Chapman and Bell, of Philadelphia, &c. This theory is attempted to be proved in my History of the Cholera of 1832.

When I adopted the Homœopathic method of treating this disease in 1849, I soon discovered that in addition to Camphor, a medicine was needed to check, quiet and cure this inflamed and highly irritable state of the villous surface of the stomach.

Aconite being the most specific medicine known for inflammation and for such a purpose I selected this article and used it in combination with camphor, the success attending their use is an evidence of the correctness of the choice.

The foregoing cases are selected from a great number, for the purpose of showing more fully the correctness of the plan of treatment laid down in this work, and in support of the opinions there advanced, and here repeated. It will be perceived that the symptoms in the cases were very similar, and the treatment was attended with a successful issue.

☞ Directions for preventing attacks of Cholera and for curing the first stage of the disease, or Cholerene, will be found at page 81 in the book mentioned.

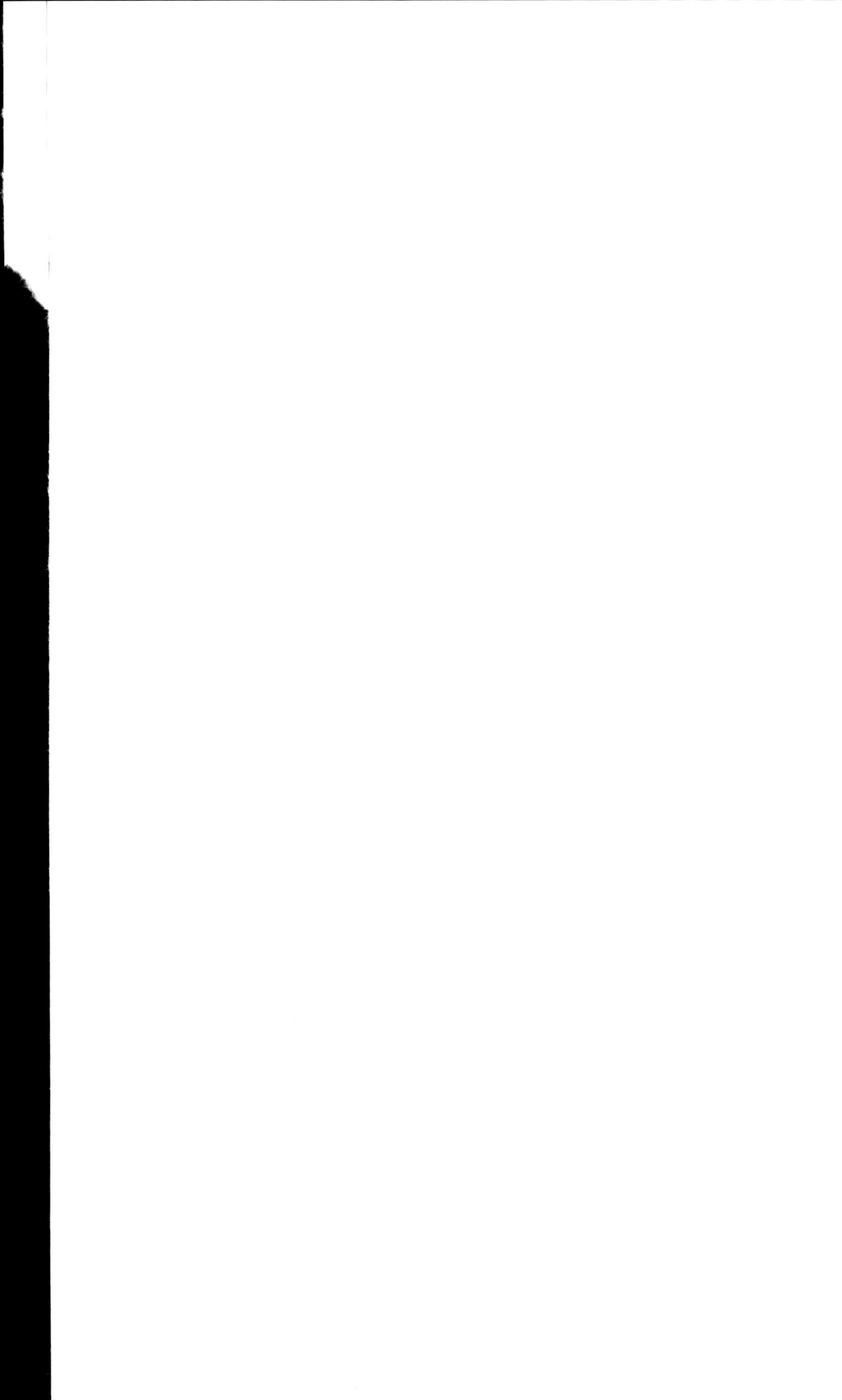

www.ingramcontent.com/pod-product-compliance
Lightning Source LLC
LaVergne TN
LVHW021130110826
845150LV00005B/980